AMERICAN JOINT COMMITTEE ON CANCER

AJCC CANCER STAGING HANDBOOK

Sixth Edition

Please visit www.cancerstaging.net for related product information for the *AJCC Cancer Staging Handbook*, including coding updates and important clarifications to the chapters on Purposes and Principles of Staging, Cancer of the Lip and Oral Cavity, Soft Tissue Sarcoma, and Retinoblastoma.

Springer

New York
Berlin
Heidelberg
Hong Kong
London
Milan
Paris
Tokyo

EDITORS

FREDERICK L. GREENE, M.D.
Chair, Department of General Surgery
Carolinas Medical Center
Charlotte, North Carolina

DAVID L. PAGE, M.D.
Professor of Pathology and Epidemiology
Vanderbilt University Medical Center
Nashville, Tennessee

IRVIN D. FLEMING, M.D.
Professor, Department of Surgery
University of Tennessee Health Science Center
Memphis, Tennessee

APRIL G. FRITZ, C.T.R., R.H.I.T.
Division of Cancer Control and Population Sciences
National Cancer Institute
Bethesda, Maryland

CHARLES M. BALCH, M.D.
Professor of Surgery and Oncology
The Johns Hopkins School of Medicine
Baltimore, Maryland

DANIEL G. HALLER, M.D.
Professor of Medicine
Associate Chief for Clinical Affairs
University of Pennsylvania Health System
Philadelphia, Pennsylvania

MONICA MORROW, M.D.
Professor of Surgery and Director, Lynn Sage Breast Center
Northwestern University
School of Medicine
Chicago, Illinois

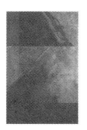

AJCC CANCER STAGING HANDBOOK

From the
AJCC Cancer Staging Manual,
Sixth Edition

AMERICAN JOINT COMMITTEE ON CANCER
Executive Office
633 North Saint Clair Street
Chicago, Illinois 60611

FOUNDING ORGANIZATIONS
American Cancer Society
American College of Physicians
American College of Radiology
American College of Surgeons
College of American Pathologists
National Cancer Institute

SPONSORING ORGANIZATIONS
American Cancer Society
American College of Surgeons
American Society of Clinical Oncology
Centers for Disease Control and Prevention

LIAISON ORGANIZATIONS
American Urological Association
Association of American Cancer Institutes
National Cancer Registrars Association
North American Association of Central Cancer Registries
American Society of Colon and Rectal Surgeons
Society of Gynecologic Oncologists
Society of Urologic Oncology

This manual was prepared and published through the support of the American Cancer Society, the American College of Surgeons, the American Society of Clinical Oncology, the Centers for Disease Control and Prevention, and the International Union Against Cancer.

Springer

American Joint Committee on Cancer
Executive Office
633 North Saint Clair Street
Chicago, IL 60611, USA

Editors:

Frederick L. Greene, M.D.   Charles M. Balch, M.D.
David L. Page, M.D.   Daniel G. Haller, M.D.
Irvin D. Fleming, M.D.   Monica Morrow, M.D.
April G. Fritz, C.T.R., R.H.I.T.

Cover illustration: Joan Greenfield, Good Design Resource, 2001.

Library of Congress Cataloging-in-Publication Data
AJCC cancer staging handbook / American Joint Committee on Cancer.—6th ed.
    p. cm.
  Frederick L. Greene and others, editors.
  Founding organizations, American Cancer Society and others.
  Includes bibliographical references and index.
  ISBN 0-387-95270-5 (softcover : alk. paper)
  1. Tumors—Classification—Handbooks, manuals, etc.   I. Greene, Frederick L.
II. American Joint Committee on Cancer.   III. American Cancer Society.
  [DNLM: 1. Neoplasm Staging.   2. Neoplasms—classification. QZ 241 A312 2001]
RC258 .A33 2002
616.99′4--dc21   2001057593

Printed on acid-free paper.

Production managed by Jenny Wolkowicki; manufacturing supervised by Joe Quatela.
Typeset by Impressions Book and Journal Services, Inc., Madison, WI.
Printed and bound by Hamilton Press.
Printed in the United States of America.

9 8 7 6 5 4 3 2   SPIN 10968468

Springer-Verlag is a part of *Springer Science+Business Media*

springeronline.com

Preface

The *AJCC Cancer Staging Handbook* is an excerpt from the *AJCC Cancer Staging Manual, Sixth Edition,* published by Springer-Verlag New York, Inc. It includes the text from that manual only and not the staging forms. Because the text was taken verbatim from the manual, some references to the forms still remain. The forms are available in the manual and from a CD-ROM packaged with each manual. It is hoped that providing the text of the manual in a practical format will facilitate its use and serve to further the uniform description of the neoplastic diseases in different parts, systems or organs.

The handbook brings together all currently available information on staging of cancer at various anatomic sites as developed by the American Joint Committee on Cancer (AJCC) with support from the American Cancer Society, American College of Surgeons, the American Society of Clinical Oncology, and the International Union Against Cancer. All of the schemes included here are uniform between the AJCC and the International Union Against Cancer.

Proper classification and staging of cancer will allow the physician to determine treatment more appropriately, to evaluate results of management more reliably, and to compare worldwide statistics reported from various institutions on a local, regional, and national basis more confidently.

Frederick L. Greene, M.D.
David L. Page, M.D.
Irvin D. Fleming, M.D.
April G. Fritz, C.T.R., R.H.I.T.

Charles M. Balch, M.D.
Daniel G. Haller, M.D.
Monica Morrow, M.D.

Editors
March 2002

Brief Contents by Part

Contents

Part IX................................329
Genitourinary Sites

Part X................................381
Ophthalmic Sites

Part XI................................415
Central Nervous System

Part XII................................425
Lymphoid Neoplasms

Part XIII................................449
Personnel and Contributors

Introduction
and Historical Overview

The Sixth Edition of the *AJCC Cancer Staging Manual* is a compendium of all currently available information on the staging of cancer for most clinically important anatomic sites. It has been developed by the American Joint Committee on Cancer (AJCC) in cooperation with the TNM Committee of the International Union Against Cancer (UICC). The two organizations have worked together at every level to create a staging schema that remains uniform throughout. The current climate that allows for a consistency of staging worldwide has been made possible by the mutual respect and diligence of those working in the staging area for both the AJCC and the UICC.

Classification and staging of cancer enable the physician and cancer registrar to stratify patients, which will lead to better treatment decisions and the development of a common language that will aid in the creation of clinical trials for the future testing of cancer treatment strategies. A common language of cancer staging is mandatory in order to realize the important contributions from many institutions throughout the world. This need for appropriate nomenclature was the driving force that led to clinical classification of cancer by the League of Nations Health Organization in 1929 and later by the UICC and its TNM Committee.

The AJCC was first organized on January 9, 1959, as the American Joint Committee for Cancer Staging and End-Results Reporting (AJC). The driving force behind the organization of this body was a desire to develop a system of clinical staging for cancer that was acceptable to the American medical profession. The founding organizations of the AJCC are the American College of Surgeons, the American College of Radiology, the College of American Pathologists, the American College of Physicians, the American Cancer Society, and the National Cancer Institute. The governance of the AJCC is represented by designees from the sponsoring organizations. In addition to the sponsoring organizations represented by the American Cancer Society, the American Society of Clinical Oncology, and the Centers for Disease Control and Prevention, the American College of Surgeons has served effectively as the administrative sponsor of the AJCC, and the Medical Director of the Commission on Cancer has served as the Executive Director of the AJCC. Fostering the work of the AJCC has been undertaken by subcommittees called task forces, which have been established along specific anatomic sites of cancer. In preparation for each new edition of the *Cancer Staging Manual,* the task forces are convened and serve as consensus panels to review scholarly material related to cancer staging and make recommendations to the AJCC regarding potential changes in the staging taxonomy.

During the last 45 years of activity related to the AJCC, a large group of consultants and liaison organization representatives have worked with the AJCC leadership. These representatives have been selected by the

American Society of Clinical Oncology, the Centers for Disease Control and Prevention, the American Urological Association, the Association of American Cancer Institutes, the National Cancer Registrars Association, the Society of Gynecologic Oncologists, the Society of Urologic Oncology, the SEER Program of the NCI, the North American Association of Central Cancer Registries (NAACCR), and the American Society of Colon and Rectal Surgeons.

Chairing the AJCC have been Murray Copeland, M.D. (1959–1969), W. A. D. Anderson, M.D. (1969–1974), Oliver H. Beahrs, M.D. (1974–1979), David T. Carr, M.D. (1979–1982), Harvey W. Baker, M.D. (1982–1985), Robert V. P. Hutter, M.D. (1985–1990), Donald E. Henson, M.D. (1990–1995), Irvin D. Fleming, M.D. (1995–2000), and currently Frederick L. Greene, M.D.

The initial work on the clinical classification of cancer was instituted by the League of Nations Health Organization (1929), the International Commission on Stage Grouping and Presentation of Results (ICPR) of the International Congress of Radiology (1953), and the International Union Against Cancer (UICC). The latter organization became most active in the field through its Committee on Clinical Stage Classification and Applied Statistics (1954). This committee was later known as the UICC TNM Committee, which now includes the Chairman of the AJCC.

Since its inception, the AJCC has embraced the TNM system in order to describe the anatomic extent of cancer at the time of initial diagnosis and before the application of definitive treatment. In addition, a classification into the stages of cancer was utilized as a guide for treatment and prognosis and for comparison of the end results of cancer management. In 1976 the AJC sponsored a National Cancer Conference on Classification and Staging. The deliberation at this conference led directly to the development of the First Edition of the *Cancer Staging Manual,* which was published in 1977. With the publication of the First Edition, the AJCC broadened its scope by recognizing its leadership role in the staging of cancer for American physicians and registrars. The Second Edition of the manual (1983) updated the earlier edition and included additional sites. This edition also served to enhance conformity with the staging espoused by the TNM Committee of the UICC.

The expanding role of the American Joint Committee in a variety of cancer classifications suggested that the original name was no longer applicable. In June 1980 the new name, the American Joint Committee on Cancer, was selected. Since the early 1980s, the close collaboration of the AJCC and the UICC has resulted in uniform and identical definitions and stage groupings of cancers for all anatomic sites so that a universal system is now available. This worldwide system was espoused by Robert V. P. Hutter, M.D., in his Presidential Address at the combined meeting of the Society of Surgical Oncology and the British Association of Surgical Oncology in London in 1987.

During the 1990s, the importance of TNM staging of cancer in the United States was heightened by the mandatory requirement that in order to meet the criteria of the Commission on Cancer of the American College of Surgeons, hospitals use the AJCC-TNM system as a major language in cancer reporting. This requirement has stimulated education of all physicians and registrars in utilization of the TNM system, and credit goes to the Approvals Program of the Commission on Cancer for this insightful recognition. The AJCC recognizes that with this Sixth Edition of the *Cancer Staging Manual,* a goal for the education of medical students, resident physicians, physicians in practice, and cancer registrars is paramount. As the 21st century unfolds, new methods of education will complement the Sixth Edition of the *AJCC Cancer Staging Manual* and will ensure that all those who care for cancer patients will be trained in the language of cancer staging.

AJCC CANCER STAGING HANDBOOK

Sixth Edition

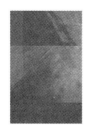

PART I
General Information on Cancer Staging and End-Results Reporting

Purposes and Principles of Staging

PHILOSOPHY OF CLASSIFICATION AND STAGING BY THE TNM SYSTEM

A clinically useful classification scheme for cancer must encompass the attributes of the tumor that define its behavior. The American Joint Committee on Cancer (AJCC) classification is based on the premise that cancers of the same anatomic site and histology share similar patterns of growth and similar outcomes.

As the size of the untreated primary cancer (T) increases, regional lymph node involvement (N) and/or distant metastasis (M) become more frequent. A simple classification scheme, which can be incorporated into a form for staging and can be universally applied, is the goal of the TNM system as proposed by the AJCC. This classification is identical to that of the *International Union Against Cancer* (UICC).

The three significant events in the life history of a cancer—local tumor growth (T), spread to regional lymph nodes (N), and metastasis (M)—are used as they appear (or do not appear) on clinical examination, before definitive therapy begins, to indicate the anatomic extent of the cancer. This shorthand method of indicating the extent of disease (TNM) at a particular designated time is an expression of the stage of the cancer at that time in its progression.

Spread to regional lymph nodes and/or distant metastasis occur before they are discernible by clinical examination. Thus, examination during the surgical procedure and histologic examination of the surgically removed tissues may identify significant additional indicators of the prognosis of the patient (T, N, and M) as different from what could be discerned clinically before therapy. Because this is the pathologic (pTNM) classification and stage grouping (based on examination of a surgically resected specimen with sufficient tissue to evaluate the highest T, N, or M classification), it is recorded in addition to the clinical classification. It does not replace the clinical classification. Both should be maintained in the patient's permanent medical record. The clinical stage is used as a guide to the selection of primary therapy. The pathologic stage can be used as a guide to the need for adjuvant therapy, to estimation of prognosis, and to reporting end results.

Therapeutic procedures, even if not curative, may alter the course and life history of a cancer patient. Although cancers that recur after therapy may be staged with the same criteria that are used in pretreatment clinical staging, the significance of these criteria may not be the same. Hence, the "restage" classification of recurrent cancer (rTNM) is considered separately for therapeutic guidance, estimation of prognosis, and end-results reporting at that time in the patient's clinical course.

The significance of the criteria for defining anatomic extent of disease differs for tumors at different anatomic sites and of different histologic types. Therefore, the criteria for T, N, and M must be defined for tumors of each anatomic site to attain validity. With certain types of tumors, such as Hodgkin's disease and lymphomas, a different system for designating the extent of the disease and its prognosis, and for classifying its stage grouping, is necessary to achieve validity. In these exceptional circumstances, other symbols or descriptive criteria are used in place of T, N, and M.

The combination of the T, N, and M classifications into stage groupings is thus a method of designating the anatomic extent of a cancer and is related to the natural history of the particular type of cancer. It is intended to provide a means by which this information can readily be communicated to others, to assist in therapeutic decisions, and to help estimate prognosis. Ultimately, it provides a mechanism for comparing similar groups of patients when evaluating different potential therapies.

For most cancer sites, the staging recommendations in this manual are concerned only with the anatomic extent of disease, but in several instances, histologic grade (soft-tissue sarcoma) and age (thyroid carcinoma) are factors that significantly influence prognosis and must be considered. In the future, biologic markers or genetic mutations may have to be included along with those of anatomic extent in classifying cancer, but at present they are supplements to, and not necessarily components of, the TNM stage based on anatomic extent of the cancer.

In addition to anatomic extent, the histologic type and histologic grade of the tumor may be important prognostic determinants in the classification for staging. These factors are also important variables affecting choices of treatment. For sarcomas, the tumor grade may prove to be the most important variable.

Philosophy of changes: The introduction of new types of therapeutic interventions or new technologies may require modification of the classification and staging systems. These dynamic processes may alter treatment and outcomes. It is essential to recognize the kinetics of change of staging systems. However, changes in the staging system make it difficult to compare outcomes of current therapy with those of past treatment. Because of this, changes to the staging system must be undertaken with caution. In this edition, only factors validated in multiple large studies have been incorporated into the staging system.

NOMENCLATURE OF THE MORPHOLOGY OF CANCER

Cancer therapy decisions are made after an assessment of the patient and the tumor, using many methods that often include sophisticated technical procedures. For most types of cancer, the anatomic extent to which the disease has spread is probably the most important factor determining prognosis and must be given prime consideration in evaluating and comparing different therapeutic regimens.

Staging classifications are based on documentation of the anatomic extent of disease, and their design requires a thorough knowledge of the natural history of each type of cancer. Such knowledge has been and continues to be derived primarily from morphologic studies, which also provide us with the definitions and classifications of tumor types.

No acceptable staging system has yet been developed for primary tumors of the central nervous system. Pediatric tumors are not included in this manual.

An accurate histologic diagnosis, therefore, is an essential element in a meaningful evaluation of the tumor. In certain types of cancer, biochemical, molecular, genetic, or immunologic measurements of normal or abnormal cellular function have become important elements in classifying tumors precisely. Increasingly, definitions and classifications should include function as a component of the pathologist's anatomic diagnosis. One may also anticipate that special techniques such as immunohistochemistry, cytogenetics, and molecular markers will be used more routinely for characterizing tumors and their behavior.

The most comprehensive and best-known English-language compendium of the macroscopic and microscopic characteristics of tumors and their associated behavior is the *Atlas of Tumor Pathology* series, published in many volumes by the Armed Forces Institute of Pathology in Washington, DC. These are revised periodically and are used as a basic reference by pathologists throughout the world.

RELATED CLASSIFICATIONS

Since 1958 the World Health Organization (WHO) has had a program aimed at providing internationally acceptable criteria for the histologic classification of tumors of various anatomic sites. This has resulted in the *International Histological Classification of Tumours*, which contains, in an illustrated 25-volume series, definitions, descriptions, and multiple illustrations of tumor types and proposed nomenclature.

The WHO International Classification of Diseases for Oncology (ICD-O), Third Edition, is a numerical coding system for neoplasms by topography and morphology. The coded morphology nomenclature is identical to the morphology field for neoplasms in the *Systematized Nomenclature of Medicine* (SNOMED) published by the College of American Pathologists.

In the interest of promoting national and international collaboration in cancer research, and specifically to facilitate appropriate comparison of data among different clinical investigations, use of the *International Histological Classification of Tumours* for classification and definition of tumor types, and use of the ICD-O codes for storage and retrieval of data, are recommended.

BIBLIOGRAPHY

Atlas of tumor pathology, 3rd series. Washington, DC: Armed Forces Institute of Pathology, 1991–2002

International Union Against Cancer (UICC): prognostic factors in cancer, 2nd ed. Gospodarowicz MK, Henson DE, Hutter RVP, O'Sullivan B, Sobin LH, Wittekind Ch (Eds.). New York: Wiley-Liss, 2001

International Union Against Cancer (UICC) TNM supplement: a commentary on uniform use, 2nd ed. Wittekind Ch, Henson DE, Hutter RVP, Sobin LH (Eds.). New York: Wiley-Liss, 2001

World Health Organization: ICD-O International classification of diseases for oncology, 3rd ed. Geneva: WHO, 2000

World Health Organization: International histological classification of tumours, 2nd ed. Berlin-Heidelberg-New York: Springer-Verlag, 1988–1997

GENERAL RULES FOR STAGING OF CANCER

The practice of dividing cancer cases into groups according to stage arose from the observation that survival rates were higher for cases in which the disease was localized than for those in which the disease had extended beyond the organ or site of origin. These groups were often referred to as "early cases" and "late cases," implying some regular progression with time. Actually, the stage of disease at the time of diagnosis may be a reflection not only of the rate of growth and extension of the neoplasm, but also of the type of tumor and of the tumor-host relationship.

The staging of cancer is used to analyze and compare groups of patients. It is preferable to reach agreement on the recording of accurate information about the anatomic extent of the disease for each site, because the precise clinical description and histopathologic classification of malignant neoplasms may serve a number of related objectives, such as (1) selection of primary and adjuvant therapy, (2) estimation of prognosis, (3) assistance in evaluation of the results of treatment, (4) facilitation of the exchange of information among treatment centers, and (5) contribution to the continuing investigation of human cancers.

The principal purpose served by international agreement on the classification of cancer cases by anatomic extent of disease, however, is to provide a method of conveying clinical experience to others without ambiguity.

There are many classification schemes: the clinical and pathologic anatomic extent of disease; the reported duration of symptoms or signs; the sex and age of the patient; and the histologic type and grade. All of these represent variables that are known to affect or can predict the outcome of the patient. Classification by anatomic extent of disease as determined clinically and histopathologically (when possible) is the classification to which the attention of the AJCC and the UICC is primarily directed.

The clinician's immediate task is to select the most effective course of treatment and estimate the prognosis. This decision and this judgment require, among other things, an objective assessment of the anatomic extent of the disease.

To meet these stated objectives, a system of classification is needed that (1) has basic principles applicable to all anatomic sites regardless of treatment, and (2) allows the clinical appraisal to be supplemented by later information derived from surgery, histopathology, and other staging studies. The TNM system fulfills these requirements.

GENERAL RULES OF THE TNM SYSTEM

The TNM system is an expression of the anatomic extent of disease and is based on the assessment of three components:

T   The extent of the primary tumor
N   The absence or presence and extent of regional lymph node metastasis
M   The absence or presence of distant metastasis

The use of numerical subsets of the TNM components indicates the progressive extent of the malignant disease.

T0, T1, T2, T3, T4
N0, N1, N2, N3
M0, M1

In effect, the system is a shorthand notation for describing the clinical and pathologic anatomic extent of a particular malignant tumor. The following general rules apply to all sites.

1. All cases should use the following time guidelines for evaluating stage: through the first course of surgery or 4 months, whichever is longer.
2. All cases should be confirmed microscopically for TNM classification (including clinical classification). Rare cases that do not have biopsy or cytology of the tumor can be staged but should be analyzed separately and should not be included in survival analyses.
3. Four classifications are described for each site:
   - *Clinical classification*, designated **cTNM** or **TNM**
   - *Pathologic classification*, designated **pTNM**
   - *Retreatment classification*, designated **rTNM**
   - *Autopsy classification*, designated **aTNM**

Clinical classification is based on evidence acquired before primary treatment. Clinical assessment uses information available prior to first definitive treatment, including but not limited to physical examination, imaging, endoscopy, biopsy, and surgical exploration. Clinical stage is assigned prior to any cancer-directed treatment and is not changed on the basis of subsequent information. Clinical staging ends if a decision is made not to treat the patient. The clinical stage is essential to selecting and evaluating primary therapy.

Pathologic classification uses the evidence acquired before treatment, supplemented or modified by the additional evidence acquired during and from surgery, particularly from pathologic examination. The pathologic stage provides additional precise data used for estimating prognosis and calculating end results.

- The pathologic assessment of the primary tumor (pT) entails resection of the primary tumor sufficient to evaluate the highest pT category and, with several partial removals, may necessitate an effort at reasonable reconstruction to approximate the native size prior to manipulation.
- The complete pathologic assessment of the regional lymph nodes (pN) ideally entails removal of a sufficient number of lymph nodes to evaluate the highest pN category.

Exception: Sentinel node assessment may be appropriate for some sites and is clarified in chapter guidelines for those sites.*

*Note: The sentinel lymph node is the first lymph node to receive lymphatic drainage from a primary tumor. If it contains metastatic tumor, this indicates that other lymph nodes may contain tumor. If it does not contain metastatic tumor, other lymph nodes are not likely to contain tumor. Occasionally there is more than one sentinel lymph node.

- If pathologic assessment of lymph nodes reveals negative nodes but the number of examined lymph nodes is less than the suggested number for lymph node dissection, classify the N category as pN0.
- Isolated tumor cells (ITC) are single tumor cells or small clusters of cells not more than 0.2 mm in greatest dimension that are usually detected by immunohistochemistry or molecular methods. Cases with ITC in lymph nodes or at distant sites should be classified as N0 or M0, respectively. The same applies to cases with findings suggestive of tumor cells or their components by nonmorphologic techniques such as flow cytometry or DNA analysis. These cases should be analyzed separately and have special recording rules in the specific organ site.
- The pathologic assessment of metastases may be either clinical or pathologic when the T and/or N categories meet the criteria for pathologic staging (pT, pN, cM, or pM).

Pathologic classification of the extent of the primary tumor (T) and lymph nodes (N) is essential. Pathologic staging depends on the proven anatomic extent of disease, whether or not the primary lesion has been completely removed. If a biopsied primary tumor technically cannot be removed, or when it is unreasonable to remove it, and if the highest T and N categories or the M1 category of the tumor can be confirmed microscopically, the criteria for pathologic classification and staging have been satisfied without total removal of the primary cancer.

Retreatment classification is assigned when further treatment (such as chemotherapy) is planned for a cancer that recurs after a disease-free interval. All information available at the time of retreatment should be used in determining the stage of the recurrent tumor (**rTNM**). Biopsy confirmation of the recurrent cancer is useful if clinically feasible, but with pathologic proof of the primary site, clinical evidence of distant metastases (usually by radiographic or related methodologies) may be used.

Autopsy classification occurs when classification of a cancer by postmortem examination is done after the death of a patient (cancer was not evident prior to death). The classification of the stage is identified as **aTNM** and includes all pathologic information obtained at the time of death.

4. **Stage grouping.** After the assignment of cT, cN, and cM and/or pT, pN, and pM categories, these may be grouped into stages. Both TNM classifications and stage groupings, once established, remain in the medical record. If there is doubt concerning the T, N, or M classifi-

cation to which a particular case should be assigned, then the lower (less advanced) category should be assigned. The same principle applies to the stage grouping. Carcinoma *in situ* (CIS) is an exception to the stage grouping guidelines. By definition, CIS has not involved any structures in the primary organ that would allow tumor cells to spread to regional nodes or distant sites. Therefore, pTis, cN0, cM0, clinical stage group 0 is appropriate.

5. **Multiple tumors.** In the case of multiple, simultaneous tumors in one organ, the tumor with the highest T category is the one selected for classification and staging, and the multiplicity or the number of tumors is indicated in parentheses: for example, T2(m) or T2(5). For simultaneous bilateral cancers in paired organs, the tumors are classified separately as independent tumors in different organs. In the case of tumors of the thyroid, liver, and ovary, multiplicity is a criterion of T classification.

6. **Subsets of TNM.** Definitions of TNM categories and stage grouping may be telescoped (expanded as subsets of existing classifications) for research purposes as long as the original definitions are not changed. For instance, any of the published T, N, or M classifications can be divided into subgroups for testing and, if validated, may be submitted to the American Joint Committee on Cancer or the TNM Process Subcommittee of the UICC to be evaluated for inclusion in the classification system.

7. **Unknown primary.** In the case of a primary of unknown origin, staging can only be based on clinical suspicion of the primary origin (e.g., T0 N1 M0).

ANATOMIC REGIONS AND SITES

The sites in this classification are listed by code number of the *International Classification of Diseases for Oncology*, Third Edition (ICD-O Third Edition, World Health Organization, 2000). Most chapters are constructed according to the following outline:

Introduction
Anatomy
    Primary site
    Regional lymph nodes
    Metastatic sites
Rules for classification
    Clinical (TNM or cTNM)
    Pathologic (pTNM)
Definitions of TNM for each specific anatomic site
    T: Primary tumor size/extent
    N: Regional lymph node involvement: number/extent
    M: Distant metastasis absent/present
Stage grouping
Histopathologic type
Histologic grade

DEFINITIONS OF TNM

Primary Tumor (T)

TX	Primary tumor cannot be assessed
T0	No evidence of primary tumor
Tis	Carcinoma *in situ*
T1, T2, T3, T4	Increasing size and/or local extent of the primary tumor

Regional Lymph Nodes (N)

NX	Regional lymph nodes cannot be assessed
N0	No regional lymph node metastasis
N1, N2, N3	Increasing involvement of regional lymph nodes

Note: Direct extension of the primary tumor into a lymph node(s) is classified as a lymph node metastasis.

Note: Metastasis in any lymph node other than regional is classified as a distant metastasis.

Distant Metastasis (M)

MX	Distant metastasis cannot be assessed
M0	No distant metastasis
M1	Distant metastasis

Note: For pathologic stage grouping, if sufficient tissue to evaluate the highest T and N categories has been removed for pathologic examination, M1 may be either clinical (cM1) or pathologic (pM1). If only a metastasis has had microscopic confirmation, the classification is pathologic (pM1) and the stage is pathologic.

The category M1 may be further specified according to the following notation:

Pulmonary	PUL
Osseous	OSS
Hepatic	HEP
Brain	BRA
Lymph nodes	LYM
Bone marrow	MAR
Pleura	PLE
Peritoneum	PER
Adrenals	ADR
Skin	SKI
Other	OTH

Subdivisions of TNM. Subdivisions of some main categories are available for those who need greater specificity (e.g., T1a, 1b or N2a, 2b as with breast and prostate).

HISTOPATHOLOGIC TYPE

The histopathologic type is a *qualitative* assessment whereby a tumor is categorized (typed) according to the normal tissue type or cell type it most closely resembles (e.g., hepatocellular or cholangiocarcinoma, osteosarcoma, squamous cell carcinoma). In general, the *World Health Organiza-*

tion International Histological Classification of Tumours published in numerous anatomic site-specific editions, may be used for histopathologic typing. A list of applicable ICD-0-3 histopathologic codes, including numerical codes and alpha names, is presented at the end of each chapter following the bibliography. If a specific histology is not listed, the case cannot be staged using the AJCC classification in that chapter.

HISTOLOGIC GRADE (G)

The histologic grade is a qualitative assessment of the differentiation of the tumor expressed as the extent to which a tumor resembles the normal tissue at that site. Grade is expressed in numerical grades of differentiation from most differentiated (Grade 1) to least differentiated (Grade 4), e.g., squamous cell carcinoma, moderately differentiated, Grade 2. The term *grade* is also used when other predictive, tissue-based parameters are used for prediction, particularly nuclear grade and mitotic count.

GX   Grade cannot be assessed
G1   Well differentiated
G2   Moderately differentiated
G3   Poorly differentiated
G4   Undifferentiated

Other grading systems are in development with more precise guidelines adding features of nuclear grade and mitotic activity to the evaluation of tissue differentiation. If there is evidence of more than one grade or of differentiation of the tumor, the least differentiated is recorded as the histopathologic grade, using only G2 through G4. For example, a colonic adenocarcinoma that is partially well differentiated and partially moderately differentiated is coded as grade 2 (G2). The growing edge of a tumor is not generally assessed in grading because it may appear to be a high grade—except in breast, where that is the best reflection of prognosis.

For some anatomic sites, Grade 3 and Grade 4 are combined into a single grade—for example, poorly differentiated to undifferentiated (G3–4). The combination is valid for carcinomas of the uterine corpus, ovary, prostate, urinary bladder, kidney, renal pelvis, ureter, urethra, and breast. Only three grades are used for melanoma of the conjunctiva and uvea. Grading does not apply to carcinomas of the thyroid, eyelids, and retinoblastoma or to malignant testicular tumors and melanoma of the skin.

The use of G4 is reserved for those tumors that show no specific differentiation that would identify the cancer as arising from its site of origin. In some sites, the WHO histologic classification includes undifferentiated carcinomas—for example, in the stomach or gallbladder. In these cases, the tumor is graded as undifferentiated (G4).

Some histologic tumor types are by definition listed as G4 for staging purposes and are not to be assigned a grade of undifferentiated in ICD-O-3 coding for cancer registry purposes. These include

Small cell carcinoma, any site
Large cell carcinoma of lung

Ewing's sarcoma of bone and soft tissue
Rhabdomyosarcoma of soft tissue

Traditionally, and as discussed above, histologic stratification of solid tumors has been dominated by concerns of differentiation. Other systems have validated more complex stratifications, using other data and demonstrating different patient outcomes for three tiers supported by histologic schemes of evaluation that include relatively valid and validated criteria. In this edition, the grading systems proposed for prostate and breast cancers are in the latter group. Although manifestly different, they have been multiply validated. One uses patterns of differentiation, cellularity, and invasiveness (prostate); the other uses nuclear grading (shape and size of nuclei) and formal counts of mitotic figures as a reflection of the proliferation rate. It is clear and relevant that these systems have taken advantage of the very different natural histories of cancers in these two organs.

DESCRIPTORS

For identification of special cases of TNM or pTNM classifications, the m suffix and "y," "r," and "a" prefixes are used. Although they do not affect the stage grouping, they indicate cases that require separate analysis.

m Suffix.   Indicates the presence of multiple primary tumors in a single site and is recorded in parentheses: pT(m)NM.

y Prefix.   Indicates those cases in which classification is performed during or following initial multimodality therapy. The cTNM or pTNM category is identified by a "y" prefix. The ycTNM or ypTNM categorizes the extent of tumor actually present at the time of that examination. The "y" categorization is not an estimate of the extent of tumor prior to multimodality therapy.

r Prefix.   Indicates a recurrent tumor when staged after a disease-free interval, and is identified by the "r" prefix: rTNM. (See reclassification, r above as rTNM).

a Prefix.   Designates the stage determined at autopsy: aTNM.

OTHER DESCRIPTORS

Lymphatic Vessel Invasion (L)
LX   Lymphatic vessel invasion cannot be assessed
L0   No lymphatic vessel invasion
L1   Lymphatic vessel invasion

Venous Invasion (V)

VX   Venous invasion cannot be assessed
V0   No venous invasion
V1   Microscopic venous invasion
V2   Macroscopic venous invasion

Residual Tumor (R)

The absence or presence of residual tumor after treatment is described by the symbol R.

TNM and pTNM describe the anatomic extent of cancer in general without consideration of treatment. TNM and pTNM can be supplemented by the R classification, which deals with the tumor status after treatment. It reflects the effects of therapy, influences further therapeutic procedures, and is a strong predictor of prognosis.

The R categories are

RX   Presence of residual tumor cannot be assessed
R0   No residual tumor
R1   Microscopic residual tumor
R2   Macroscopic residual tumor

STAGE GROUPING

Classification by the TNM system achieves reasonably precise description and recording of the anatomic extent of disease. A tumor with 4 categories of T, 3 categories of N, and 2 categories of M has 24 TNM combinations. For purposes of tabulation and analysis, except in very large series, it is necessary to condense these combinations into a convenient number of TNM stage groupings.

The grouping adopted ensures, as far as possible, that each stage group is relatively homogeneous with respect to survival and that the survival rates of these stage groupings for each cancer site are distinct. Carcinoma *in situ* is categorized Stage 0; for most sites, a case with distant metastasis is categorized Stage IV. Stages I, II, and III indicate relatively greater anatomic extent of cancer within the range from Stage 0 to Stage IV.

Cancer Staging Data Form.   Each site chapter includes staging forms to be used to record the TNM classification and the stage of the cancer. The specific anatomic site of the cancer is recorded, as well as the histologic type and grade. The appropriate staging basis or classification must be recorded, such as at the time of primary therapy or at the time of recurrence. If a cancer is staged at several points, a separate form is used for each or if all are recorded in a single form, the staging basis for each, is clearly identified.

The T, N, and M classifications can be checked opposite the appropriate definitions of the extent of the primary tumor, the regional lymph nodes, and distant metastasis. The lesion(s) can be marked on a diagram, and finally, the stage grouping can be checked. In some instances, information regarding other characteristics of the tumor (not included in the stage) might be requested. These data may be pertinent in deciding management of the patient.

The cancer staging form is a specific additional document in the patient record indicating anatomic extent of disease. It is not a substitute for history, treatment, or follow-up records. The data forms in this manual may be duplicated for individual or institutional use without permission from the AJCC or the publisher.

Cancer Survival Analysis

Analyses of cancer survival data and related outcomes are quantitative tools commonly used to assess cancer treatment programs and to monitor the progress of regional and national cancer control programs. In this chapter the most common survival analysis methodology will be illustrated, basic terminology will be defined, and the essential elements of data collection and reporting will be described. Although the underlying principles are applicable to both, the focus of this discussion will be on the use of survival analysis to describe data typically available in cancer registries rather than to analyze research data obtained from clinical trials or laboratory experimentation. Discussion of statistical principles and methodology will be limited. Persons interested in statistical underpinnings or research applications are referred to textbooks that explore these topics at length (Cox and Oakes, 1984; Fleming and Harrington, 1991; Kalbfleisch and Prentice, 1980; Kleinbaum, 1996; Lee, 1992).

BASIC CONCEPTS

A *survival rate* is a statistical index that summarizes the probable frequency of specific outcomes for a group of patients at a particular point in time. A *survival curve* is a summary display of the pattern of survival rates over time. The basic concept is simple. For example, for a certain category of patient, one might ask what proportion are likely to be alive at the end of a specified interval, such as 5 years. The greater the proportion surviving, the more effective the program. Survival analysis, however, is somewhat more complicated than it first might appear. If one were to measure the length of time between diagnosis and death or record the vital status when last observed for every patient in a selected patient group, one might be tempted to describe the survival of the group as the proportion alive at the end of the period under investigation. This simple measure will be informative, however, only if all of the patients were observed for the same length of time.

In most real situations, it is not the case that all members of the group are observed for the same amount of time. Patients diagnosed near the end of the study period are more likely to be alive at last contact and will have been followed for less time than those diagnosed earlier. Even though it was not possible to follow these persons as long as the others, their survival might eventually have proved to be just as long or longer. Another difficulty is that it usually is not possible to know the outcome status of all of the persons who were in the group at the beginning. People move or change names and are lost to follow-up. Some of these persons may have died and others could be still living. Thus, if a survival rate is to describe the outcomes for an entire group accurately, there must be some means to deal with the fact that different persons in the group are observed for different lengths of time and that for others, their vital status is not known at the time of analysis. In the language of survival analysis, subjects who are observed until they reach the endpoint of interest (e.g., death) are called *uncensored* cases, and those who survive beyond the end of the follow-up or who are lost to follow-up at some point are termed *censored* cases.

Two basic survival procedures that enable one to determine overall group survival, taking into account both censored and uncensored observations, are the life table method (Berkson and Gage, 1950) and the Kaplan-Meier method (Kaplan and Meier, 1958). The life table method was the first method generally used to describe cancer survival results, and it came to be known as the actuarial method because of its similarity to the work done by actuaries in the insurance industry. The specific method of computation, i.e., life table or Kaplan-Meier, should always be indicated to avoid any confusion associated with the use of less precise terminology. Rates computed by different methods are not directly comparable, and when the survival experiences of different patient groups are compared, the different rates must be computed by the same method.

The illustrations in this chapter are based on data obtained from the public-use files of the National Cancer Institute Surveillance, Epidemiology, and End Results (SEER) program. The cases selected are a 1% random sample of the total number for the selected sites and years of diagnosis. Follow-up of these patients continued through the end of 1999. Thus, for the earliest patients, there can be as much as 16 years of follow-up, but for those diagnosed at the end of the study period, there can be as little as 1 year of follow-up. These data are used both because they are realistic in terms of the actual survival rates they yield and because they encompass a number of cases that might be seen in a single large tumor registry over a comparable number of years. They are intended only to illustrate the methodology. SEER results from 1973 to 1997 are more fully described elsewhere (Ries et al., 2000) and these illustrations should not be regarded as an adequate description of the total or current United States patterns of breast or lung cancer survival.

THE LIFE TABLE METHOD

The life table method involves dividing the total period over which a group is observed into fixed intervals, usually months or years. For each interval, the proportion surviving to the end of the interval is calculated on the basis of the number known to have experienced the endpoint event (e.g., death) during the interval and the number estimated to have been at risk at the start of the interval. For each succeeding interval, a cumulative survival rate may be calculated. The cumulative survival rate is the probability of surviving the most recent interval multiplied by the probabilities of surviving all of the prior intervals. Thus, if the percent of the patients surviving the first interval is 90% and is the same for the second and third intervals, the cumulative survival percentage is 72.9% (.9 × .9 × .9 = .729).

Results from the life table method for calculating survival for the breast cancer illustration are shown in Figure 2.1. Two thousand eight hundred nineteen (2,819) patients diagnosed between 1983 and 1998 were followed through 1999. Following the life table calculation method for each

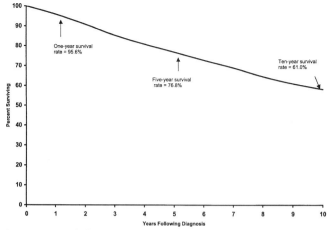

FIG 2.1. Survival of 2,819 breast cancer patients from the Surveillance, Epidemiology, and End Results Program of the National Cancer Institute, 1983–1998. Calculated by the life table method.

year after diagnosis, the 1-year survival rate is 95.6%. The 5-year cumulative survival rate is 76.8%. At 10 years, the cumulative survival is 61.0 %.

The lung cancer data show a much different survival pattern (Fig. 2.2). At 1 year following diagnosis, the survival rate is only 41.8%. By 5 years it has fallen to 12.0%, and only 6.8% of lung cancer patients are estimated to have survived for 10 years following diagnosis. For lung cancer patients the *median survival time* is 10.0 months. Median survival time is the amount of time required to pass so that half the patients have experienced

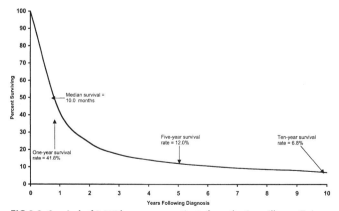

FIG 2.2. Survival of 2,347 lung cancer patients from the Surveillance, Epidemiology, and End Results Program of the National Cancer Institute, 1983–1998. Calculated by the life table method.

the endpoint event and half the patients remain event-free. If the cumulative survival does not fall below 50% it is not possible to estimate median survival from the data, as is the case in the breast cancer data.

In the case of breast cancer, the 10-year survival rate is important because such a large proportion of patients live more than 5 years past their diagnosis. The 10-year time frame for lung cancer is less meaningful because such a large proportion of this patient group dies well before that much time passes.

An important assumption of all actuarial survival methods is that censored cases do not differ from the entire collection of uncensored cases in any systematic manner that would affect their survival. For example, if the more recently diagnosed cases in Figure 2.1, i.e., those who were most likely not to have died yet, tended to be detected with earlier-stage disease than the uncensored cases; or if they were treated differently, the assumption about comparability of censored and uncensored cases would not be met, and the result for the group as a whole would be inaccurate. Thus it is important, when patients are included in a life table analysis, that one be reasonably confident that differences in the amount of information available about survival are not related to differences that might affect survival.

THE KAPLAN-MEIER METHOD

These same data can be analyzed using the Kaplan-Meier method (Kaplan and Meier, 1958). It is similar to the life table method but provides for calculating the proportion surviving to each point in time that a death occurs, rather than at fixed intervals. The principal difference evident in a survival curve is that the stepwise changes in the cumulative survival rate appear to occur independently of the intervals on the Years Following Diagnosis axis.

PATIENT-, DISEASE-, AND TREATMENT-SPECIFIC SURVIVAL

Although overall group survival is informative, comparisons of the overall survival between two groups often are confounded by differences in the patients, their tumors, or the treatments they received. For example, it would be misleading to compare the overall survival depicted in Figure 2.1 with the overall survival of other breast cancer patients who tend to be diagnosed with more advanced disease, whose survival would be presumed to be poorer. The simplest approach to accounting for possible differences between groups is to provide survival results that are specific to the categories of patient, disease, or treatment that may affect results. In most cancer applications the most important variable by which survival results should be subdivided is the stage of disease. Figure 2.3 shows the *stage-specific* 5-year survival curves of the same breast cancer patients described earlier. These data show that breast cancer patient survival differs markedly according to the stage of the tumor at the time of diagnosis.

Almost any variable can be used to subclassify survival rates, but some are more meaningful than others. For example, it would be possible to

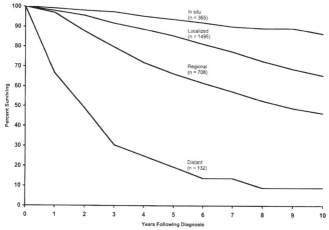

FIG 2.3. Survival of 2,819 breast cancer patients from the Surveillance, Epidemiology, and End Results Program of the National Cancer Institute, 1983–1998. Calculated by the life table method and stratified by historic stage of disease. *Note:* Excludes 119 patients with unknown stage of disease. SEER uses extent of disease (EOD) staging.

provide season-of-diagnosis-specific (i.e., spring, summer, winter, fall) survival rates, but the season of diagnosis probably has no biologic association with the length of a breast cancer patient's survival. On the other hand, the race-specific and age-specific survival rates shown in Figures 2.4

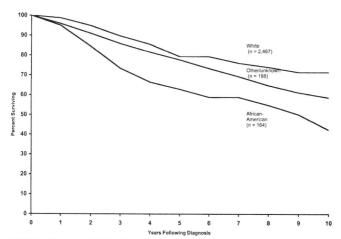

FIG 2.4. Survival of 2,819 breast cancer patients from the Surveillance, Epidemiology, and End Results Program of the National Cancer Institute, 1983–1998. Calculated by the life table method and stratified by race.

and 2.5 suggest that both of these variables are related to breast cancer survival. Whites have the highest survival rates and African-Americans the lowest. In the case of age, these data suggest that only the oldest patients experience poor survival and that it would be helpful to consider the effects of other causes of death that affect older persons using adjustments to be described.

Although the factors that affect survival may be unique to each type of cancer, it has become conventional that a basic description of survival for a specific cancer should include stage, age, and race-specific survival results. Treatment is a factor by which survival is commonly subdivided but it must be kept in mind that selection of treatment is usually related to some other factors which exert influence on survival. For example, in cancer care the choice of treatment is often dependent on the stage of disease at diagnosis.

ADJUSTED SURVIVAL RATE

The survival rates depicted in the illustrations account for all deaths, regardless of cause. This is known as *observed survival rate*. Although observed survival is a true reflection of total mortality in the patient group, we frequently are interested in describing mortality attributable only to the disease under investigation. The *adjusted survival rate* is the proportion of the initial patient group that escaped death due to a specific cause (e.g., cancer) if no other cause of death was operating. Whenever reliable information on cause of death is available, an adjustment can be made for deaths due to causes other than the disease under study. This is accomplished by treating patients who died without the disease of interest as censored observations.

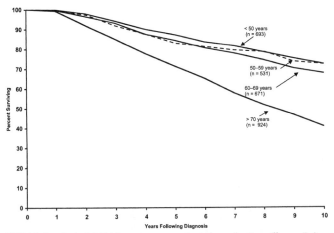

FIG 2.5. Survival of 2,819 breast cancer patients from the Surveillance, Epidemiology, and End Results Program of the National Cancer Institute, 1983–1998. Calculated by the life table method and stratified by age at diagnosis.

If adjusted survival rates were calculated for lung cancer, the pattern of survival would show little difference between observed and adjusted rates, because lung cancer usually is the cause of death for patients with the diagnosis. For diseases with more favorable survival patterns, such as breast cancer, patients live long enough to be at risk of other causes of death, and in these instances, adjusted survival rates will tend to be higher than observed survival rates and to give a clearer picture of the specific effects of the diagnosis under investigation. Adjusted rates can be calculated for either life table or Kaplan-Meier results.

RELATIVE SURVIVAL

Information on cause of death is sometimes unavailable or unreliable. Under such circumstances, it is not possible to compute an adjusted survival rate. However, it is possible to adjust partially for differences in the risk of dying from causes other than the disease under study. This can be done by means of the *relative survival rate*, which is the ratio of the observed survival rate to the expected rate for a group of people in the general population similar to the patient group with respect to race, sex, and age. The relative survival rate is calculated using a procedure described by Ederer, Axtell, and Cutler (1961).

The relative survival rate represents the likelihood that a patient will not die from causes associated specifically with their cancer at some specified time after diagnosis. It is always larger than the observed survival rate for the same group of patients. If the group is sufficiently large and the patients are roughly representative of the population of the United States (taking race, sex, and age into account), the relative survival rate provides a useful estimate of the probability of escaping death from the specific cancer under study. However, if reliable information on cause of death is available, it is preferable to use the adjusted rate. This is particularly true when the series is small or when the patients are largely drawn from a particular socioeconomic segment of the population. Relative survival rates may be derived from life table or Kaplan-Meier results.

REGRESSION METHODS

Examining survival within specific patient, disease, or treatment categories is the simplest way of studying multiple factors possibly associated with survival. This approach, however, is limited to factors into which patients may be broadly grouped. This approach does not lend itself to studying the effects of measures that vary on an interval scale. There are many examples of interval variables in cancer, such as number of positive nodes, cell counts, and laboratory marker values. If the patient population were to be divided up into each interval value, too few subjects would be in each analysis to be meaningful. In addition, when more than one factor is considered, the number of curves that result provide so many comparisons that the effects of the factors defy interpretation.

Conventional multiple regression analysis investigates the joint effects of multiple variables on a single outcome, but it is incapable of dealing with censored observations. For this reason, other statistical methods have had to be developed to assess the relationship of survival time to a number of variables simultaneously. The most commonly used is the Cox proportional hazards regression model (Cox, 1972). This model provides a method for estimating the influence of multiple covariates on the survival distribution from data that include censored observations. Covariates are the multiple factors to be studied in association with survival. In the Cox proportional hazards regression model, the covariates may be categorical variables such as race, interval measures such as age, or laboratory test results.

Specifics of these methods are beyond the scope of this chapter. Fortunately, many readily accessible computer packages for statistical analysis now permit the methods to be applied quite easily by the knowledgeable analyst. Although much useful information can be derived from multivariate survival models, they generally do require additional assumptions about the shape of the survival curve and the nature of the effects of the covariates. One must always examine the appropriateness of the model that is used relative to the assumptions required.

STANDARD ERROR OF A SURVIVAL RATE

Survival rates that describe the experience of the specific group of patients are frequently used to generalize to larger populations. The existence of true population values is postulated, and these values are estimated from the group under study, which is only a sample of the larger population. If a survival rate were calculated from a second sample taken from the same population, it is unlikely that the results would be exactly the same. The difference between the two results is called the sampling variation (chance variation or sampling error). The *standard error* is a measure of the extent to which sampling variation influences the computed survival rate. In repeated observations under the same conditions, the true or population survival rate will lie within the range of two standard errors on either side of the computed rate about 95 times in 100. This range is called the *95% confidence interval.*

COMPARISON OF SURVIVAL BETWEEN PATIENT GROUPS

In comparing survival rates of two patient groups, the statistical significance of the observed difference is of interest. The essential question is "What is the probability that the observed difference may have occurred by chance?" The standard error of the survival rate provides a simple means for answering this question. If the 95% confidence intervals of two survival rates do not overlap, the observed difference would customarily be considered statistically significant—that is, unlikely to be due to chance.

It is possible that the differences between two groups at each comparable time of follow-up do not differ significantly but that when the survival curves are considered in their entirety, the individual insignificant differences combine to yield a significantly different pattern of survival. The most common statistical test that examines the whole pattern of differences between survival curves is the *log rank test.* This test equally weights the effects of differences occurring throughout the follow-up and is the appropriate choice for most situations. Other tests weight the differences according to the numbers of persons at risk at different points and can yield different results depending on whether deaths tend more to occur early or later in the follow-up.

Care must be exercised in the interpretation of tests of statistical significance. For example, if differences exist in the patient and disease characteristics of two treatment groups, a statistically significant difference in survival results may primarily reflect differences between the two patient series, rather than differences in efficacy of the treatment regimens. The more definitive approach to therapy evaluation requires a randomized clinical trial that helps to ensure comparability of the patient characteristics and the disease characteristics of the two treatment groups.

DEFINITION OF STUDY STARTING POINT

The starting time for determining survival of patients depends on the purpose of the study. For example, the starting time for studying the natural history of a particular cancer might be defined in reference to the appearance of the first symptom. Various reference dates are commonly used as starting times for evaluating the effects of therapy. These include (1) date of diagnosis, (2) date of first visit to physician or clinic, (3) date of hospital admission, and (4) date of treatment initiation. If the time to recurrence of a tumor after apparent complete remission is being studied, the starting time is the date of apparent complete remission. The specific reference date used should be clearly specified in every report.

The date of initiation of therapy should be used as the starting time for evaluating therapy. For untreated patients, the most comparable date is the time at which it was decided that no tumor-directed treatment would be given. For both treated and untreated patients, the above times from which survival rates are calculated will usually coincide with the date of the initial staging of cancer.

VITAL STATUS

At any given time, the vital status of each patient is defined as alive, dead, or unknown (i.e., lost to follow-up). The endpoint of each patient's participation in the study is (1) a specified "terminal event" such as death, (2) survival to the completion of the study, or (3) loss to follow-up. In each case, the observed follow-up time is the time from the starting point to the terminal event, to the end of the study, or to the date of last observation. This observed follow-up may be further described in terms of patient status at the endpoint, such as

Alive; tumor-free; no recurrence
Alive; tumor-free; after recurrence
Alive with persistent, recurrent, or metastatic disease
Alive with primary tumor
Dead; tumor-free
Dead; with cancer (primary, recurrent, or metastatic disease)
Dead; postoperative
Unknown; lost to follow-up

Completeness of the follow-up is crucial in any study of survival, because even a small number of patients lost to follow-up may lead to inaccurate or biased results. The maximum possible effect of bias from patients lost to follow-up may be ascertained by calculating a maximum survival rate, assuming that all lost patients lived to the end of the study. A minimum survival rate may be calculated by assuming that all patients lost to follow-up died at the time they were lost.

TIME INTERVALS

The total survival time is often divided into intervals in units of weeks, months, or years. The survival curve for these intervals provides a description of the population under study with respect to the dynamics of survival over a specified time. The time interval used should be selected with regard to the natural history of the disease under consideration. In diseases with a long natural history, the duration of study could be 5 to 20 years, and survival intervals of 6 to 12 months will provide a meaningful description of the survival dynamics. If the population being studied has a very poor prognosis (e.g., patients with carcinoma of the esophagus or pancreas), the total duration of study may be 2 to 3 years, and the survival intervals may be described in terms of 1 to 3 months. In interpreting survival rates, one must also take into account the number of individuals entering a survival interval.

SUMMARY

This chapter has reviewed the rudiments of survival analysis as it is often applied to cancer registry data. Complex analysis of data and exploration of research hypotheses demand greater knowledge and expertise than could be conveyed herein. Survival analysis is now performed automatically in many different registry data management and statistical analysis programs available for use on personal computers. Persons with access to these programs are encouraged to explore the different analysis features available to demonstrate for themselves the insight on cancer registry data that survival analysis can provide.

BIBLIOGRAPHY

American Joint Committee on Cancer: AJCC Cancer Staging Manual, 5th ed. Fleming ID, Cooper JS, Henson DE et al (Eds.). Philadelphia: Lippincott-Raven, 1997

Berkson J, Gage RP: Calculation of survival rates for cancer. Proc Staff Meet Mayo Clin 25:270–286, 1950

Cox DR: Regression models and life tables. J R Stat Soc B 34:187–220, 1972

Cox DR, Oakes D: Analysis of survival data. London: Chapman and Hall, 1984

Ederer F, Axtell LM, Cutler SJ: The relative survival rate: a statistical methodology. Natl Cancer Inst Monogr 6:101–121, 1961

Fleming TR, Harrington DP: Counting processes and survival analysis. New York: John Wiley, 1991

Kalbfleisch JD, Prentice RL: The statistical analysis of failure time data. New York: John Wiley, 321, 1980

Kaplan EL, Meier P: Nonparametric estimation from incomplete observations. J Am Stat Assn 53:457–481, 1958

Kleinbaurn DG: Survival analysis: a self learning text. New York: Springer-Verlag, 1996

Lee ET: Statistical methods for survival data analysis. New York: John Wiley, 1992

Mantel N: Evaluation of survival data and two new rank order statistics arising in its consideration. Cancer Chemother Rep 50:163–170, 1966

Ries LAG, Eisner MP, Kosary CL, et al (Eds.): SEER cancer statistics review, 1973–1997: tables and graphs, National Cancer Institute. Bethesda, MD: National Institutes of Health, NIH Pub. No. 00-2789, 2000

PART II
Head and Neck Sites

SUMMARY OF CHANGES

- Across the board for all head and neck sites, a uniform description of advanced tumors has been recommended whereby T4 lesions are divided into T4a (resectable) and T4b (unresectable). This will allow assignment of patients with advanced stage disease to three categories: Stage IVA, advanced resectable disease; Stage IVB, advanced unresectable disease; and Stage IVC, advanced distant metastatic disease.

- In general, every effort has been made to bring the stage groupings to a relatively uniform combination of T, N, and M categories for all sites, including paranasal sinuses, salivary tumors, and thyroid tumors.

- No changes have been made in the N staging for any sites except that a descriptor has been added for nodal metastasis in the upper neck or in the lower neck, designated by (U) and (L), respectively. This descriptor will not influence nodal staging.

INTRODUCTION

Cancers of the head and neck may arise from any of the lining membranes of the upper aerodigestive tract. The T classifications indicating the extent of the primary tumor are generally similar but differ in specific details for each site because of anatomic considerations. The N classification for cervical lymph node metastasis is uniform for all mucosal sites except nasopharynx. The N classification for thyroid and nasopharynx are unique to those sites and are based on tumor behavior and prognosis. The staging systems presented in this section are all clinical staging, based on the best possible estimate of the extent of disease before first treatment. Imaging techniques (computed tomography [CT], magnetic resonance imaging [MRI], and ultrasonography) may be applied and, in more advanced tumor stages, have added to the accuracy of primary (T) and nodal (N) staging, especially in the nasopharyngeal, paranasal sinuses, and regional lymph nodal areas. Appropriate imaging studies should be obtained whenever the clinical findings are uncertain. Similarly, endoscopic evaluation of the primary tumor, when appropriate, is desirable for detailed assessment of the primary tumor for accurate T staging. Fine-needle aspiration biopsy (FNAB) may confirm the presence of tumor and its histopathologic nature, but it cannot rule out the presence of tumor.

Any diagnostic information that contributes to the overall accuracy of the pretreatment assessment should be considered in clinical staging and treatment planning. When surgical treatment is carried out, cancer of the head and neck can be staged—(pathologic stage [pTNM]) using all information available from clinical assessment, as well as from the pathologic study of the resected specimen. The pathologic stage does not replace the clinical stage, which should be reported as well.

In reviewing the staging systems, several changes in the T classifications as well as stage groupings are made to reflect current practices of treatment, clinical relevance, and contemporary data. Uniform T staging for oral cavity, oropharynx, salivary, and thyroid cancers greatly simplifies the system and will improve compliance by clinicians. T4 tumors are subdivided into advanced resectable (T4a) and advanced unresectable (T4b) categories. Regrouping of Stage IV disease for all sites into advanced resectable (Stage IVA), advanced unresectable (Stage IVB), and distant metastatic (Stage IVC) also simplifies advanced-disease staging.

This section presents the staging classification for six major head and neck sites: the oral cavity, the pharynx (nasopharynx, oropharynx, and hypopharynx), the larynx, the paranasal sinuses, the salivary glands, and the thyroid gland.

Regional Lymph Nodes. The status of the regional lymph nodes in head and neck cancer is of such prognostic importance that the cervical nodes must be assessed for each patient and tumor. The lymph nodes may be subdivided into specific anatomic subsites and grouped into seven levels for ease of description.

Level I:	Submental
	Submandibular
Level II:	Upper jugular
Level III:	Mid-jugular
Level IV:	Lower jugular
Level V:	Posterior triangle (spinal accessory and transverse cervical) (upper, middle, and lower, corresponding to the levels that define upper, middle, and lower jugular nodes)
Level VI:	Prelaryngeal (Delphian)
	Pretracheal
	Paratracheal
Level VII:	Upper mediastinal
Other groups:	Sub-occipital
	Retropharyngeal
	Parapharyngeal
	Buccinator (facial)
	Preauricular
	Periparotid and intraparotid

The location of the lymph node levels conforms to the following clinical descriptions, which also correlate with surgical landmarks at the time of surgical neck exploration (Fig. 2.1).

Level I: Contains the submental and submandibular triangles bounded by the anterior and posterior bellies of the digastric muscle, and the hyoid bone inferiorly, and the body of the mandible superiorly.

Level II: Contains the upper jugular lymph nodes and extends from the level of the skull base superiorly to the hyoid bone inferiorly.

Level III: Contains the middle jugular lymph nodes from the hyoid bone superiorly to the level of the lower border of the cricoid cartilage inferiorly.

Level IV: Contains the lower jugular lymph nodes from the level of the cricoid cartilage superiorly to the clavicle inferiorly.

Level V: Contains the lymph nodes in the posterior triangle bounded by the anterior border of the trapezius muscle posteriorly, the posterior border of the sternocleidomastoid muscle anteriorly, and the clavicle inferiorly. For descriptive purposes, Level V may be further subdivided into upper, middle, and lower levels corresponding to the superior and inferior planes that define Levels II, III, and IV.

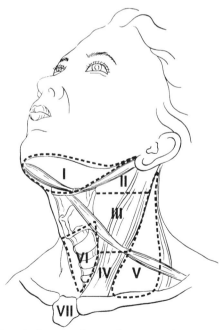

FIG 2.1. Schematic diagram indicating the location of the lymph node levels in the neck as described in the text.

Level VI: Contains the lymph nodes of the anterior central compart-
             ment from the hyoid bone superiorly to the suprasternal
             notch inferiorly. On each side, the lateral boundary is formed
             by the medial border of the carotid sheath.
Level VII: Contains the lymph nodes inferior to the suprasternal notch
             in the superior mediastinum.

The pattern of the lymphatic drainage varies for different anatomic sites. However, the location of the lymph node metastases has prognostic significance in patients with squamous cell carcinoma of the head and neck. Survival is significantly worse when metastases involve lymph nodes beyond the first echelon of lymphatic drainage and, particularly, lymph nodes in the lower regions of the neck, i.e., Level IV and Level V (supra-clavicular region). Consequently, it is recommended that each N staging category be recorded to show, in addition to the established parameters, whether the nodes involved are located in the upper (U) or lower (L) regions of the neck, depending on their location above or below the lower border of the cricoid cartilage.

The natural history and response to treatment of cervical nodal me-tastases from nasopharynx primary sites are different, in terms of their impact on prognosis, so they justify a different N classification scheme. Regional node metastases from well-differentiated thyroid cancer do not significantly affect the ultimate prognosis and therefore also justify a unique staging system for thyroid cancers.

Histopathologic examination is necessary to exclude the presence of tumor in lymph nodes. No imaging study (as yet) can identify microscopic tumor foci in regional nodes or distinguish between small reactive nodes and small malignant nodes.

When enlarged lymph nodes are detected, the actual size of the nodal mass(es) should be measured. It is recognized that most masses over 3 cm in diameter are not single nodes but are confluent nodes or tumor in soft tissues of the neck. Imaging studies showing amorphous spiculated mar-gins of involved nodes or involvement of internodal fat resulting in loss of normal oval to round nodal shape strongly suggest extracapsular (ex-tranodal) tumor spread. Pathologic examination is necessary for docu-mentation of tumor extent in terms of the location or level of the lymph node(s) involved, the number of nodes that contain metastases, and the presence or absence of extracapsular spread of tumor.

Metastatic Sites.   The most common sites of distant spread are in the lungs and bones; hepatic and brain metastases occur less often. Mediastinal lymph node metastases are considered distant metastases.

Regional Lymph Nodes (N)
NX   Regional lymph nodes cannot be assessed
N0   No regional lymph node metastasis
*N1   Metastasis in a single ipsilateral lymph node, 3 cm or less in great-
         est dimension

*N2   Metastasis in a single ipsilateral lymph node, more than 3 cm but not more than 6 cm in greatest dimension; or in multiple ipsilateral lymph nodes, none more than 6 cm in greatest dimension; or in bilateral or contralateral lymph nodes, none more than 6 cm in greatest dimension

*N2a   Metastasis in single ipsilateral lymph node more than 3 cm but not more than 6 cm in greatest dimension

*N2b   Metastasis in multiple ipsilateral lymph nodes, none more than 6 cm in greatest dimension

*N2c   Metastasis in bilateral or contralateral lymph nodes, none more than 6 cm in greatest dimension

*N3   Metastasis in a lymph node more than 6 cm in greatest dimension

*Note: A designation of "U" or "L" may be used to indicate metastasis above the lower border of the cricoid (U) or below the lower border of the cricoid (L).

Distant Metastasis (M)

MX   Distant metastasis cannot be assessed
M0   No distant metastasis
M1   Distant metastasis

OUTCOME RESULTS

The survival curves shown for each anatomic site were constructed using head and neck cancer cases extracted from the National Cancer Data Base (NCDB) Call 9 data set, which represents patients diagnosed between 1985 and 1996. Survival analyses were performed on 1985–1991 cases that, as a result of the methodology of data collection, have at least 5 years of follow-up. The survival methods, performed using SPSS software, included observed survival (death from all causes) and relative survival (representing death from the cancer derived from observed survival rates adjusted for expected deaths based on age, race, and gender).

Anatomic sites and histologic types were coded on the NCDB according to the second edition of the *International Classification of Diseases for Oncology* (ICD-O-2). The subsites to be included in each analysis were chosen on the basis of those listed in the fourth edition of the AJCC's *Manual for Staging of Cancer*. Survival analyses for the lip, oral cavity, oropharynx, nasopharynx, hypopharynx, and the larynx's subsites included squamous cell carcinomas only (M8050, 8051–8082). Survival analyses for the maxillary sinus and major salivary glands included all histologic types. Survival analyses for the thyroid gland included papillary adenocarcinoma (M8050, 8260, 8340, 8503–8604), follicular adenocarcinoma (M8330–8332), medullary carcinoma (M8510–8512), and anaplastic carcinoma (M8021).

Only cases that were staged according to the third or fourth editions of the AJCC's *Manual for Staging of Cancer* were included. The survival analyses for the different sites were stratified by AJCC "combined" stage (representing pathologic stage, when available, and only clinical stage when pathological stage was not available). The 95% confidence intervals are provided for each year-5 survival rate, so that significance differences between the year-5 survival rates of the different stages can be determined.

BIBLIOGRAPHY

Beahrs O, Henson DE, Hutter RVP, Kennedy BJ (Eds.): American Joint Committee on Cancer: Manual for Staging of Cancer, 4th ed. Philadelphia: JB Lippincott, 1992

Cerezo L, Millan I, Torre A, Aragon G, Otero J.: Prognostic factors for survival and tumor control in cervical lymph node metastases from head and neck cancer: a multivariate study of 492 cases. Cancer 69:1224–1234, 1992

Cooper JS, Farnan NC, Asbell SO, et al: Recursive partitioning analysis of 2105 patients treated in Radiation Therapy Oncology Group studies of head and neck cancer. Cancer 77:1905–1911, 1996

Deleyiannis FW, Thomas DB, Vaughan TL, et al: Alcoholism: independent predictor of survival in patients with head and neck cancer. J Natl Cancer Inst 88:542–549, 1996

Faye-Lund H, Abdelnoor M: Prognostic factors of survival in a cohort of head and neck cancer patients in Oslo. Eur J Cancer B Oral Oncol 2:83–90, 1996

Grandi C, Alloisio M, Moglia D, et al: Prognostic significance of lymphatic spread in head and neck carcinomas: therapeutic implications. Head Neck Surg 8:67–73, 1985

Harnsberger HR: Squamous cell carcinoma: nodal staging. In Handbook of head and neck imaging, 2nd ed. St. Louis: Mosby, 283–298, 1995

Hillsamer PJ, Schuller DE, McGhee RB, et al: Improving diagnostic accuracy of cervical metastases with CT and MRI imaging. Arch Otolaryngo Head Neck Surg, 116:2297–1301, 1990

Jones AS, Roland NJ, Field JK, Phillips DE: The level of cervical lymph node metastases: their prognostic relevance and relationship with head and neck squamous carcinoma primary sites. Clin Otolaryngol 19:63–69, 1994

Kalnins IK, Leonard AG, Sako K et al: Correlation between prognosis and degree of lymph node involvement in carcinoma of the oral cavity. Am J Surg 34:450–454, 1977

Kowalski LP, Bagietto R, Lara JR, et al: Prognostic significance of the distribution of neck node metastasis from oral carcinoma. Head Neck 22:207–214, 2000

Mancuso AA, Harnsberger HR, Muraki AS, et al: Computed tomography of cervical and retropharyngeal lymph nodes: normal anatomy, variants of normal, and application in staging head and neck cancer. II. Pathology. Radiology 148:715–723, 1983

Medina JE: A rational classification of neck dissections. Otolaryngol Head Neck Surg 100:169–176, 1989

Percy C, Van Holten V, Muir C (Eds.): International classification of disease for oncology, 2nd ed. Geneva: World Health Organization, 1990

Piccirillo JF: Inclusion of comorbidity in a staging system for head and neck cancer. Oncology 9:831–836, 1995

Richard JM, Sancho-Garnier H, Michaeu C, et al: Prognostic factors in cervical lymph node metastasis in upper respiratory and digestive tract carcinomas: study of 1713 cases during a 15-year period. Laryngoscope 97:97–101, 1987

Robbins KT: Neck dissection: classification and incisions. In Shockley WW, Pillsbury HC (Eds.): The neck: diagnosis and surgery. St. Louis: Mosby, 381–391, 1994

Singh B, Alfonso A, Sabin S, et al: Outcome differences in younger and older patients with laryngeal cancer: a retrospective case-control study. Am J Otolaryngol, 21:92–97, 2000

Singh B, Bhaya M, Zimbler M, et al: Impact of comorbidity on outcome of young patients with head and neck squamous cell carcinoma. Head Neck 20:1–7, 1998

Som PM: Detection of metastasis in cervical lymph nodes: CT and MR criteria and differential diagnosis. Am J Radiol 158:961–969, 1992

Stell PM, Morton RP, Singh SD: Cervical lymph node metastases: the significance of the level of the lymph node. Clin Oncol 9:101–107, 1983

Stevens MH, Harnsberger HR, Mancuso AA: Computed tomography of cervical lymph nodes: staging and management of head and neck cancer. Arch Otolaryngol 111(11):735–739, 1985

Strong EW, Kasdorf H, Henk JM: Squamous cell carcinoma of the head and neck. In Hermanek P, Gospodarowicz MK, Henson DE, et al (Eds.): Prognostic factors in cancer, UICC Geneva. Berlin-New York: Springer-Verlag, 23–27, 1995

Yousem DM, Som PM, Hackney DB, et al: Central nodal necrosis and extracapsular neoplastic spread in cervical lymph nodes: MR imaging versus CT. Radiology 182:753–759, 1992

2

3

Lip and Oral Cavity

(Nonepithelial tumors such as those of lymphoid tissue, soft tissue, bone, and cartilage are not included.)

C00.0 External upper lip
C00.1 External lower lip
C00.2 External lip, NOS
C00.3 Mucosa of upper lip
C00.4 Mucosa of lower lip
C00.5 Mucosa of lip, NOS
C00.6 Commissure of lip
C00.8 Overlapping lesion of lip
C00.9 Lip, NOS
C02.0 Dorsal surface of tongue, NOS
C02.1 Border of tongue

C02.2 Ventral surface of tongue, NOS
C02.3 Anterior two-thirds of tongue, NOS
C02.8 Overlapping lesion of tongue
C02.9 Tongue, NOS
C03.0 Upper gum
C03.1 Lower gum
C03.9 Gum, NOS
C04.0 Anterior floor of mouth
C04.1 Lateral floor of mouth
C04.8 Overlapping lesion of floor of mouth

C04.9 Floor of mouth, NOS
C05.0 Hard palate
C05.8 Overlapping lesion of palate
C05.9 Palate, NOS
C06.0 Cheek mucosa
C06.1 Vestibule of mouth
C06.2 Retromolar area
C06.8 Overlapping lesion of other and unspecified parts of mouth
C06.9 Mouth, NOS

SUMMARY OF CHANGES

- T4 lesions have been divided into T4a (resectable) and T4b (unresectable), leading to the division of Stage IV into Stage IVA, Stage IVB, and Stage IVC.

ANATOMY

Primary Site. The oral cavity extends from the skin-vermilion junction of the lips to the junction of the hard and soft palate above and to the line of circumvallate papillae below and is divided into the following specific areas:

Mucosal Lip. The lip begins at the junction of the vermilion border with the skin and includes only the vermilion surface or that portion of the lip that comes into contact with the opposing lip. It is well defined into an upper and lower lip joined at the commissures of the mouth.

Buccal Mucosa. This includes all the membrane lining of the inner surface of the cheeks and lips from the line of contact of the opposing lips to the line of attachment of mucosa of the alveolar ridge (upper and lower) and pterygomandibular raphe.

Lower Alveolar Ridge. This refers to the mucosa overlying the alveolar process of the mandible which extends from the line of attachment of mucosa in the buccal gutter to the line of free mucosa of the floor of the mouth. Posteriorly it extends to the ascending ramus of the mandible.

Upper Alveolar Ridge. This refers to the mucosa overlying the alveolar process of the maxilla which extends from the line of attachment of mucosa in the upper gingival buccal gutter to the junction of the hard palate. Its posterior margin is the upper end of the pterygopalatine arch.

Retromolar Gingiva (Retromolar Trigone). This is the attached mucosa overlying the ascending ramus of the mandible from the level of the posterior surface of the last molar tooth to the apex superiorly, adjacent to the tuberosity of the maxilla.

Floor of the Mouth. This is a semilunar space over the myelohyoid and hyoglossus muscles, extending from the inner surface of the lower alveolar ridge to the undersurface of the tongue. Its posterior boundary is the base of the anterior pillar of the tonsil. It is divided into two sides by the frenulum of the tongue and contains the ostia of the submaxillary and sublingual salivary glands.

Hard Palate. This is the semilunar area between the upper alveolar ridge and the mucous membrane covering the palatine process of the maxillary palatine bones. It extends from the inner surface of the superior alveolar ridge to the posterior edge of the palatine bone.

Anterior Two-Thirds of the Tongue (Oral Tongue). This is the freely mobile portion of the tongue that extends anteriorly from the line of circumvallate papillae to the undersurface of the tongue at the junction of the floor of the mouth. It is composed of four areas: the tip, the lateral borders, the dorsum, and the undersurface (nonvillous ventral surface of the tongue). The undersurface of the tongue is considered a separate category by the World Health Organization (WHO).

Regional Lymph Nodes. Mucosal cancer of the oral cavity may spread to regional lymph node(s). Tumors of each anatomic site have their own predictable patterns of regional spread. The risk of regional metastasis is generally related to the T category and, probably more important, to the depth of infiltration of the primary tumor. Cancer of the lip carries a low metastatic risk and initially involves adjacent submental and submandibular nodes, then jugular nodes. Cancers of the hard palate and alveolar ridge likewise have a low metastatic potential and involve buccinator, submandibular, jugular, and occasionally retropharyngeal nodes. Other oral cancers will spread primarily to submandibular and jugular nodes and uncommonly to posterior triangle/supraclavicular nodes. Cancer of the anterior oral tongue may spread directly to lower jugular nodes. The closer to the midline the primary, the greater the risk of bilateral cervical nodal spread. Any previous treatment to the neck, surgical and/or radiation, may alter normal lymphatic drainage patterns, resulting in unusual distribution of regional spread of disease to the cervical lymph nodes. In general, cervical lymph node involvement from oral cavity primary sites is predictable and orderly, spreading from the primary to upper, then middle, and subsequently lower cervical nodes. However, disease in the anterior oral cavity may also spread directly to the mid-cervical lymph nodes. The risk of distant metastasis is more dependent on the N than on the T status of the head and neck cancer. Midline nodes are considered ipsilateral. In addition to the components to describe the N category, regional lymph nodes should also be described according to the level of the neck that is involved. It is recognized that the level of involved nodes in the neck is prognostically significant (lower is worse), as is the presence of extracapsular extension of metastatic tumor from individual nodes. Imaging studies showing amorphous spiculated margins of involved nodes or involvement of internodal fat resulting in loss of normal oval-to-round nodal shape strongly suggest extracapsular (extranodal) tumor spread; however, pathologic examination is necessary for documentation of the extent of such disease. No imaging study (as yet) can identify microscopic foci of cancer in regional nodes or distinguish between small reactive nodes and small malignant nodes (unless central radiographic inhomogeneity is present). For pN, a selective neck dissection will ordinarily include six or more lymph nodes, and a radical or modified radical neck dissection will ordinarily include ten or more lymph nodes. Negative pathologic examination of a lesser number of nodes still mandates a pN0 designation.

Metastatic Sites. The lungs are the commonest site of distant metastases; skeletal and hepatic metastases occur less often. Mediastinal lymph node metastases are considered distant metastases.

RULES FOR CLASSIFICATION

Clinical Staging. The assessment of the primary tumor is based on inspection and palpation of the oral cavity and neck. Additional studies may include CT or MRI. When imaging is utilized, one study will generally suffice to evaluate primary and nodal tumor extent. Clinical assessment of the extent of mucosal involvement is more accurate than radiographic assessment. The radiographic estimate of deep tissue extent and of regional lymph node involvement is usually more accurate than clinical assessment. MRI is generally more revealing of extent of soft tissue, perivascular, and perineural spread, skull base involvement, and intracranial tumor extension. On the other hand, high-resolution CT with contrast will often provide similar information if carefully done, will provide better images of bone and larynx detail, and is minimally affected by motion. CT or MR imaging may be more useful in evaluation of advanced tumors for assessment of bone invasion (mandible or maxilla) and deep tissue invasion (deep extrinsic tongue muscles, midline tongue, soft tissues of neck). Clinical examination supplemented with dental films or panoramic X-rays may be helpful in determining cortical bone involvement. If CT or MR imaging is undertaken for primary tumor evaluation, radiologic assessment of nodal involvement should be done simultaneously. For lesions of an advanced extent, appropriate screening for distant metastases should be considered. Ultrasonography may be helpful in assessment of major vascular invasion as an adjunctive test. The tumor must be confirmed histologically. All clinical, imaging, and pathologic data available prior to first definitive treatment may be used for clinical staging.

Pathologic Staging. Complete resection of the primary site and/or regional nodal dissections, followed by pathologic examination of the resected specimen(s), allows the use of this designation for pT and/or pN, respectively. Specimens that are resected after radiation or chemotherapy need to be identified and considered in context. pT is derived from the actual measurement of the unfixed tumor in the surgical specimen. It should be noted, however, that up to 30% shrinkage of soft tissues may ocur in the resected specimen. Pathologic staging represents additional and important information and should be included as such in staging, but it does not supplant clinical staging as the primary staging scheme.

DEFINITION OF TNM

Primary Tumor (T)

TX	Primary tumor cannot be assessed
T0	No evidence of primary tumor
Tis	Carcinoma *in situ*
T1	Tumor 2 cm or less in greatest dimension
T2	Tumor more than 2 cm but not more than 4 cm in greatest dimension
T3	Tumor more than 4 cm in greatest dimension
T4 (lip)	Tumor invades through cortical bone, inferior alveolar nerve, floor of mouth, or skin of face, i.e., chin or nose
T4a	(oral cavity) Tumor invades adjacent structures (e.g., through cortical bone, into deep [extrinsic] muscle of tongue [genioglossus, hyoglossus, palatoglossus, and styloglossus], maxillary sinus, skin of face)
T4b	Tumor invades masticator space, pterygoid plates, or skull base and/or encases internal carotid artery

Note: Superficial erosion alone of bone/tooth socket by gingival primary is not sufficient to classify a tumor as T4.

Regional Lymph Nodes (N)

NX	Regional lymph nodes cannot be assessed
N0	No regional lymph node metastasis
N1	Metastasis in a single ipsilateral lymph node, 3 cm or less in greatest dimension
N2	Metastasis in a single ipsilateral lymph node, more than 3 cm but not more than 6 cm in greatest dimension; or in multiple ipsilateral lymph nodes, none more than 6 cm in greatest dimension; or in bilateral or contralateral lymph nodes, none more than 6 cm in greatest dimension
N2a	Metastasis in single ipsilateral lymph node more than 3 cm but not more than 6 cm in greatest dimension
N2b	Metastasis in multiple ipsilateral lymph nodes, none more than 6 cm in greatest dimension
N2c	Metastasis in bilateral or contralateral lymph nodes, none more than 6 cm in greatest dimension
N3	Metastasis in a lymph node more than 6 cm in greatest dimension

Distant Metastasis (M)

MX	Distant metastasis cannot be assessed
M0	No distant metastasis
M1	Distant metastasis

STAGE GROUPING

Stage 0	Tis	N0	M0
Stage I	T1	N0	M0
Stage II	T2	N0	M0
Stage III	T3	N0	M0
	T1	N1	M0
	T2	N1	M0
	T3	N1	M0
Stage IVA	T4a	N0	M0
	T4a	N1	M0
	T1	N2	M0
	T2	N2	M0
	T3	N2	M0
	T4a	N2	M0
Stage IVB	Any T	N3	M0
	T4b	Any N	M0
Stage IVC	Any T	Any N	M1

HISTOPATHOLOGIC TYPE

The predominant cancer is squamous cell carcinoma. The staging guidelines are applicable to all forms of carcinoma. Nonepithelial tumors such as those of lymphoid tissue, soft tissue, and bone and cartilage (i.e., lymphoma, melanoma, and sarcoma) are not included. Histologic confirmation of diagnosis is required. Histopathologic grading of squamous carcinoma is recommended; the grade is subjective and uses a descriptive as well as numerical form, i.e., well, moderately well, and poorly differentiated, depending on the degree of closeness to, or deviation from, squamous epithelium in mucosal sites. Also recommended is a quantitative evaluation of depth of invasion of the primary tumor and the presence or absence of vascular invasion and perineural invasion.

CHARACTERISTICS OF TUMOR (SEE FIG. 3.1A, B, C)

Endophytic. The measurement using an ocular micrometer is taken perpendicular from the surface of the invasive squamous cell carcinoma (A) to the deepest area of involvement (B) and recorded in millimeters. The measurement should not be done on tangential sections or in lesions without a clearly recognizable surface component.

Exophytic. The measurement that is better characterized as tumor thickness rather than depth of invasion, is taken from the surface (A) to the deepest area (B).

Ulcerated. The measurement is taken from the ulcer base (A) to the deepest area (B), as well as from the surface of the most lateral extent of the invasive carcinoma (C) to the deepest area (D).

Depth of tumor invasion (mm) should be recorded. Depth is *not* used for T staging.

Although the grade of the tumor does not enter into staging of the tumor, it should be recorded. The pathologic description of any lymphadenectomy specimen should describe the size, number, and position of involved lymph node(s) and the presence or absence of extracapsular extension.

HISTOLOGIC GRADE (G)

GX   Grade cannot be assessed
G1   Well differentiated
G2   Moderately differentiated
G3   Poorly differentiated

PROGNOSTIC FACTORS

In addition to the importance of the TNM factors outlined previously, the overall health of these patients clearly influences outcome. Comorbidity can be classified by more general measures, such as the Karnofsky Performance Status (KPS), or by more specific measures, such as the Kaplan-Feinstein Index. The KPS provides a uniform, objective assessment of an individual's functional status. The scale, in 10-point increments from 0 (dead) to 100 (normal, no complaints, no evidence of disease), was devised in 1948 by David A. Karnofsky. The KPS is a reliable, independent predictor of survival outcome for patients with solid tumors, so it is a required baseline assessment in clinical protocols in head and neck and other cancers. The AJCC strongly recommends recording of KPS along with standard staging information.

Karnofsky Scale: Criteria of Performance Status (PS)

100   Normal; no complaints; no evidence of disease
90   Able to carry on normal activity; minor signs or symptoms of disease
80   Able to carry on normal activity with effort; some signs or symptoms of disease
70   Cares for self; unable to carry on normal activity or do active work
60   Requires occasional assistance but is able to care for most of own needs
50   Requires considerable assistance and frequent medical care
40   Disabled; requires special care and assistance

Diagnosis and treatment of depression may also aid in symptom control and improved quality of life. Continued exposure to carcinogens, such as alcohol and tobacco smoke, probably affects patients' outcomes adversely.

Figures 3.2A, 3.2B, 3.3A, and 3.3B show observed and relative survival rates for patients with squamous cell carcinoma of the lip and squamous cell carcinoma of the oral cavity for the years 1985–1991, classified by the AJCC staging classification.

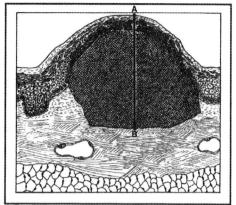

A. Exophytic

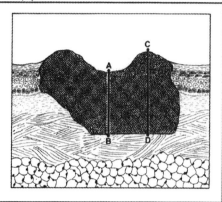

B. Ulcerated

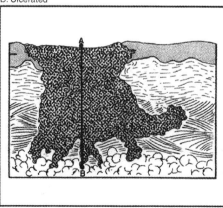

C Endophytic

FIG. 3.1. Characteristics of lip and oral cavity tumors. A: Exophytic; B: Ulcerated; C: Endophytic.

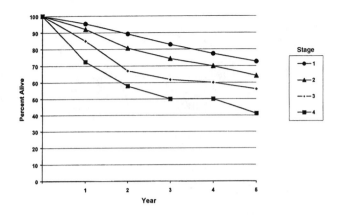

OBSERVED SURVIVAL BY STAGE	1	2	3	4	5	95% CIs*	CASES
1	95.2	89.2	82.9	77.3	72.6	70.1 – 75.0	1543
2	82.0	80.6	71.3	69.9	64.1	57.6 – 70.6	248
3	85.0	67.0	61.8	60.0	56.0	43.3 – 68.6	69
4	72.4	57.9	50.0	50.0	41.1	27.8 – 54.5	65

FIG. 3.2A. Five-year, observed survival by "combined" AJCC stage for squamous cell carcinoma of the lip, 1985–1991. (*95% confidence intervals correspond to year-5 survival rates.)

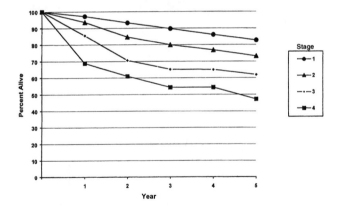

RELATIVE SURVIVAL BY STAGE	1	2	3	4	5	95% CIs*	CASES
1	97.2	93.2	89.7	86.1	82.8	80.1 – 85.6	1552
2	93.6	84.7	79.9	76.8	73.1	65.6 – 80.5	252
3	85.6	70.6	65.1	64.9	61.9	47.2 – 76.7	69
4	68.9	61.0	54.3	54.3	47.2	31.8 – 62.6	66

FIG. 3.2B. Five-year, relative survival by "combined" AJCC stage for squamous cell carcinoma of the lip, 1985–1991. (*95% confidence intervals correspond to year-5 survival rates.)

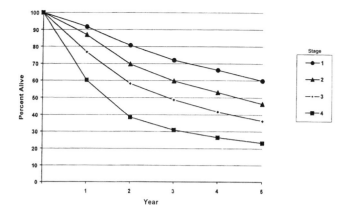

OBSERVED SURVIVAL BY STAGE	1	2	3	4	5	95% CIs*	CASES
1	91.6	80.6	72.0	66.1	59.8	57.7 – 61.8	2511
2	87.0	69.6	59.7	53.0	46.3	43.8 – 48.7	1839
3	76.7	58.1	48.7	41.6	36.3	33.6 – 38.9	1431
4	60.2	38.4	30.9	26.5	23.3	21.5 – 25.0	2433

FIG. 3.3A. Five-year, observed survival by "combined" AJCC stage for squamous cell carcinoma of the oral cavity, 1985–1991. (*95% confidence intervals correspond to year-5 survival rates.)

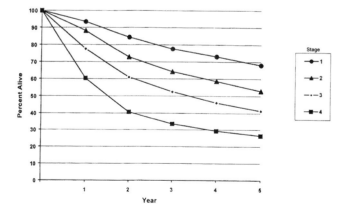

RELATIVE SURVIVAL BY STAGE	1	2	3	4	5	95% CIs*	CASES
1	93.3	84.4	77.5	73.0	68.1	65.7 – 70.4	2528
2	88.1	72.7	64.2	58.6	52.9	50.2 – 55.7	1858
3	77.5	60.9	52.5	46.0	41.3	38.3 – 44.4	1445
4	60.3	40.6	33.5	29.3	26.5	24.5 – 28.6	2459

FIG. 3.3B. Five-year, relative survival by "combined" AJCC stage for squamous cell carcinoma of the oral cavity, 1985–1991. (*95% confidence intervals correspond to year-5 survival rates.)

BIBLIOGRAPHY

Byers RM, Weber RS, Andrews T, et al: Frequency and therapeutic implications of "skip metastases" in the neck from squamous carcinoma of the oral tongue. Head Neck 19:14–19, 1997

Cooper JS, Farnan NC, Asbell SO, et al: Recursive partitioning analysis of 2105 patients treated in Radiation Therapy Oncology Group studies of head and neck cancer. Cancer 77:1905–1911, 1996

Cruse CW, Radocha RF: Squamous carcinoma of the lip. Plast Reconst Surg 80:787–791, 1987

de Leeuw JRJ, de Graeff A, Ros WJG, et al: Prediction of depressive symptomatology after treatment of head and neck cancer: the influence of pretreatment physical and depressive symptoms, coping, and social support. Head and Neck 22:799–807, 2000

Deleyiannis FW, Thomas DB, Vaughan TL, et al: Alcoholism: independent predictor of survival in patients with head and neck cancer. J Natl Cancer Inst 88:542–549, 1996

Evans JF, Shah JP: Epidermoid carcinoma of the palate. Am J Surg 142:451–455, 1981

Faye-Lund H, Abdelnoor M: Prognostic factors of survival in a cohort of head and neck cancer patients in Oslo. Eur J Cancer B Oral Oncol 2:83–90, 1996

Franceschi D, Gupta R, Spiro RH, et al: Improved survival in the treatment of squamous carcinoma of the oral tongue. Am J Surg 166:360–365, 1992

Kaplan MH, Feinstein AR: The importance of classifying initial co-morbidity in evaluating the outcome of diabetes mellitus. J Chron Dis 27:387–404, 1974

Karnofsky DA, Abelman WH, Craver LF, Burchenal JH: The use of the nitrogen mustards in the palliative treatment of carcinoma. Cancer 1:634–656, 1948

Krishnan-Nair M, Sankaranarayanan N, Padmanabhan T: Evaluation of the role of radiotherapy in the management of carcinoma of the buccal mucosa. Cancer 61:1326–1331, 1988

McDaniel JS, Dominique L, Musselman L, et al: Depression in patients with cancer. Psychiatry 52:89–99, 1995

Petrovich Z, Krusk H, Tobochnik N, et al: Carcinoma of the lip. Arch Otolaryngol 105:187–191, 1979

Piccirillo JF: Inclusion of comorbidity in a staging system for head and neck cancer. Oncology 9:831–836, 1995

Rodgers LW, Stringer SP, Mendenhall WH, et al: Management of squamous carcinoma of the floor of the mouth. Head Neck 15:16–19, 1993

Shaha AR, Spiro RH, Shah JP, et al: Squamous carcinoma of the floor of the mouth. Am J Surg 148:455–459, 1984

Soo KC, Spiro RH, King W, et al: Squamous carcinoma of the gums. Am J Surg 156:281–285, 1988

Spiro RH, Spiro JD, Strong EW: Surgical approaches to squamous carcinoma confined to the tongue and floor of the mouth. Head Neck 9:27–31, 1986

Totsuka Y, Usui Y, Tei K, et al: Mandibular involvement by squamous cell carcinoma of the lower alveolus: analysis and comparative study of the histologic and radiologic features. Head Neck 13:40–50, 1991

Urist M, O'Brien CJ, Soong SJ, et al: Squamous cell carcinoma of the buccal mucosa: analysis of prognostic factors. Am J Surg 154:411–414, 1987

Wendt CD, Peters LJ, Delclos L, et al: Primary radiotherapy in the treatment of Stage I and II oral tongue cancer: importance of the proportion of therapy delivered with interstitial therapy. Int J Radiation Oncology Biol Phys 18:1287–1292, 1990

HISTOLOGIES—LIP AND ORAL CAVITY

8010/2	Carcinoma *in situ*, NOS
8010/3	Carcinoma, NOS
8012/3	Large cell carcinoma, NOS
8013/3	Large cell neuroendocrine carcinoma
8020/3	Carcinoma, undifferentiated, NOS
8021/3	Carcinoma, anaplastic, NOS
8030/3	Giant cell and spindle cell carcinoma
8031/3	Giant cell carcinoma
8032/3	Spindle cell carcinoma, NOS
8033/3	Pseudosarcomatous carcinoma
8041/3	Small cell carcinoma, NOS
8042/3	Oat cell carcinoma
8043/3	Small cell carcinoma, fusiform cell
8044/3	Small cell carcinoma, intermediate cell
8045/3	Combined small cell carcinoma
8051/3	Verrucous carcinoma, NOS
8052/2	Papillary squamous cell carcinoma, non-invasive
8052/3	Papillary squamous cell carcinoma
8070/2	Squamous cell carcinoma *in situ*, NOS
8070/3	Squamous cell carcinoma, NOS
8071/3	Squamous cell carcinoma, keratinizing, NOS
8072/3	Squamous cell carcinoma, large cell
8073/3	Squamous cell carcinoma, small cell, non-keratinizing
8074/3	Squamous cell carcinoma, spindle cell
8075/3	Squamous cell carcinoma, adenoid
8076/2	Squamous cell carcinoma *in situ* with questionable stromal invasion
8076/3	Squamous cell carcinoma, microinvasive
8082/3	Lymphoepithelial carcinoma
8083/3	Basaloid squamous cell carcinoma
8084/3	Squamous cell carcinoma, clear cell type
8090/3	Basal cell carcinoma, NOS
8091/3	Multifocal superficial basal cell carcinoma
8092/3	Infiltrating basal cell carcinoma, NOS
8093/3	Basal cell carcinoma, fibroepithelial
8094/3	Basosquamous carcinoma
8097/3	Basal cell carcinoma, nodular
8098/3	Adenoid basal carcinoma
8123/3	Basaloid carcinoma
8140/2	Adenocarcinoma *in situ*, NOS
8140/3	Adenocarcinoma, NOS
8144/3	Adenocarcinoma, intestinal type
8145/3	Carcinoma, diffuse type
8147/3	Basal cell adenocarcinoma
8200/3	Adenoid cystic carcinoma
8246/3	Neuroendocrine carcinoma, NOS
8310/3	Clear cell adenocarcinoma, NOS
8430/3	Mucoepidermoid carcinoma
8440/3	Cystadenocarcinoma, NOS
8480/3	Mucinous adenocarcinoma
8481/3	Mucin-producing adenocarcinoma
8510/3	Medullary carcinoma, NOS
8525/3	Polymorphous low-grade adenocarcinoma
8550/3	Acinar cell carcinoma
8560/3	Adenosquamous carcinoma

8562/3	Epithelial-myoepithelial carcinoma
8574/3	Adenocarcinoma with neuroendocrine differentiation
8940/3	Mixed tumor, malignant, NOS
8941/3	Carcinoma in pleomorphic adenoma

Pharynx
(Including Base of Tongue, Soft Palate, and Uvula)

*(Nonepithelial tumors such as those of lymphoid tissue, soft tissue, bone, and cartilage
are not included.)*

2

C01.9 Base of tongue, NOS	C10.9 Oropharynx, NOS	C13.1 Hypopharyngeal aspect
C02.4 Lingual tonsil	C11.0 Superior wall of	of aryepiglottic fold
C05.1 Soft palate, NOS	nasopharynx	C13.2 Posterior wall of
C05.2 Uvula	C11.1 Posterior wall of	hypopharynx
C09.0 Tonsillar fossa	nasopharynx	C13.8 Overlapping lesion
C09.1 Tonsillar pillar	C11.2 Lateral wall of	C13.9 Hypopharynx, NOS
C09.8 Overlapping lesion	nasopharynx	C14.0 Pharynx, NOS
C09.9 Tonsil, NOS	C11.3 Anterior wall of	C14.2 Waldeyer's ring
C10.0 Vallecula	nasopharynx	C14.8 Overlapping lesion of lip,
C10.2 Lateral wall of	C11.8 Overlapping lesion	oral cavity and pharynx
oropharynx	C11.9 Nasopharynx, NOS	
C10.4 Branchial cleft	C12.9 Pyriform sinus	
C10.8 Overlapping lesion	C13.0 Postcricoid region	

SUMMARY OF CHANGES

- For oropharynx and hypopharynx only, T4 lesions have been divided into
  T4a (resectable) and T4b (unresectable), leading to the division of Stage
  IV into Stage IVA, Stage IVB, and Stage IVC.

ANATOMY

Primary Sites and Subsites. The pharynx (including base of tongue, soft
palate, and uvula) is divided into three regions: nasopharynx, oropharynx
and hypopharynx (Fig. 4.1). Each region is further subdivided into specific
sites as summarized in the following:

Nasopharynx. The nasopharynx begins anteriorly at the posterior cho-
ana and extends along the plane of the airway to the level of the free border
of the soft palate. It includes the vault, the lateral walls (including the fossae
of Rosenmuller and the mucosa covering the torus tubaris forming the
eustachian tube orifice), and the posterior wall. The floor is the superior
surface of the soft palate. The posterior margins of the choanal orifices
and of the nasal septum are included in the nasal fossa.

Parapharyngeal involvement denotes posterolateral infiltration of tumor beyond the pharyngobasilar fascia. Involvement of the masticator
space denotes extension of tumor beyond the anterior surface of the lateral
pterygoid muscle, or lateral extension beyond the posterolateral wall of the
maxillary antrum, and the pterygomaxillary fissure.

Oropharynx. The oropharynx is the portion of the continuity of the
pharynx extending from the plane of the superior surface of the soft palate
to the superior surface of the hyoid bone (or floor of the vallecula). It
includes the base of the tongue, the inferior (anterior) surface of the soft
palate and the uvula, the anterior and posterior tonsillar pillars, the

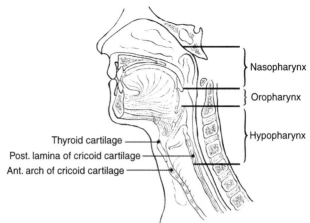

FIG. 4.1. Sagittal view of the face and neck depicting the subdivisions of the pharynx as described in the text.

glossotonsillar sulci, the pharyngeal tonsils, and the lateral and posterior pharyngeal walls.

Hypopharynx. The hypopharynx is that portion of the pharynx extending from the plane of the superior border of the hyoid bone (or floor of the vallecula) to the plane corresponding to the lower border of the cricoid cartilage. It includes the pyriform sinuses (right and left), the lateral and posterior hypopharyngeal walls, and the postcricoid region. The postcricoid area extends from the level of the arytenoid cartilages and connecting folds to the inferior border of the cricoid cartilage. It connects the two pyriform sinuses, thus forming the anterior wall of the hypopharynx. The pyriform sinus extends from the pharyngoepiglottic fold to the upper end of the esophagus at the lower border of the cricoid cartilage and is bounded laterally by the lateral pharyngeal wall and medially by the lateral surface of the aryepiglottic fold and the arytenoid and cricoid cartilages. The posterior pharyngeal wall extends from the level of the superior surface of the hyoid bone (or floor of the vallecula) to the inferior border of the cricoid cartilage and from the apex of one pyriform sinus to the other.

Regional Lymph Nodes.   The risk of regional nodal spread from cancers of the pharynx is high. Primary nasopharyngeal tumors commonly spread to retropharyngeal, upper jugular, and spinal accessory nodes, often bilaterally. Oropharyngeal cancers involve upper and mid-jugular lymph nodes and (less commonly) submental/submandibular nodes. Hypopharyngeal cancers spread to adjacent parapharyngeal, paratracheal, and mid- and lower jugular nodes. Bilateral lymphatic drainage is common.

In clinical evaluation, the maximum size of the nodal mass should be measured. Most masses over 3 cm in diameter are not single nodes but, rather, are confluent nodes or tumor in soft tissues of the neck. There are three categories of clinically involved nodes for the nasopharynx, oropharynx, and hypopharynx: N1, N2, and N3. The use of subgroups a, b, and c is not required but is recommended. Midline nodes are considered ipsilateral nodes. In addition to the components to describe the N category, regional lymph nodes should also be described according to the level of the neck that is involved. The level of involved nodes in the neck is prognostically significant (lower is worse), as is the presence of extracapsular extension of metastatic tumor from individual nodes. Imaging studies showing amorphous spiculated margins of involved nodes or involvement of internodal fat resulting in loss of normal oval-to-round nodal shape strongly suggest extracapsular (extranodal) tumor spread; however, pathologic examination is necessary for documentation of such disease extent. No imaging study (as yet) can identify microscopic foci in regional nodes or distinguish between small reactive nodes and small malignant nodes (unless central radiographic inhomogeneity is present).

For pN, a selective neck dissection will ordinarily include 6 or more lymph nodes, and a radical or modified radical neck dissection will ordinarily include 10 or more lymph nodes. Negative pathologic examination of a lesser number of nodes still mandates a pN0 designation.

Metastatic Sites. The lungs are the commonest site of distant metastases; skeletal or hepatic metastases occur less often. Mediastinal lymph node metastases are considered distant metastases.

RULES FOR CLASSIFICATION

Clinical Staging. Clinical staging is generally employed for squamous cell carcinomas of the pharynx. Assessment is based primarily on inspection and on indirect and direct endoscopy. Palpation of sites (when feasible) and of neck nodes is essential. Neurologic evaluation of all cranial nerves is required. Imaging studies are essential in clinical staging of pharynx tumors. Cross-sectional imaging in nasopharyngeal cancer is mandatory to complete the staging process. Magnetic resonance imaging (MRI) often is the study of choice because of its multiplanar capability, superior soft tissue contrast, and sensitivity for skull base and intracranial tumor spread. Computed tomography (CT) imaging with axial and coronal thin section technique with contrast is an alternative. Radiologic nodal staging should be done to assess adequately the retropharyngeal and cervical nodal status.

Cross-sectional imaging in oropharyngeal carcinoma is recommended when the deep tissue extent of the primary tumor is in question. CT or MRI may be employed. Cross-sectional imaging of hypopharyngeal carcinoma is recommended when the extent of the primary tumor is in doubt, particularly its deep extent in relationship to adjacent structures (i.e., larynx, thyroid, cervical vertebrae, and carotid sheath). CT is preferred currently because it entails less motion artifact than MRI. Radiologic nodal staging should be done simultaneously. Complete endoscopy, usually under general anesthesia, is performed after completion of other staging studies, to assess the surface extent of the tumor accurately and to assess deep involvement by palpation for muscle invasion and to facilitate biopsy. A careful search for other primary tumors of the upper aerodigestive tract is indicated because of the incidence of multiple independent primary tumors occurring simultaneously.

Pathologic Staging.   Pathologic staging requires the use of all information obtained in clinical staging and in histologic study of the surgically resected specimen. The surgeon's evaluation of gross unresected residual tumor must also be included. The pathologic description of any lymphadenectomy specimen should describe the size, number, and level of any involved nodes and the presence or absence of extracapsular extension.

DEFINITION OF TNM

Primary Tumor (T)

TX   Primary tumor cannot be assessed
T0   No evidence of primary tumor
Tis   Carcinoma *in situ*

Nasopharynx

T1   Tumor confined to the nasopharynx
T2   Tumor extends to soft tissues
     T2a Tumor extends to the oropharynx and/or nasal cavity without parapharyngeal extension*
     T2b Any tumor with parapharyngeal extension*
T3   Tumor involves bony structures and/or paranasal sinuses
T4   Tumor with intracranial extension and/or involvement of cranial nerves, infratemporal fossa, hypopharynx, orbit, or masticator space

Note: Parapharyngeal extension denotes posterolateral infiltration of tumor beyond the pharyngobasilar fascia.

Oropharynx

T1   Tumor 2 cm or less in greatest dimension
T2   Tumor more than 2 cm but not more than 4 cm in greatest dimension
T3   Tumor more than 4 cm in greatest dimension
T4a   Tumor invades the larynx, deep/extrinsic muscle of tongue, medial pterygoid, hard palate, or mandible
T4b   Tumor invades lateral pterygoid muscle, pterygoid plates, lateral nasopharynx, or skull base or encases carotid artery

Hypopharynx

T1   Tumor limited to one subsite of hypopharynx and 2 cm or less in greatest dimension
T2   Tumor invades more than one subsite of hypopharynx or an adjacent site, or measures more than 2 cm but not more than 4 cm in greatest diameter without fixation of hemilarynx
T3   Tumor more than 4 cm in greatest dimension or with fixation of hemilarynx
T4a   Tumor invades thyroid/cricoid cartilage, hyoid bone, thyroid gland, esophagus, or central compartment soft tissue*

T4b   Tumor invades prevertebral fascia, encases carotid artery, or involves mediastinal structures

Note: Central compartment soft tissue includes prelaryngeal strap muscles and subcutaneous fat.

Regional Lymph Nodes (N)

Nasopharynx
The distribution and the prognostic impact of regional lymph node spread from nasopharynx cancer, particularly of the undifferentiated type, are different from those of other head and neck mucosal cancers and justify the use of a different N classification scheme.

NX   Regional lymph nodes cannot be assessed
N0   No regional lymph node metastasis
N1   Unilateral metastasis in lymph node(s), 6 cm or less in greatest dimension, above the supraclavicular fossa*
N2   Bilateral metastasis in lymph node(s), 6 cm or less in greatest dimension, above the supraclavicular fossa*
N3   Metastasis in a lymph node(s)* >6 cm and/or to supraclavicular fossa
       N3a Greater than 6 cm in dimension
       N3b Extension to the supraclavicular fossa**

Note: Midline nodes are considered ipsilateral nodes.

   **Supraclavicular zone or fossa is relevant to the staging of nasopharyngeal carcinoma and is the triangular region originally described by Ho. It is defined by three points: (1) the superior margin of the sternal end of the clavicle, (2) the superior margin of the lateral end of the clavicle, (3) the point where the neck meets the shoulder (see Fig. 4.2). Note that this would include caudal portions of Levels IV and V. All cases with lymph nodes (whole or part) in the fossa are considered N3b.

Oropharynx and Hypopharynx
NX   Regional lymph nodes cannot be assessed
N0   No regional lymph node metastasis
N1   Metastasis in a single ipsilateral lymph node, 3 cm or less in greatest dimension
N2   Metastasis in a single ipsilateral lymph node, more than 3 cm but not more than 6 cm in greatest dimension, or in multiple ipsilateral lymph nodes, none more than 6 cm in greatest dimension, or in bilateral or contralateral lymph nodes, none more than 6 cm in greatest dimension
N2a   Metastasis in a single ipsilateral lymph node more than 3 cm but not more than 6 cm in greatest dimension
N2b   Metastasis in multiple ipsilateral lymph nodes, none more than 6 cm in greatest dimension

N2c   Metastasis in bilateral or contralateral lymph nodes, none more than 6 cm in greatest dimension

N3   Metastasis in a lymph node more than 6 cm in greatest dimension

Distant Metastasis (M)

MX   Distant metastasis cannot be assessed

M0   No distant metastasis

M1   Distant metastasis

STAGE GROUPING: NASOPHARYNX

Stage	T	N	M
Stage 0	Tis	N0	M0
Stage I	T1	N0	M0
Stage IIA	T2a	N0	M0
Stage IIB	T1	N1	M0
	T2	N1	M0
	T2a	N1	M0
	T2b	N0	M0
	T2b	N1	M0
Stage III	T1	N2	M0
	T2a	N2	M0
	T2b	N2	M0
	T3	N0	M0
	T3	N1	M0
	T3	N2	M0
Stage IVA	T4	N0	M0
	T4	N1	M0
	T4	N2	M0
Stage IVB	Any T	N3	M0
Stage IVC	Any T	Any N	M1

STAGE GROUPING: OROPHARYNX, HYPOPHARYNX

Stage	T	N	M
Stage 0	Tis	N0	M0
Stage I	T1	N0	M0
Stage II	T2	N0	M0
Stage III	T3	N0	M0
	T1	N1	M0
	T2	N1	M0
	T3	N1	M0
Stage IVA	T4a	N0	M0
	T4a	N1	M0
	T1	N2	M0
	T2	N2	M0
	T3	N2	M0
	T4a	N2	M0
Stage IVB	T4b	Any N	M0
	Any T	N3	M0
Stage IVC	Any T	Any N	M1

HISTOPATHOLOGIC TYPE

The predominant cancer type is squamous cell carcinoma for all pharyngeal sites. Non-epithelial tumors such as those of lymphoid tissue, soft tissue, bone, and cartilage are not included in this system. For nasopharyngeal carcinomas, it is recommended that the World Health Organization (WHO) classification be used (Table 4.1), p. 57. Histologic diagnosis is necessary to use this classification.

HISTOLOGIC GRADE (G): OROPHARYNX, HYPOPHARYNX

GX   Grade cannot be assessed
G1   Well differentiated
G2   Moderately differentiated
G3   Poorly differentiated

PROGNOSTIC FACTORS

In addition to the importance of the TNM factors outlined previously, the overall health of these patients clearly influences outcome. Comorbidity can be classified by more general measures, such as the Karnofsky performance score, or by more specific measures, such as the Kaplan-Feinstein Index. Continued exposure to carcinogens, such as alcohol and tobacco smoke, probably affects patients' outcomes adversely.

Figures 4.3A, 4.3B, 4.4A, 4.4B, 4.5A, and 4.5B show observed and relative survival rates for patients with squamous cell carcinoma of the Oropharynx (4.3A,B), squamous cell carcinoma of the nasopharynx (4.4A,B), and squamous cell carcinoma of the hypopharynx (4.5A,B) for the years 1985–1991, classified by the AJCC staging classification.

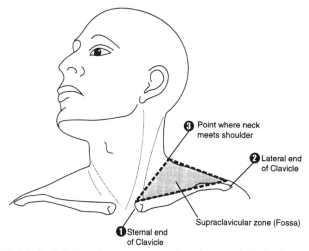

FIG. 4.2. Shaded triangular area corresponds to the supraclavicular fossa used in staging carcinoma of the nasopharynx.

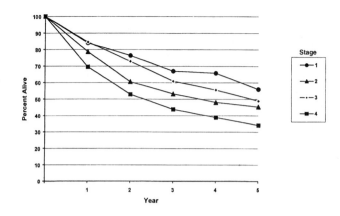

OBSERVED SURVIVAL BY STAGE	1	2	3	4	5	95% CIs*	CASES
1	84.1	76.4	66.9	65.7	56.0	45.6 – 66.3	104
2	78.7	60.5	53.2	48.1	45.4	34.8 – 56.0	96
3	84.6	72.9	60.9	55.6	49.0	41.8 – 56.0	205
4	69.6	52.9	43.9	38.8	34.1	30.2 – 37.9	665

FIG. 4.3A. Five-year, observed survival by "combined" AJCC stage for squamous cell carcinoma of the nasopharynx, 1985–1991. (*95% confidence intervals correspond to year-5 survival rates.)

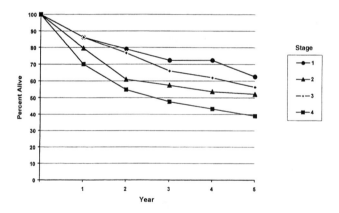

RELATIVE SURVIVAL BY STAGE	1	2	3	4	5	95% CIs*	CASES
1	86.2	79.0	72.3	72.3	62.5	50.5 – 74.5	104
2	79.6	60.9	57.4	53.6	52.1	39.9 – 64.4	96
3	86.2	76.7	65.9	61.9	56.3	48.1 – 64.4	205
4	70.1	54.8	47.6	43.3	38.9	34.6 – 43.3	669

FIG. 4.3B. Five-year, relative survival by "combined" AJCC stage for squamous cell carcinoma of the nasopharynx, 1985–1991. (*95% confidence intervals correspond to year-5 survival rates.)

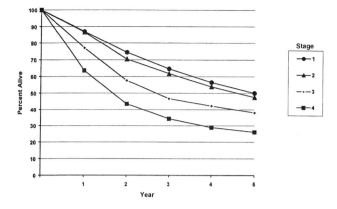

OBSERVED SURVIVAL BY STAGE	1	2	3	4	5	95% CIs*	CASES
1	87.0	74.4	64.6	56.5	50.0	46.7 – 53.4	980
2	86.6	70.4	61.8	53.9	47.5	44.3 – 50.6	1107
3	77.1	57.6	46.7	42.2	37.9	35.3 – 40.4	1529
4	63.6	43.5	34.2	28.9	26.1	24.5 – 27.6	3419

FIG. 4.4A. Five-year, observed survival by "combined" AJCC stage for squamous cell carcinoma of the oropharynx, 1985–1991. (*95% confidence intervals correspond to year-5 survival rates.)

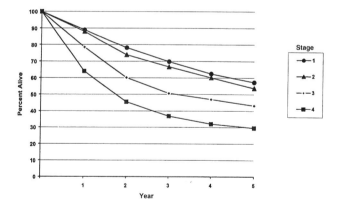

RELATIVE SURVIVAL BY STAGE	1	2	3	4	5	95% CIs*	CASES
1	88.9	78.1	69.8	62.4	57.3	53.5 – 61.2	986
2	87.9	73.8	66.6	60.1	53.7	50.1 – 57.3	1118
3	78.5	60.1	50.6	47.0	43.2	40.3 – 46.2	1541
4	64.0	45.5	36.7	32.0	29.6	27.8 – 31.3	3451

FIG. 4.4B. Five-year, relative survival by "combined" AJCC stage for squamous cell carcinoma of the oropharynx, 1985–1991. (*95% confidence intervals correspond to year-5 survival rates.)

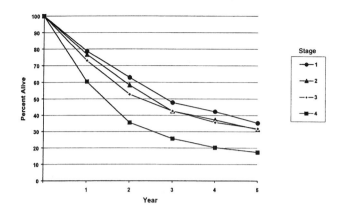

OBSERVED SURVIVAL BY STAGE	1	2	3	4	5	95% CIs*	CASES
1	78.7	62.8	47.8	42.3	35.2	29.4 – 41.0	299
2	76.7	58.2	42.6	37.1	31.3	26.1 – 36.6	345
3	73.0	52.7	42.7	35.6	31.8	27.9 – 35.6	617
4	60.4	35.5	25.7	20.2	17.4	15.5 – 19.2	1671

FIG. 4.5A. Five-year, observed survival by "combined" AJCC stage for squamous cell carcinoma of the hypopharynx, 1985–1991. (*95% confidence intervals correspond to year-5 survival rates.)

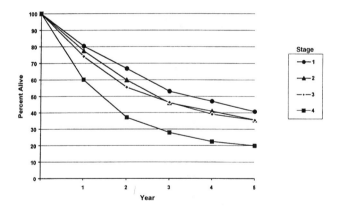

RELATIVE SURVIVAL BY STAGE	1	2	3	4	5	95% CIs*	CASES
1	80.3	66.7	53.0	47.0	40.7	31.4 – 47.4	304
2	77.5	59.8	46.0	40.9	35.6	29.6 – 41.6	350
3	74.1	55.5	46.3	39.0	35.5	31.1 – 39.8	620
4	60.1	37.1	27.9	22.4	19.9	17.7 – 22.0	1688

FIG. 4.5B. Five-year, relative survival by "combined" AJCC stage for squamous cell carcinoma of the hypopharynx, 1985–1991. (*95% confidence intervals correspond to year-5 survival rates.)

TABLE 4.1. Classification of Nasopharyngeal Carcinoma

WHO Classification	Former Terminology
Type 1. Squamous cell carcinoma	Squamous cell carcinoma
Type 2. Nonkeratinizing carcinoma	Transitional cell carcinoma
Without lymphoid stroma	Intermediate cell carcinoma
With lymphoid stroma	Lymphoepithelial carcinoma (Regaud)
Type 3. Undifferentiated carcinoma	Anaplastic carcinoma,
Without lymphoid stroma	Clear cell carcinoma
With lymphoid stroma	Lymphoepithelial carcinoma (Schminke)

2

BIBLIOGRAPHY

Boyd TS, Harari PM, Tannehill SP, Voytovich MC, Hartig GK, Ford CN, Foote RL, Campbell BH, Schultz CJ: Planned postradiotherapy neck dissection in patients with advanced head and neck cancer. Head Neck 29:132–137, 1998

Chong V, Mukherji S, Ng S-H, et al: Nasopharyngeal carcinoma; review of how imaging affects staging. J Computer Assisted Tomography 23:984–993, 1999

Chua D, Sham J, Kwong D, et al: Prognostic value of paranasopharyngeal extension of nasopharyngeal carcinoma. A significant factor in local control and distant metastasis. Cancer 78:202–210, 1996

Colangelo LA, Logemann JA, Pauloski BR, Pelzer JR, Rademaker AW: T stage and functional outcome in oral and oropharyngeal cancer patients. Head Neck 18:259–268, 1996

Cooper J, Cohen R, Stevens R: A comparison of staging systems for nasopharyngeal carcinoma. Cancer 83:213–219, 1998

Deleyiannis FW, Weymuller EA Jr, Coltrera MD: Quality of life of disease-free survivors of advanced (Stage III or IV) oropharyngeal cancer. Head Neck 19:466–473, 1997

Forastiere AA, Trotti A. Radiotherapy and concurrent chemotherapy: a strategy that improves locoregional control and survival in oropharyngeal cancer. J Nat Cancer Inst 91:2065–2066, 1999

Garden AS, Morrison WH, Clayman GL, Ang KK, Peters LJ: Early squamous cell carcinoma of the hypopharynx: outcomes of treatment with radiation alone to the primary disease. Head Neck 18:317–22, 1996

Gwozdz JT, Morrison WH, Garden AS, Weber RS, Peters LJ, Ang KK: Concomitant boost radiotherapy for squamous carcinoma of the tonsillar fossa. Int J Rad Onc Biol Phys 39:127–135, 1997

Harrison LB, Lee HJ, Pfister DG, Kraus DH, White C, Raben A, Zelefsky MJ, Strong EW, Shah JP: Long-term results of primary radiotherapy with/without neck dissection for squamous cell cancer of the base of the tongue. Head Neck 20:668–673, 1998

Ho J: Stage classification of nasopharyngeal carcinoma, etiology and control. IARC Scientific Publications 20:99–113, 1978

Hoffman HT, Karnell LH, Shah JP, Ariyan S, Brown GS, Fee WE, Glass AG, Goepfert H, Ossoff RH, Fremgen AM: Hypopharyngeal cancer patient care evaluation. Laryngoscope 107:1005–1017, 1997

Hoffman HT, Karnell LH, Funk GF, Robinson RA, Menck HR: The National Cancer Data Base report on cancer of the head and neck. Arch Otolaryngol-Head Neck Surg 951–962, 1998

Iro H, Waldfahrer F: Evaluation of the newly updated TNM classification of head and neck carcinoma with data from 3,247 patients. Cancer 83:2201–2207, 1998

Kraus DH, Zelefsky MJ, Brock HA, Huo J, Harrison LB, Shah JP: Combined surgery and radiation therapy for squamous cell carcinoma of the hypopharynx. Otolaryngol-HN Surg 116, 637–641, 1997

Lee A, Foo W, Law S, et al: N-staging of nasopharyngeal carcinoma: Discrepancy between UICC/AJCC and Ho systems. Clinical Oncology 17:377–381, 1995

Lefebvre JL, Buisset E, Coche-Dequeant B, Van JT, Prevost B, Hecquet B, Damaille A: Epilarynx: pharynx or larynx? Head Neck 17:377–381, 1995

Lefebvre JL, Chevalier D, Luboinski B, Kirkpatric A, Collette L, Sahmoud T: Larynx preservation in pyriform sinus cancer: preliminary results of a European Organization for Research Treatment of Cancer phase III trial. EORTC Head and Neck Cancer Cooperative Group. J Nat Cancer Inst 88:890–899, 1996

Mendenhall WM, Amdur RJ, Stringer SP, Villaret DB, Cassissi NJ: Stratification of stage IV squamous cell carcinoma of the oropharynx. Head Neck 22:626–628, 2000

Pauloski BR, Logemann JA, Colangelo LA, Rademaker AW, McConnel FM, Heiser MA, Carndinale S, Shedd D, Stein D, Beery Q, Myers E, Lewin J, Haxer M, Esclamado R: Surgical variables affecting speech in treated patients with oral and oropharyngeal cancer. Laryngoscope 108:908–916, 1998

Perez CA, Patel MM, Chao KS, Simpson JR, Sessions D, Spector GJ, Haughey B, Lockett MA: Carcinoma of the tonsillar fossa: prognostic factors and long-term therapy outcome. Int J Rad Onc, Biol Phys 42:1077–1084, 1998

Prehn RB, Pasic TR, Harari PM, Brown WD, Ford CN: Influence of computed tomography on pretherapeutic tumor staging of head and neck cancer patients. Otolaryngol-Head Neck Surg 199:628–633, 1998

Pugliano FA, Piccirillo JF, Zequeira MR, Emami B, Perez CA, Simpson JR, Frederickson JM: Clinical-severity staging system for oropharyngeal cancer: five-year survival rates. Arch Otolaryngol-Head Neck Surg 123:1118–1124, 1997

Righi PD, Kelley DJ, Ernst R, Deutsch MD, Gaskill-Shipley M, Wilson KM, Gluckman JL: Evaluation of prevertebral muscle invasion by squamous cell carcinoma. Can computed tomography replace open neck exploration? Arch Otolaryngol Head Neck Surg 122:660–663, 1996

Teresi L, Lufkin R, Vinuela F, et al: MR imaging of the nasopharynx and floor of the middle cranial fossa. Part II. Malignant Tumors. Radiol 164:817–821, 1987

Thabet HM, Sessions DG, Gado MY, Gnepp DA, Harvey JE, Talaat M: Comparison of clinical evaluation and computed tomographic diagnostic accuracy for tumor of the larynx and hypopharynx. Laryngoscope 106:589–594, 1996

Veneroni S, Silvestrini R, Costa A, Salvatori P, Faranda A, Monlinari R: Biological indicators of survival in patients treated by surgery for squamous cell carcinoma of the oral cavity and oropharynx. Oral Oncol 33:408–413, 1997

Wang MB, Kuber MM, Lee SP, Julliard GF, Abemayor E: Tonsillar carcinoma: analysis of treatment results. J Otolaryngol 27:263–269, 1998

Wahlberg PC, Andersson KE, Biorklund AT, Moller TR: Carcinoma of the hypopharynx: analysis of incidence and survival in Sweden over a 30-year period. Head Neck 20:714–719, 1998

Weber RS, Gidley P, Morrison WH, Peters LJ, Hankins PD, Wolf P, Guilla-mondegui OM: Treatment selection for carcinoma of the base of the tongue. Am J Surg 60:415–419, 1990

Zelefsky MJ, Kraus DH, Pfister DG, Raben A, Shah JP, Strong EW, Spiro RH, Bosl GJ, Harrison LB: Combined chemotherapy and radiotherapy versus surgical and postoperative radiotherapy for advanced hypopharyngeal cancer. Head Neck 18:405–411, 1996

HISTOLOGIES—PHARYNX

8010/2	Carcinoma *in situ*, NOS
8010/3	Carcinoma, NOS
8012/3	Large cell carcinoma, NOS
8013/3	Large cell neuroendocrine carcinoma
8020/3	Carcinoma, undifferentiated, NOS
8021/3	Carcinoma, anaplastic, NOS
8030/3	Giant cell and spindle cell carcinoma
8031/3	Giant cell carcinoma
8032/3	Spindle cell carcinoma, NOS
8033/3	Pseudosarcomatous carcinoma
8041/3	Small cell carcinoma, NOS
8042/3	Oat cell carcinoma
8043/3	Small cell carcinoma, fusiform cell
8044/3	Small cell carcinoma, intermediate cell
8045/3	Combined small cell carcinoma
8051/3	Verrucous carcinoma, NOS
8052/2	Papillary squamous cell carcinoma, non-invasive
8052/3	Papillary squamous cell carcinoma
8070/2	Squamous cell carcinoma *in situ*, NOS
8070/3	Squamous cell carcinoma, NOS
8071/3	Squamous cell carcinoma, keratinizing, NOS
8072/3	Squamous cell carcinoma, large cell
8073/3	Squamous cell carcinoma, small cell, non-keratinizing
8074/3	Squamous cell carcinoma, spindle cell
8075/3	Squamous cell carcinoma, adenoid
8076/2	Squamous cell carcinoma *in situ* with questionable stromal invasion
8076/3	Squamous cell carcinoma, microinvasive
8082/3	Lymphoepithelial carcinoma
8083/3	Basaloid squamous cell carcinoma
8084/3	Squamous cell carcinoma, clear cell type
8090/3	Basal cell carcinoma, NOS
8091/3	Multifocal superficial basal cell carcinoma
8092/3	Infiltrating basal cell carcinoma, NOS
8093/3	Basal cell carcinoma, fibroepithelial
8094/3	Basosquamous carcinoma
8097/3	Basal cell carcinoma, nodular
8098/3	Adenoid basal carcinoma
8123/3	Basaloid carcinoma
8140/2	Adenocarcinoma *in situ*, NOS
8140/3	Adenocarcinoma, NOS
8144/3	Adenocarcinoma, intestinal type
8145/3	Carcinoma, diffuse type
8147/3	Basal cell adenocarcinoma
8200/3	Adenoid cystic carcinoma
8246/3	Neuroendocrine carcinoma, NOS

8310/3	Clear cell adenocarcinoma, NOS
8430/3	Mucoepidermoid carcinoma
8440/3	Cystadenocarcinoma, NOS
8480/3	Mucinous adenocarcinoma
8481/3	Mucin-producing adenocarcinoma
8510/3	Medullary carcinoma, NOS
8525/3	Polymorphous low-grade adenocarcinoma
8550/3	Acinar cell carcinoma
8560/3	Adenosquamous carcinoma
8562/3	Epithelial-myoepithelial carcinoma
8574/3	Adenocarcinoma with neuroendocrine differentiation
8940/3	Mixed tumor, malignant, NOS
8941/3	Carcinoma in pleomorphic adenoma

5

Larynx

(Nonepithelial tumors such as those of lymphoid tissue, soft tissue, bone, and cartilage are not included.)

C10.1 Anterior (lingual) surface of epiglottis	C32.1 Supraglottis (laryngeal surface)	C32.8 Overlapping lesion of larynx
C32.0 Glottis	C32.2 Subglottis	C32.9 Larynx, NOS
	C32.3 Laryngeal cartilage	

SUMMARY OF CHANGES

- T4 lesions have been divided into T4a (resectable) and T4b (unresectable), leading to the division of Stage IV into Stage IVA, Stage IVB, and Stage IVC.

ANATOMY

Primary Site. The following anatomic definition of the larynx allows classification of carcinomas arising in the encompassed mucous membranes but excludes cancers arising on the lateral or posterior pharyngeal wall, pyriform fossa, postcricoid area, or base of tongue.

The anterior limit of the larynx is composed of the anterior or lingual surface of the suprahyoid epiglottis, the thyrohyoid membrane, the anterior commissure, and the anterior wall of the subglottic region, which is composed of the thyroid cartilage, the cricothyroid membrane, and the anterior arch of the cricoid cartilage.

The posterior and lateral limits include the laryngeal aspect of the aryepiglottic folds, the arytenoid region, the interarytenoid space, and the posterior surface of the subglottic space, represented by the mucous membrane covering the surface of the cricoid cartilage.

The superolateral limits are composed of the tip and the lateral borders of the epiglottis. The inferior limits are made up of the plane passing through the inferior edge of the cricoid cartilage.

For purposes of this clinical stage classification, the larynx is divided into three regions: supraglottis, glottis, and subglottis. The supraglottis is composed of the epiglottis (both its lingual and laryngeal aspects), aryepiglottic folds (laryngeal aspect), arytenoids, and ventricular bands (false cords). The epiglottis is divided for staging purposes into suprahyoid and infrahyoid portions by a plane at the level of the hyoid bone. The inferior boundary of the supraglottis is a horizontal plane passing through the lateral margin of the ventricle at its junction with the superior surface of the vocal cord. The glottis is composed of the superior and inferior surfaces of the true vocal cords, including the anterior and posterior commissures. It occupies a horizontal plane 1 cm in thickness, extending inferiorly from the lateral margin of the ventricle. The subglottis is the region extending from the lower boundary of the glottis to the lower margin of the cricoid cartilage.

The division of the larynx is summarized as follows:

Site	Subsite
Supraglottis	Suprahyoid epiglottis
	Infrahyoid epiglottis
	Aryepiglottic folds (laryngeal aspect)
	Arytenoids
	Ventricular bands (false cords)
Glottis	True vocal cords, including anterior and posterior commissures
Subglottis	Subglottis

Regional Lymph Nodes. The incidence and distribution of cervical nodal metastases from cancer of the larynx vary with the site of origin and the T classification of the primary tumor. The true vocal cords are nearly devoid of lymphatics, and tumors of that site alone rarely spread to regional nodes. By contrast, the supraglottis has a rich and bilaterally interconnected lymphatic network, and primary supraglottic cancers are commonly accompanied by regional lymph node spread. Glottic tumors may spread directly to adjacent soft tissues and prelaryngeal, pretracheal, paralaryngeal, and paratracheal nodes, as well as to upper, mid-, and lower jugular nodes. Supraglottic tumors commonly spread to upper and midjugular nodes, considerably less commonly to submental or submandibular nodes, and occasionally to retropharyngeal nodes. The rare subglottic primary tumors spread first to adjacent soft tissues and prelaryngeal, pretracheal, paralaryngeal, and paratracheal nodes, then to mid- and lower jugular nodes. Contralateral lymphatic spread is common.

In clinical evaluation, the physical size of the nodal mass should be measured. Most masses over 3 cm in diameter are not single nodes but, rather, are confluent nodes or tumor in soft tissues of the neck. There are three categories of clinically positive nodes: N1, N2, and N3. Midline nodes are considered ipsilateral nodes. In addition to the components to describe the N category, regional lymph nodes should also be described according to the level of the neck that is involved. Pathologic examination is necessary for documentation of such disease extent. Imaging studies showing amorphous spiculated margins of involved nodes or involvement of internodal fat resulting in loss of normal oval-to-round nodal shape strongly suggest extracapsular (extranodal) tumor spread. No imaging study (as yet) can identify microscopic foci in regional nodes or distinguish between small reactive nodes and small malignant nodes without central radiographic inhomogeneity.

Metastatic Sites. Distant spread is common only for patients who have bulky regional lymphadenopathy. When distant metastases occur, spread to the lungs is most common; skeletal or hepatic metastases occur less often. Mediastinal lymph node metastases are considered distant metastases.

RULES FOR CLASSIFICATION

Clinical Staging. The assessment of the larynx is accomplished primarily by inspection, using indirect mirror and direct endoscopic examination with a fiberoptic nasolaryngoscope. The tumor must be confirmed histologically, and any other data obtained by biopsies may be included. Cross-sectional imaging in laryngeal carcinoma is recommended when the primary tumor extent is in question on the basis of clinical examination. Radiologic nodal staging should be done simultaneously to supplement clinical examination.

Complete endoscopy under general anesthesia is usually performed after completion of other diagnostic studies to accurately assess, document, and biopsy the tumor.

Pathologic Staging. Pathologic staging requires the use of all information obtained in clinical staging and in histologic study of the surgically resected specimen. The surgeon's evaluation of gross unresected residual tumor must also be included. Specimens that are resected after radiation or chemotherapy need to be identified and considered in context. The pathologic description of any lymphadenectomy specimen should describe the size, number, and position of the involved node(s) and the presence or absence of extracapsular extension.

DEFINITION OF TNM

Primary Tumor (T)

TX   Primary tumor cannot be assessed
T0   No evidence of primary tumor
Tis   Carcinoma *in situ*

Supraglottis

T1   Tumor limited to one subsite of supraglottis with normal vocal cord mobility
T2   Tumor invades mucosa of more than one adjacent subsite of supraglottis or glottis or region outside the supraglottis (e.g., mucosa of base of tongue, vallecula, medial wall of pyriform sinus) without fixation of the larynx
T3   Tumor limited to larynx with vocal cord fixation and/or invades any of the following: postcricoid area, pre-epiglottic tissues, para-glottic space, and/or minor thyroid cartilage erosion (e.g., inner cortex)
T4a   Tumor invades through the thyroid cartilage and/or invades tissues beyond the larynx (e.g., trachea, soft tissues of neck including deep extrinsic muscle of the tongue, strap muscles, thyroid, or esophagus)
T4b   Tumor invades prevertebral space, encases carotid artery, or invades mediastinal structures

Glottis

T1   Tumor limited to the vocal cord(s) (may involve anterior or posterior commissure) with normal mobility
T1a   Tumor limited to one vocal cord
T1b   Tumor involves both vocal cords

T2	Tumor extends to supraglottis and/or subglottis, and/or with impaired vocal cord mobility
T3	Tumor limited to the larynx with vocal cord fixation and/or invades paraglottic space, and or minor thyroid cartilage erosion (e.g., inner cortex)
T4a	Tumor invades through the thyroid cartilage and/or invades tissues beyond the larynx (e.g., trachea, soft tissues of neck including deep extrinsic muscle of the tongue, strap muscles, thyroid, or esophagus)
T4b	Tumor invades prevertebral space, encases carotid artery, or invades mediastinal structures

Subglottis

T1	Tumor limited to the subglottis
T2	Tumor extends to vocal cord(s) with normal or impaired mobility
T3	Tumor limited to larynx with vocal cord fixation
T4a	Tumor invades cricoid or thyroid cartilage and/or invades tissues beyond the larynx (e.g., trachea, soft tissues of neck including deep extrinsic muscles of the tongue, strap muscles, thyroid, or esophagus)
T4b	Tumor invades prevertebral space, encases carotid artery, or invades mediastinal structures

Regional Lymph Nodes (N)

NX	Regional lymph nodes cannot be assessed
N0	No regional lymph node metastasis
N1	Metastasis in a single ipsilateral lymph node, 3 cm or less in greatest dimension
N2	Metastasis in a single ipsilateral lymph node, more than 3 cm but not more than 6 cm in greatest dimension, or in multiple ipsilateral lymph nodes, none more than 6 cm in greatest dimension, or in bilateral or contralateral lymph nodes, none more than 6 cm in greatest dimension
N2a	Metastasis in a single ipsilateral lymph node, more than 3 cm but not more than 6 cm in greatest dimension
N2b	Metastasis in multiple ipsilateral lymph nodes, none more than 6 cm in greatest dimension
N2c	Metastasis in bilateral or contralateral lymph nodes, none more than 6 cm in greatest dimension
N3	Metastasis in a lymph node, more than 6 cm in greatest dimension

Distant Metastasis (M)

MX	Distant metastasis cannot be assessed
M0	No distant metastasis
M1	Distant metastasis

HISTOPATHOLOGIC TYPE

The predominant cancer is squamous cell carcinoma. The staging guidelines are applicable to all forms of carcinoma. Nonepithelial tumors such as those of lymphoid tissue, soft tissue, bone, and cartilage (i.e., lymphoma, melanoma, and sarcoma) are not included. Histologic confirmation of diagnosis is required. Histopathologic grading of squamous carcinoma is recommended. The grade is subjective and uses a descriptive as well as numerical form (i.e., well differentiated, moderately differentiated, and poorly differentiated), depending on the degree of closeness to or deviation from squamous epithelium in mucosal sites. Also recommended where feasible is a quantitative evaluation of depth of invasion of the primary tumor and the presence or absence of vascular invasion and perineural invasion. Although the grade of tumor does not enter into the staging of the tumor, it should be recorded. The pathologic description of any lymphadenectomy specimen should describe the size, number, and position of the involved node(s) and the presence or absence of extracapsular extension.

HISTOLOGIC GRADE (G)

GX   Grade cannot be assessed
G1   Well differentiated
G2   Moderately differentiated
G3   Poorly differentiated

Figures 5.1A, 5.1B, 5.2A, 5.2B, 5.3A, 5.3B, 5.4A, and 5.4B show observed and relative survival rates for patients with squamous cell carcinoma of the larynx (5.1A,B), squamous cell carcinoma of the supraglottis (5.2A,B), squamous cell carcinoma of the glottis (5.3A,B), and squamous cell carcinoma of the subglottis (5.4A,B) for the year 1985–1991, classified by the AJCC staging classification.

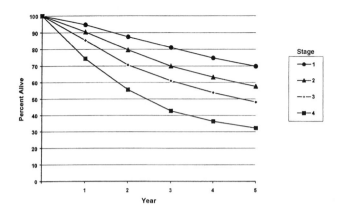

OBSERVED SURVIVAL BY STAGE	1	2	3	4	5	95% CIs*	CASES
1	94.6	87.5	81.0	74.8	69.8	68.6 – 71.1	5750
2	90.4	79.6	69.9	63.2	57.5	55.5 – 59.9	2763
3	85.4	70.6	61.0	53.8	48.1	46.1 – 50.1	2661
4	74.4	55.6	42.8	36.3	32.2	30.4 – 33.9	3064

FIG. 5.1A. Five-year, observed survival by "combined" AJCC stage for squamous cell carcinoma of the larynx, 1985–1991. (*95% confidence intervals correspond to year-5 survival rates.)

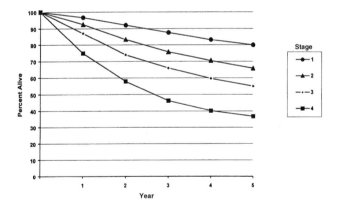

RELATIVE SURVIVAL BY STAGE	1	2	3	4	5	95% CIs*	CASES
1	96.7	92.0	87.6	83.2	79.9	78.4 – 81.3	5775
2	92.5	83.3	75.7	70.4	65.7	63.5 – 68.0	2779
3	87.1	73.9	65.9	59.6	55.0	52.6 – 57.3	2675
4	74.9	57.9	46.3	40.2	36.7	34.7 – 38.7	3095

FIG. 5.1B. Five-year, relative survival by "combined" AJCC stage for squamous cell carcinoma of the larynx, 1985–1991. (*95% confidence intervals correspond to year-5 survival rates.)

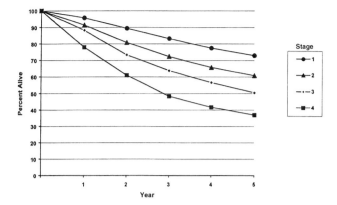

OBSERVED SURVIVAL BY STAGE	1	2	3	4	5	95% CIs*	CASES
1	95.7	89.4	83.3	77.4	72.9	71.5 – 74.3	4508
2	91.4	80.8	72.3	65.7	60.8	57.9 – 63.6	1333
3	88.3	73.3	63.8	56.6	50.5	46.9 – 54.0	868
4	78.0	61.0	48.4	41.7	36.9	32.6 – 41.1	581

FIG. 5.2A. Five-year, observed survival by "combined" AJCC stage for squamous cell carcinoma of the supraglottis, 1985–1991. (*95% confidence intervals correspond to year-5 survival rates.)

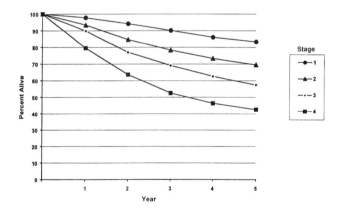

RELATIVE SURVIVAL BY STAGE	1	2	3	4	5	95% CIs*	CASES
1	97.8	94.1	90.1	86.1	83.4	81.8 – 85.0	4528
2	93.4	84.7	78.3	73.3	69.5	66.3 – 72.7	1340
3	89.9	77.0	69.1	62.6	57.4	53.3 – 61.5	872
4	79.6	63.6	52.5	46.4	42.6	37.7 – 47.4	587

FIG. 5.2B. Five-year, relative survival by "combined" AJCC stage for squamous cell carcinoma of the supraglottis, 1985–1991. (*95% confidence intervals correspond to year-5 survival rates.)

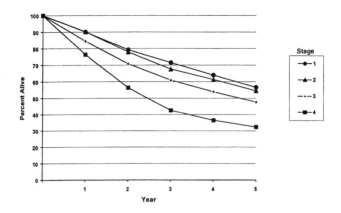

OBSERVED SURVIVAL BY STAGE	1	2	3	4	5	95% CIs*	CASES
1	90.1	79.2	71.5	63.9	56.6	53.0 – 60.2	823
2	90.2	77.9	67.5	61.3	54.5	51.3 – 57.7	1044
3	84.5	70.8	60.9	53.9	47.7	44.7 – 50.7	1203
4	76.4	56.4	42.6	36.4	32.3	29.9 – 34.7	1657

FIG. 5.3A. Five-year, observed survival by "combined" AJCC stage for squamous cell carcinoma of the glottis, 1985–1991. (*95% confidence intervals correspond to year-5 survival rates.)

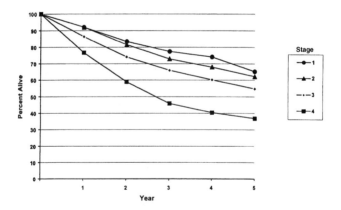

RELATIVE SURVIVAL BY STAGE	1	2	3	4	5	95% CIs*	CASES
1	92.0	83.5	77.4	71.0	65.1	61.0 – 69.3	826
2	92.0	81.5	72.9	67.9	62.1	58.5 – 65.8	1049
3	86.4	74.1	65.9	60.1	54.7	51.3 – 58.2	1208
4	76.7	58.9	45.9	40.4	36.8	34.1 – 39.6	1672

FIG. 5.3B. Five-year, relative survival by "combined" AJCC stage for squamous cell carcinoma of the glottis, 1985–1991. (*95% confidence intervals correspond to year-5 survival rates.)

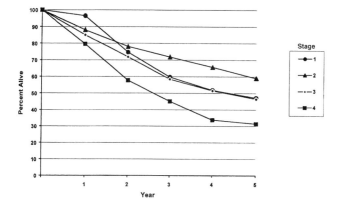

OBSERVED SURVIVAL BY STAGE	1	2	3	4	5	95% CIs*	CASES
1	96.5	74.6	59.7	51.8	47.3	28.0 – 66.5	29
2	88.1	78.0	71.8	65.6	59.0	45.1 – 72.9	51
3	85.1	71.8	58.4	51.5	46.5	31.7 – 61.2	48
4	79.6	57.7	45.1	33.8	31.4	18.1 – 44.7	56

FIG. 5.4A. Five-year, observed survival by "combined" AJCC stage for squamous cell carcinoma of the subglottis, 1985–1991. (*95% confidence intervals correspond to year-5 survival rates.)

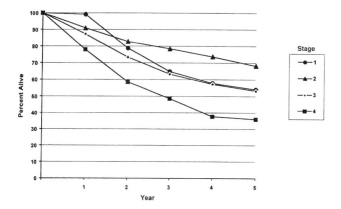

RELATIVE SURVIVAL BY STAGE	1	2	3	4	5	95% CIs*	CASES
1	99.1	79.7	64.7	57.8	54.1	31.9 – 76.4	29
2	90.9	82.8	78.4	73.6	68.2	52.3 – 84.1	53
3	87.3	73.3	63.2	57.2	53.2	36.2 – 70.2	48
4	78.0	58.5	48.6	37.6	36.0	20.7 – 51.2	56

FIG. 5.4B. Five-year, relative survival by "combined" AJCC stage for squamous cell carcinoma of the subglottis, 1985–1991. (*95% confidence intervals correspond to year-5 survival rates.)

BIBLIOGRAPHY

Archer CR, Yeager VL, Herbold DR: CT versus histology of laryngeal cancer: the value in predicting laryngeal cartilage invasion. Laryngoscope 93:140–147, 1983

Cooper JS, Farnan NC, Asbell SO, et al: Recursive partitioning analysis of 2,105 patients treated in Radiation Therapy Oncology Group studies of head and neck cancer. Cancer 77:1905–1911, 1996

Deleyiannis FW, Thomas DB, Vaughan TL, et al: Alcoholism: independent predictor of survival in patients with head and neck cancer. J Natl Cancer Inst 88:542–549, 1996

Eibaud JD, Elias EG, Suter CM, et al: Prognostic factors in squamous cell carcinoma of the larynx. Am J Surg 58:314–317, 1989

Faye-Lund H, Abdelnoor M: Prognostic factors of survival in a cohort of head and neck cancer patients in Oslo. Eur J Cancer B Oral Oncol 2:83–90, 1996

Isaacs JJ, Mancuso AA, Mendenhall WM, et al: Deep spread patterns in CT staging of t2–4 squamous cell laryngeal carcinoma. Otolaryngol Head Neck Surg 99:455–464, 1988

Kaplan MH, Feinstein AR: The importance of classifying initial co-morbidity in evaluating the outcome of diabetes mellitus. J Chron Dis 37:387–404, 1974

Karnofsky DA, Abelman WH, Craver LF, Burchenal JH: The use of nitrogen mustards in the palliative treatment of carcinoma. Cancer 1:634–656, 1948

Mafee MF, Schield JA, Valvassori GE, et al: CT of the larynx: correlation with anatomic and pathologic studies in cases of laryngeal carcinoma. Radiology 147:123–128, 1983

Mendenhall WM, Parsons JT, Stringer SP, et al: Carcinoma of the supraglottic larynx: a basis for comparing the results of radiotherapy and surgery. Head Neck 12:204–209, 1990

Piccirillo JF. Inclusion of comorbidity in a staging system for head and neck cancer. Oncology 9:831–836, 1995

Rozack MS, Maipang T, Sabo K, et al: Management of advanced glottic carcinomas. Am J Surg 158:318–320, 1989

Singh B, Alfonso A, Sabin S, et al: Outcome differences in younger and older patients with laryngeal cancer: a retrospective case-control study. Am J Otolaryngol 21:92–97, 2000

Singh B, Bhaya M, Zimbler M, et al: Impact of comorbidity on outcome of young patients with head and neck squamous cell carcinoma. Head Neck 20:1–7, 1998

Strong EW. Cancer of the larynx and hypopharynx. Prob Gen Surg 5:166–189, 1988

Van Nostrand AWP, Brodarec I: Laryngeal carcinoma: modification of surgical techniques based upon an understanding of tumor growth characteristics. J Otolaryngol 11:186–192, 1982

Veterans Administration Laryngeal Study Group: Induction chemotherapy plus radiation compared to surgery plus radiation in patients with advanced laryngeal cancer. N Engl J Med 324:1685–1690, 1991

HISTOLOGIES—LARYNX

8010/2	Carcinoma *in situ*, NOS
8010/3	Carcinoma, NOS
8012/3	Large cell carcinoma, NOS
8013/3	Large cell neuroendocrine carcinoma
8020/3	Carcinoma, undifferentiated, NOS
8021/3	Carcinoma, anaplastic, NOS

8030/3	Giant cell and spindle cell carcinoma
8031/3	Giant cell carcinoma
8032/3	Spindle cell carcinoma, NOS
8033/3	Pseudosarcomatous carcinoma
8041/3	Small cell carcinoma, NOS
8042/3	Oat cell carcinoma
8043/3	Small cell carcinoma, fusiform cell
8044/3	Small cell carcinoma, intermediate cell
8045/3	Combined small cell carcinoma
8051/3	Verrucous carcinoma, NOS
8052/2	Papillary squamous cell carcinoma, non-invasive
8052/3	Papillary squamous cell carcinoma
8070/2	Squamous cell carcinoma *in situ*, NOS
8070/3	Squamous cell carcinoma, NOS
8071/3	Squamous cell carcinoma, keratinizing, NOS
8072/3	Squamous cell carcinoma, large cell
8073/3	Squamous cell carcinoma, small cell, non-keratinizing
8074/3	Squamous cell carcinoma, spindle cell
8075/3	Squamous cell carcinoma, adenoid
8076/2	Squamous cell carcinoma *in situ* with questionable stromal invasion
8076/3	Squamous cell carcinoma, microinvasive
8082/3	Lymphoepithelial carcinoma
8083/3	Basaloid squamous cell carcinoma
8084/3	Squamous cell carcinoma, clear cell type
8090/3	Basal cell carcinoma, NOS
8091/3	Multifocal superficial basal cell carcinoma
8092/3	Infiltrating basal cell carcinoma, NOS
8093/3	Basal cell carcinoma, fibroepithelial
8094/3	Basosquamous carcinoma
8097/3	Basal cell carcinoma, nodular
8098/3	Adenoid basal carcinoma
8123/3	Basaloid carcinoma
8140/2	Adenocarcinoma *in situ*, NOS
8140/3	Adenocarcinoma, NOS
8144/3	Adenocarcinoma, intestinal type
8145/3	Carcinoma, diffuse type
8147/3	Basal cell adenocarcinoma
8200/3	Adenoid cystic carcinoma
8246/3	Neuroendocrine carcinoma, NOS
8310/3	Clear cell adenocarcinoma, NOS
8430/3	Mucoepidermoid carcinoma
8440/3	Cystadenocarcinoma, NOS
8480/3	Mucinous adenocarcinoma
8481/3	Mucin-producing adenocarcinoma
8510/3	Medullary carcinoma, NOS
8525/3	Polymorphous low-grade adenocarcinoma
8550/3	Acinar cell carcinoma
8560/3	Adenosquamous carcinoma
8562/3	Epithelial-myoepithelial carcinoma
8574/3	Adenocarcinoma with neuroendocrine differentiation
8940/3	Mixed tumor, malignant, NOS
8941/3	Carcinoma in pleomorphic adenoma

Nasal Cavity and Paranasal Sinuses

(Nonepithelial tumors such as those of lymphoid tissue, soft tissue, bone, and cartilage are not included)

C30.0 Nasal cavity   C31.0 Maxillary sinus   C31.1 Ethmoid sinus

---

SUMMARY OF CHANGES

- A new site has been added for inclusion into the staging system. In addition to maxillary sinus, the nasoethmoid complex is described as a second site with two regions within this site: nasal cavity and ethmoid sinuses.

- The nasal cavity region is further divided into four subsites: septum, floor, lateral wall, and vestibule. The ethmoid sinus region is divided into two subsites: right and left.

- The T staging of ethmoid lesions has been revised to reflect nasoethmoid tumors, and appropriate description for the T staging has been added.

- For maxillary sinus, T4 lesions have been divided into T4a (resectable) and T4b (unresectable), leading to the division of Stage IV into Stage IVA, Stage IVB, and Stage IVC.

ANATOMY

Primary Sites.   Cancer of the maxillary sinus is the most common of the sinonasal malignancies. Ethmoid sinus and nasal cavity cancers are equal in frequency but considerably less common than maxillary sinus cancers. Tumors of the sphenoid and frontal sinuses are rare.

The location as well as the extent of the mucosal lesion within the maxillary sinus has prognostic significance. Historically, Ohngren's line, connecting the medial canthus of the eye to the angle of the mandible, is used to divide the maxillary sinus into an anteroinferior portion (infrastructure), which is associated with a good prognosis, and a superoposterior portion (suprastructure), which has a poor prognosis (Fig. 6.1A,B). The poorer outcome associated with superoposterior cancers reflects early access of these tumors to critical structures, including the eye, skull base, pterygoids, and infratemporal fossa.

For the purpose of staging, the nasoethmoidal complex is divided into two sites: nasal cavity and ethmoid sinuses. The ethmoids are further subdivided into two subsites: left and right, separated by the nasal septum. The nasal cavity is divided into four subsites: the septum, floor, lateral wall, and vestibule.

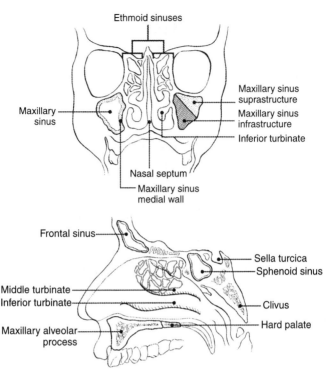

FIG. 6.1A, B. Sites of origin of tumors of the paranasal sinuses.

Site	Subsite
Maxillary Sinus	Left/Right
Nasal Cavity	Septum
	Floor
	Lateral wall
	Vestibule
Ethmoid sinus	Left
	Right

Regional Lymph Nodes. Regional lymph node spread from cancer of nasal cavity and paranasal sinuses is relatively uncommon. Involvement of buccinator, submandibular, upper jugular, and (occasionally) retropharyngeal nodes may occur with advanced maxillary sinus cancer, particularly those extending beyond the sinus walls to involve adjacent structures, including soft tissues of the cheek, upper alveolus, palate, and buccal mucosa. Ethmoid sinus cancers are less prone to regional lymphatic spread. When only one side of the neck is involved, it should be considered ipsilateral. Bilateral spread may occur with advanced primary cancer, particularly with spread of the primary beyond the midline.

In clinical evaluation, the physical size of the nodal mass should be measured. Most masses over 3 cm in diameter are not single nodes but, rather, are confluent nodes or tumor in soft tissues of the neck. There are three categories of clinically positive nodes: N1, N2, and N3. The use of subgroups a, b, and c is not required but is recommended. Midline nodes are considered ipsilateral nodes. In addition to the components to describe the N category, regional lymph nodes should also be described according to the level of the neck that is involved. Pathologic examination is necessary for documentation of such disease extent. Imaging studies showing amorphous spiculated margins of involved nodes or involvement of internodal fat resulting in loss of normal oval-to-round nodal shape strongly suggest extracapsular (extranodal) tumor spread. No imaging study (as yet) can identify microscope foci in regional nodes or distinguish between small reactive nodes and small malignant nodes without central radiographic inhomogeneity.

For pN, a selective neck dissection will ordinarily include 6 or more lymph nodes, and a radical or modified radical neck dissection will ordinarily include 10 or more lymph nodes. Negative pathologic examination of a lesser number of lymph nodes still mandates a pN0 designation.

Metastatic Sites.   Distant spread usually occurs to lungs but occasionally there is spread to bone.

RULES FOR CLASSIFICATION

Clinical Staging.   The assessment of primary maxillary sinus, nasal cavity, and ethmoid tumors is based on inspection and palpation, including examination of the orbits, nasal and oral cavities, and nasopharynx, and neurologic evaluation of the cranial nerves. Nasal endoscopy with rigid or fiberoptic flexible instruments is recommended. Radiologic assessment with magnetic resonance imaging (MRI) or computed tomography (CT) is mandatory for accurate pretreatment staging of malignant tumor of the sinuses. If available, MRI more accurately depicts skull base and intracranial involvement and the differentiation of fluid from solid tumor. Neck nodes are assessed by palpation $+ / -$ imaging. Imaging for possible nodal metastases is probably unnecessary in the presence of a clinically negative neck. Examinations for distant metastases include appropriate radiographs, blood chemistries, blood count, and other routine studies as indicated.

Pathologic Staging.   Pathologic staging requires the use of all information obtained in clinical staging and histologic study of the surgically resected specimen. The surgeon's evaluation of gross unresected residual tumor must also be included. Specimens that are resected after radiation or chemotherapy need to be identified and considered in context. The pathologic description of the lymphadenectomy specimen should describe the size, number, and position of the involved node(s) and the presence or absence of extracapsular extension.

DEFINITION OF TNM

Primary Tumor (T)

TX   Primary tumor cannot be assessed
T0   No evidence of primary tumor
Tis   Carcinoma *in situ*

Maxillary Sinus

T1   Tumor limited to maxillary sinus mucosa with no erosion or destruction of bone
T2   Tumor causing bone erosion or destruction including extension into the hard palate and/or middle nasal meatus, except extension to posterior wall of maxillary sinus and pterygoid plates
T3   Tumor invades any of the following: bone of the posterior wall of maxillary sinus, subcutaneous tissues, floor or medial wall of orbit, pterygoid fossa, ethmoid sinuses
T4a   Tumor invades anterior orbital contents, skin of cheek, pterygoid plates, infratemporal fossa, cribriform plate, sphenoid or frontal sinuses
T4b   Tumor invades any of the following: orbital apex, dura, brain, middle cranial fossa, cranial nerves other than maxillary division of trigeminal nerve (V_2), nasopharynx, or clivus

Nasal Cavity and Ethmoid Sinus

T1   Tumor restricted to any one subsite, with or without bony invasion
T2   Tumor invading two subsites in a single region or extending to involve an adjacent region within the nasoethmoidal complex, with or without bony invasion
T3   Tumor extends to invade the medial wall or floor of the orbit, maxillary sinus, palate, or cribriform plate
T4a   Tumor invades any of the following: anterior orbital contents, skin of nose or cheek, minimal extension to anterior cranial fossa, pterygoid plates, sphenoid or frontal sinuses
T4b   Tumor invades any of the following: orbital apex, dura, brain, middle cranial fossa, cranial nerves other than (V_2), nasopharynx, or clivus

Regional Lymph Nodes (N)

NX   Regional lymph nodes cannot be assessed
N0   No regional lymph node metastasis
N1   Metastasis in a single ipsilateral lymph node, 3 cm or less in greatest dimension
N2   Metastasis in a single ipsilateral lymph node, more than 3 cm but not more than 6 cm in greatest dimension, or in multiple ipsilateral lymph nodes, none more than 6 cm in greatest dimension, or in bilateral or contralateral lymph nodes, none more than 6 cm in greatest dimension
N2a   Metastasis in a single ipsilateral lymph node, more than 3 cm but not more than 6 cm in greatest dimension
N2b   Metastasis in multiple ipsilateral lymph nodes, none more than 6 cm in greatest dimension

N2c   Metastasis in bilateral or contralateral lymph nodes, none more than 6 cm in greatest dimension
N3   Metastasis in a lymph node, more than 6 cm in greatest dimension

Distant Metastasis (M)
MX   Distant metastasis cannot be assessed
M0   No distant metastasis
M1   Distant metastasis

STAGE GROUPING			
Stage 0	Tis	N0	M0
Stage I	T1	N0	M0
Stage II	T2	N0	M0
Stage III	T3	N0	M0
	T1	N1	M0
	T2	N1	M0
	T3	N1	M0
Stage IVA	T4a	N0	M0
	T4a	N1	M0
	T1	N2	M0
	T2	N2	M0
	T3	N2	M0
	T4a	N2	M0
Stage IVB	T4b	Any N	M0
	Any T	N3	M0
Stage IVC	Any T	Any N	M1

HISTOPATHOLOGIC TYPE

The predominant cancer is squamous cell carcinoma. The staging guidelines are applicable to all forms of carcinoma. Nonepithelial tumors such as those of lymphoid tissue, soft tissue, bone, and cartilage are not included. Histologic confirmation of diagnosis is required. Histopathologic grading of squamous carcinoma is recommended. The grade is subjective and uses a descriptive as well as a numerical form (i.e., well differentiated, moderately differentiated, and poorly differentiated), depending on the degree of closeness to or deviation from squamous epithelium in mucosal sites. Also recommended where feasible is a quantitative evaluation of depth of invasion of the primary tumor and the presence or absence of vascular invasion and perineural invasion. Although the grade of the tumor does not enter into the staging of the tumor, it should be recorded. The pathologic description of any lymphadenectomy specimen should describe the size, number, and position of the involved node(s) and the presence or absence of extracapsular extension.

HISTOLOGIC GRADE (G)

GX   Grade cannot be assessed
G1   Well differentiated
G2   Moderately differentiated
G3   Poorly differentiated

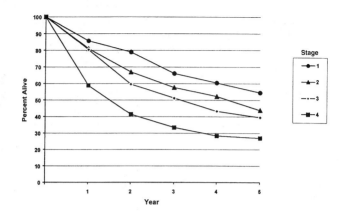

OBSERVED SURVIVAL BY STAGE	1	2	3	4	5	95% CIs*	CASES
1	85.7	78.9	66.0	60.4	54.5	41.4 – 67.6	65
2	81.0	66.9	57.6	52.2	43.8	32.6 – 54.9	87
3	80.4	59.6	51.2	43.2	39.5	31.5 – 47.5	162
4	58.9	51.4	33.4	28.4	27.0	22.2 – 31.8	364

FIG. 6.2A. Five-year, observed survival by "combined" AJCC stage for cancer of the maxillary sinus, 1985–1991. (*95% confidence intervals correspond to year-5 survival rates.)

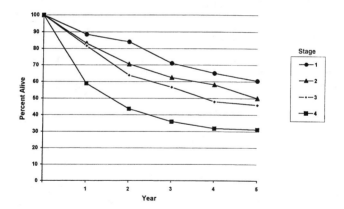

RELATIVE SURVIVAL BY STAGE	1	2	3	4	5	95% CIs*	CASES
1	88.5	84.0	71.0	65.0	60.4	45.5 – 75.3	67
2	83.1	70.5	62.4	58.1	50.0	37.1 – 62.9	87
3	81.6	63.8	56.6	47.9	45.9	36.8 – 55.0	167
4	58.9	43.6	35.9	31.8	31.1	25.5 – 36.7	370

FIG. 6.2B. Five-year, relative survival by "combined" AJCC stage for cancer of the maxillary sinus, 1985–1991. (*95% confidence intervals correspond to year-5 survival rates.)

PROGNOSTIC FACTORS

In addition to the importance of the TNM factors outlined previously, the overall health of these patients clearly influences outcome. Comorbidity can be classified by more general measures, such as the Karnofsky performance score, or by more specific measures, such as the Kaplan-Feinstein Index or the Charlson Index, and it can increase in incidence and severity with increasing age. Continued exposure to carcinogens, such as alcohol and tobacco smoke, probably affects patients' outcomes adversely.

Figures 6.2A and 6.2B show observed and relative survival rates for patients with cancer of the maxillary sinus for the years 1985–1991, classified by the AJCC staging classification.

BIBLIOGRAPHY

Bridger GP, Mendelsohn MS, Baldwinn M, et al: Paranasal sinus cancer. Aust N Z J Surg 61:290–294, 1991

Cantu G, Solero CL, Mariani L, et al: A new classification for malignant tumors involving the anterior skull base. Arch Otolaryngol Head Neck Surg 125:1252–1257, 1999

Jiang GL, Ang KA, Peters LJ, et al: Maxillary sinus carcinomas: natural history and results of postoperative radiotherapy. Radiother Oncol 21:194–200, 1991

Jiang GL, Morrison WH, Garden AS, et al: Ethmoid sinus carcinoma: natural history and treatment results. Radiother Oncol 49:21–27 1998

Kondo M, Horiuchi M, Shiga H, et al: CT of malignant tumors of the nasal cavity and paranasal sinuses. Cancer 50:226–231, 1982

Le QT, Fu KK, Kaplan M, et al: Treatment of maxillary sinus carcinoma. A comparison of the 1997 and 1977 American Joint Committee on Cancer Staging Systems. Cancer 86:1700–1711, 1999

Paulino AFG, Singh B, Carew J, et al: Epstein-Barr virus in squamous carcinoma of the anterior nasal cavity. Ann Diagn Pathol 4:7–10, 2000

Piccirillo JF. Inclusion of comorbidity in a staging system for head and neck cancer. Oncology 9:831–836, 1995

Shah JP, Kraus DH, Bilsky MH, et al: Craniofacial resection for malignant tumors involving the anterior skull base. Arch Otolaryngol Head Neck Surg 13:1312–1317, 1997

Singh B, Bhaya M, Zimbler M. et al: Impact of cormorbidity on outcome of young patients with head and neck squamous cell carcinoma. Head Neck 20:1–7, 1998

Sisson GA, Toriumi DM, Atiyah RH: Paranasal sinus malignancy: a comprehensive update. Laryngoscope 99:143–150, 1989

Som PM, Dillon WP, Sze G, et al: Benign and malignant sinonasal lesions with intracranial extension: differentiation with MRI imaging. Radiology 172:763–766, 1989

Van Tassel P, Lee YY: GD-DTPA enhanced MR for detecting intracranial extension of sinonasal malignancies. JCAT 15:387–392, 1991

HISTOLOGIES—PARANASAL SINUSES

8010/2	Carcinoma *in situ*, NOS
8010/3	Carcinoma, NOS
8012/3	Large cell carcinoma, NOS
8013/3	Large cell neuroendocrine carcinoma
8020/3	Carcinoma, undifferentiated, NOS

8021/3	Carcinoma, anaplastic, NOS
8030/3	Giant cell and spindle cell carcinoma
8031/3	Giant cell carcinoma
8032/3	Spindle cell carcinoma, NOS
8033/3	Pseudosarcomatous carcinoma
8041/3	Small cell carcinoma, NOS
8042/3	Oat cell carcinoma
8043/3	Small cell carcinoma, fusiform cell
8044/3	Small cell carcinoma, intermediate cell
8045/3	Combined small cell carcinoma
8051/3	Verrucous carcinoma, NOS
8052/2	Papillary squamous cell carcinoma, non-invasive
8052/3	Papillary squamous cell carcinoma
8070/2	Squamous cell carcinoma *in situ*, NOS
8070/3	Squamous cell carcinoma, NOS
8071/3	Squamous cell carcinoma, keratinizing, NOS
8072/3	Squamous cell carcinoma, large cell
8073/3	Squamous cell carcinoma, small cell, non-keratinizing
8074/3	Squamous cell carcinoma, spindle cell
8075/3	Squamous cell carcinoma, adenoid
8076/2	Squamous cell carcinoma *in situ* with questionable stromal invasion
8076/3	Squamous cell carcinoma, microinvasive
8082/3	Lymphoepithelial carcinoma
8083/3	Basaloid squamous cell carcinoma
8084/3	Squamous cell carcinoma, clear cell type
8090/3	Basal cell carcinoma, NOS
8091/3	Multifocal superficial basal cell carcinoma
8092/3	Infiltrating basal cell carcinoma, NOS
8093/3	Basal cell carcinoma, fibroepithelial
8094/3	Basosquamous carcinoma
8097/3	Basal cell carcinoma, nodular
8098/3	Adenoid basal carcinoma
8123/3	Basaloid carcinoma
8140/2	Adenocarcinoma *in situ*, NOS
8140/3	Adenocarcinoma, NOS
8144/3	Adenocarcinoma, intestinal type
8145/3	Carcinoma, diffuse type
8147/3	Basal cell adenocarcinoma
8200/3	Adenoid cystic carcinoma
8246/3	Neuroendocrine carcinoma, NOS
8310/3	Clear cell adenocarcinoma, NOS
8430/3	Mucoepidermoid carcinoma
8440/3	Cystadenocarcinoma, NOS
8480/3	Mucinous adenocarcinoma
8481/3	Mucin-producing adenocarcinoma
8510/3	Medullary carcinoma, NOS
8525/3	Polymorphous low-grade adenocarcinoma
8550/3	Acinar cell carcinoma
8560/3	Adenosquamous carcinoma
8562/3	Epithelial-myoepithelial carcinoma
8574/3	Adenocarcinoma with neuroendocrine differentiation
8940/3	Mixed tumor, malignant, NOS
8941/3	Carcinoma in pleomorphic adenoma

Major Salivary Glands

(Parotid, Submandibular, and Sublingual)

C07.9 Parotid gland	C08.8 Overlapping lesion of	C08.9 Major salivary gland,
C08.0 Submandibular gland	major salivary glands	NOS
C08.1 Sublingual gland		

SUMMARY OF CHANGES

- In order to maintain internal consistency of T staging across all sites, the description for T3 has been revised. In addition to tumors having extra-parenchymal extension, all tumors larger than 4 cm are considered T3.

- T4 lesions have been divided into T4a (resectable) and T4b (unresectable), leading to the division of Stage IV into Stage IVA, Stage IVB, and Stage IVC.

This staging system is based on an extensive retrospective review of the world literature regarding malignant tumors of the major salivary glands. Numerous factors affect patient survival, including the histologic diagnosis, cellular differentiation of the tumor (grade), site, size, degree of fixation or local extension, facial nerve involvement, and the status of regional lymph nodes as well as distant metastases. The classification involves the four dominant clinical variables: tumor size, local extension of the tumor, nodal metastasis, and distant metastasis. The T4 category has been divided into T4a and T4b. T4a indicates advanced lesions that are resectable with grossly clear margins; T4b reflects extension to areas that preclude resection with clear margins. Histologic grade, patient age, and tumor site are important additional factors that should be recorded for future analysis and potential inclusion in the staging system.

ANATOMY

Primary Site. The major salivary glands include the parotid, submandibular, and sublingual glands. Tumors arising in minor salivary glands (mucus-secreting glands in the lining membrane of the upper aerodigestive tract) are staged according to the anatomic site of origin (e.g., oral cavity, sinuses, etc.).

Primary tumors of the parotid constitute the largest proportion of salivary gland tumors. Sublingual primary cancers are rare and may be difficult to distinguish with certainty from minor salivary gland primary tumors of the anterior floor of the mouth.

Regional Lymph Nodes. Regional lymphatic spread from salivary gland cancer is less common than from head and neck mucosal squamous cancers and varies according to the histology and size of the primary tumor. Most nodal metastases will be clinically apparent on initial evaluation.

Low-grade tumors rarely metastasize to regional nodes, whereas the risk of regional spread is substantially higher from high-grade cancers. Regional dissemination tends to be orderly, progressing from intraglandular to adjacent (periparotid, submandibular) nodes, then to upper and midjugular nodes, and occasionally to retropharyngeal nodes. Bilateral lymphatic spread is rare.

For pathologic reporting (pN), histologic examination of a selective neck dissection will ordinarily include 6 or more lymph nodes and a radical or modified radical neck dissection will ordinarily include 10 or more lymph nodes. Negative pathologic evaluation of a lesser number of nodes still mandates a pN0 designation.

Metastatic Sites.   Distant spread is most frequently to the lungs.

RULES FOR CLASSIFICATION

Clinical Staging.   The assessment of primary salivary gland tumors includes a pertinent history (pain, trismus, etc.), inspection, palpation, and evaluation of the cranial nerves. Radiologic studies may add information valuable for staging. The soft tissues of the neck from the skull base to the hyoid bone must be studied, with the lower neck included whenever lymph node metastases are suspected. Images of the intratemporal facial nerve are critical to the identification of perineural tumor in this area. Cancers of the submandibular and sublingual salivary glands merit cross-sectional imaging. Computed tomography (CT) or MRI may be useful in assessing the extent of deep extraglandular tumor, bone invasion, and deep tissue extent (extrinsic tongue muscle and/or soft tissues of the neck).

Pathologic Staging.   The surgical pathology report and all other available data should be used to assign a pathologic classification to those patients who have resection of the cancer.

DEFINITION OF TNM

Primary Tumor (T)

TX   Primary tumor cannot be assessed

T0   No evidence of primary tumor

T1   Tumor 2 cm or less in greatest dimension without extraparenchymal extension*

T2   Tumor more than 2 cm but not more than 4 cm in greatest dimension without extraparenchymal extension*

T3   Tumor more than 4 cm and/or tumor having extraparenchymal extension*

T4a   Tumor invades skin, mandible, ear canal, and/or facial nerve

T4b   Tumor invades skull base and/or pterygoid plates and/or encases carotid artery

Note: Extraparenchymal extension is clinical or macroscopic evidence of invasion of soft tissues. Microscopic evidence alone does not constitute extraparenchymal extension for classification purposes.

Regional Lymph Nodes (N)

NX Regional lymph nodes cannot be assessed
N0 No regional lymph node metastasis
N1 Metastasis in a single ipsilateral lymph node, 3 cm or less in greatest dimension
N2 Metastasis in a single ipsilateral lymph node, more than 3 cm but not more than 6 cm in greatest dimension, or in multiple ipsilateral lymph nodes, none more than 6 cm in greatest dimension, or in bilateral or contralateral lymph nodes, none more than 6 cm in greatest dimension
N2a Metastasis in a single ipsilateral lymph node, more than 3 cm but not more than 6 cm in greatest dimension
N2b Metastasis in multiple ipsilateral lymph nodes, none more than 6 cm in greatest dimension
N2c Metastasis in bilateral or contralateral lymph nodes, none more than 6 cm in greatest dimension
N3 Metastasis in a lymph node, more than 6 cm in greatest dimension

Distant Metastasis (M)

MX Distant metastasis cannot be assessed
M0 No distant metastasis
M1 Distant metastasis

STAGE GROUPING			
Stage I	T1	N0	M0
Stage II	T2	N0	M0
Stage III	T3	N0	M0
	T1	N1	M0
	T2	N1	M0
	T3	N1	M0
Stage IVA	T4a	N0	M0
	T4a	N1	M0
	T1	N2	M0
	T2	N2	M0
	T3	N2	M0
	T4a	N2	M0
Stage IVB	T4b	Any N	M0
	Any T	N3	M0
Stage IVC	Any T	Any N	M1

HISTOPATHOLOGIC TYPE

The suggested histopathologic typing is that proposed by the World Health Organization.

Acinic cell carcinoma
Mucoepidermoid carcinoma
Adenoid cystic carcinoma
Polymorphous low-grade adenocarcinoma

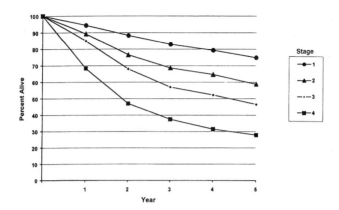

OBSERVED SURVIVAL BY STAGE	1	2	3	4	5	95% CIs*	CASES
1	94.3	88.3	83.0	79.3	74.9	72.1 – 77.6	1124
2	89.2	76.6	68.7	64.6	58.7	53.9 – 63.4	476
3	85.0	68.0	57.0	52.2	46.5	41.7 – 51.3	470
4	68.4	47.0	37.4	31.4	27.9	24.0 – 31.8	576

FIG. 7.1A. Five-year, observed survival by "combined" AJCC stage for cancer of the major salivary glands, 1985–1991. (*95% confidence intervals correspond to year-5 survival rates.)

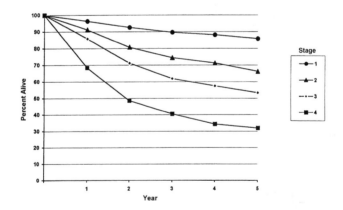

RELATIVE SURVIVAL BY STAGE	1	2	3	4	5	95% CIs*	CASES
1	96.3	92.5	89.6	88.1	85.8	82.7 – 89.0	1130
2	91.1	80.7	74.4	71.2	66.2	60.8 – 71.7	478
3	85.8	71.2	61.9	57.4	53.3	47.8 – 58.7	477
4	68.4	48.5	40.5	34.3	31.9	7.5 – 36.4	580

FIG. 7.1B. Five-year, relative survival by "combined" AJCC stage for cancer of the major salivary glands, 1985–1991. (*95% confidence intervals correspond to year-5 survival rates.)

Epithelial-myoepithelial carcinoma
Basal cell adenocarcinoma
Sebaceous carcinoma
Papillary cystadenocarcinoma
Mucinous adenocarcinoma
Oncocytic carcinoma
Salivary duct carcinoma
Adenocarcinoma
Myoepithelial carcinoma
Carcinoma in pleomorphic adenoma
Squamous cell carcinoma
Small cell carcinoma
Other carcinomas

HISTOLOGIC GRADE (G)

Histologic grading is applicable only to some types of salivary cancer: mucoepidermoid carcinoma, adenocarcinoma not otherwise specified, or when either of these is the carcinomatous element of carcinoma in pleomorphic adenoma.

In most instances, the histologic type defines the grade (i.e., salivary duct carcinoma is high grade; basal cell adenocarcinoma is low grade).

Figures 7.1A and 7.1B show relative and observed survival rates for patients with cancer of the major salivary glands for the years 1985–1991, classified by the AJCC staging classification.

BIBLIOGRAPHY

Batsakis JG, Luna MA: Histopathologic grading of salivary gland neoplasms: I. Mucoepidermoid carcinomas. Ann Otol Rhinol Laryngol 99:835–838, 1990

Beckhardt RN, Weber RS, Zane R, et al: Minor salivary gland tumors of the palate: clinical and pathologic correlates of outcome. Laryngoscope 105:1155–1160, 1995

Calearo C, Pastore A, Storchi OF, et al: Parotid gland carcinoma: analysis of prognostic factors. Ann Otol Rhinol Laryngol 107:969–973, 1998

Frankenthaler RA, Luna MA, Lee SS, et al: Prognostic variables in parotid gland cancer. Arch Otolaryngol Head Neck Surg 11:1251–1256, 1991

Gallo O, Franchi A, Bottai GV, et al: Risk factors for distant metastases from carcinoma of the parotid gland. Cancer 80:844–851, 1977

Goepfert H, Luna MA, Lindberg RH, et al: Malignant salivary gland tumors of the paranasal sinuses and nasal cavity. Arch Otolaryngol 109:662–668, 1983

Hicks MJ, el-Naggar AK, Byers RM, et al: Prognostic factors in mucoepidermoid carcinomas of major salivary glands: a clinicopathologic and flow cytometric study. Eur J Cancer B Oral Oncol 30B:329–334, 1994

Hoffman HT, Karnell LH, Robinson RA, et al: National Cancer Data Base report on cancer of the head and neck: acinic cell carcinoma. Head Neck 21:297–309, 1999

Iro H, Waldfahrer F. Evaluation of the newly updated TNM classification of head and neck carcinoma with data from 3,247 patients. Cancer 83:2201–2207, 1998

Kane WJ, McCaffrey TV, Olsen KD, et al: Primary parotid malignancies: a clinical and pathologic review. Arch Otolaryngol Head and Neck Surg 117:307–315, 1991

Lopes MA, Santos GC, Kowalski LP: Multivariate survival analysis of 128 cases of oral cavity minor salivary gland carcinomas. Head Neck 20:699–706, 1998

Overgaard PD, Sogaard H, Elbrond O, et al: Malignant parotid tumors in 110 consecutive patients: treatment results and prognosis. Laryngoscope 102:1064–1069, 1992

Renehan A, Gleave EN, Hancock BD et al: Long-term follow-up of over 1,000 patients with salivary gland tumours treated in a single centre. Br J Surg 83:1750–1754, 1996

Seifert G, Sobin LH: Histological typing of salivary gland tumours. WHO international histological classification of tumours, 2nd ed. Berlin-Heidelberg-New York: Springer-Verlag, 1991

Spiro RH: Salivary neoplasms: Overview of a 35-year experience with 2,807 patients. Head Neck Surg 8:177–184, 1986

Spiro RH, Hajdu SI, Strong EW: Tumors of the submaxillary gland. Am J Surg 132:463–468, 1976

Spiro RH, Huvos AG: Stage means more than grade in adenoid cystic carcinoma. Am J Surg 164:623–628, 1992

Therkildsen MH, Christensen M, Andersen LJ, et al: Salivary gland carcinomas—prognostic factors. Acta Oncol 37:701–713, 1998

Vander Poorten VL, Balm AJ, Hilgers FJ, et al: The development of a prognostic score for patients with parotid carcinoma. Cancer 85:2057–2067, 1999

Vander Poorten VL, Balm AJ, Hilgers FJ, et al: Prognostic factors for long-term results of the treatment of patients with malignant submandibular gland tumors. Cancer 85:2255–2264, 1999

HISTOLOGIES—MAJOR SALIVARY GLANDS

8010/3	Carcinoma, NOS
8013/3	Large cell neuroendocrine carcinoma
8020/3	Carcinoma, undifferentiated, NOS
8021/3	Carcinoma, anaplastic, NOS
8032/3	Spindle cell carcinoma, NOS
8033/3	Pseudosarcomatous carcinoma
8041/3	Small cell carcinoma, NOS
8042/3	Oat cell carcinoma
8043/3	Small cell carcinoma, fusiform cell
8044/3	Small cell carcinoma, intermediate cell
8045/3	Combined small cell carcinoma
8070/3	Squamous cell carcinoma, NOS
8076/3	Squamous cell carcinoma, microinvasive
8082/3	Lymphoepithelial carcinoma
8083/3	Basaloid squamous cell carcinoma
8140/3	Adenocarcinoma
8147/3	Basal cell adenocarcinoma
8200/3	Adenoid cystic carcinoma
8246/3	Neuroendocrine carcinoma, NOS
8290/3	Oncocytic carcinoma
8310/3	Clear cell adenocarcinoma, NOS
8410/3	Sebaceous carcinoma
8430/3	Mucoepidermoid carcinoma
8440/3	Cystadenocarcinoma, NOS
8441/3	Serous cystadenocarcinoma, NOS
8450/3	Papillary cystadenocarcinoma
8480/3	Mucinous adenocarcinoma

8525/3	Polymorphous low-grade adenocarcinoma
8550/3	Acinar cell carcinoma
8560/3	Adenosquamous carcinoma
8562/3	Epithelial-myoepithelial carcinoma
8940/3	Mixed tumor, malignant, NOS
8941/3	Carcinoma in pleomorphic adenoma
8982/3	Malignant myoepithelioma

2

Thyroid

C73.9 Thyroid gland

SUMMARY OF CHANGES

- Tumor staging (T) has been revised and the categories redefined.

- T4 is now divided into T4a and T4b.

- Nodal staging (N) has been revised.

- All anaplastic carcinomas are considered T4. The T4 category for anaplastic carcinomas is divided into T4a (intrathyroidal anaplastic carcinoma—surgically resectable) and T4b (extrathyroidal anaplastic carcinoma—surgically unresectable).

- For papillary and follicular carcinomas, the stage grouping for patients older than 45 has been revised. Stage III includes tumors with minimal extrathyroid extension. Stage IVA includes tumors of any size extending beyond the thyroid capsule to invade subcutaneous soft tissues, larynx, trachea, esophagus OR recurrent laryngeal nerve. Stage IVB includes tumors that invade prevertebral fascia, carotid artery, or mediastinal vessels. Stage IVC includes advanced tumors with distant metastasis.

Although staging for cancers in other head and neck sites is based entirely on the anatomic extent of disease, it is not possible to follow this pattern for the unique group of malignant tumors that arise in the thyroid gland. Both the *histologic diagnosis* and the *age* of the patient are of such importance in the behavior and prognosis of thyroid cancer that these factors are included in this staging system.

ANATOMY

Primary Site. The thyroid gland ordinarily is composed of a right and a left lobe lying adjacent and lateral to the upper trachea and esophagus. An isthmus connects the two lobes, and in some cases a pyramidal lobe is present extending upward anterior to the thyroid cartilage.

Regional Lymph Nodes. Regional lymph node spread from thyroid cancer is common but of less prognostic significance in patients with well-differentiated tumors (papillary, follicular) than in medullary cancers. The adverse prognostic influence of lymph node metastasis in patients with differentiated carcinomas is observed, only in the older age group. The first echelon of nodal metastasis consists of the paralaryngeal, paratracheal, and prelaryngeal (Delphian) nodes adjacent to the thyroid gland in the central compartment of the neck generally described as Level VI. Metastases secondarily involve the mid- and lower jugular, the supraclavicular, and (much less commonly) the upper deep jugular and spinal accessory lymph nodes. Lymph node metastasis to submandibular and submental lymph nodes is very rare. Upper mediastinal (Level VII) nodal spread occurs frequently both anteriorly and posteriorly. Retropharyngeal nodal metastasis may be seen, usually in the presence of extensive lateral cervical metastasis. Bilateral nodal spread is common. The components of the N category are described as follows: first echelon (central compartment/Level VI), or N1a, and lateral cervical and/or superior mediastinal or N1b. The lymph node metastasis should also be described according to the level of the neck that is involved. Nodal metastases from medullary thyroid cancer carry a much more ominous prognosis, although they follow a similar pattern of spread.

For pN, histologic examination of a selective neck dissection will ordinarily include 6 or more lymph nodes, whereas histologic examination of a radical or a modified radical comprehensive neck dissection will ordinarily include 10 or more lymph nodes. Negative pathologic evaluation of a lesser number of nodes still mandates a pN0 designation.

Metastatic Sites.   Distant spread occurs by hematogenous routes—for example to lungs and bones—but many other sites may be involved.

RULES FOR CLASSIFICATION

Clinical Staging.   The assessment of a thyroid tumor depends on inspection and palpation of the thyroid gland and regional lymph nodes. Indirect laryngoscopy to evaluate vocal cord motion is essential. A variety of imaging procedures can provide additional useful information. These include radioisotope thyroid scans, ultrasonography, computed tomography scans (CT), and magnetic resonance imaging (MRI) scans. When cross-sectional imaging is utilized, MRI is recommended so as to avoid contamination of the body with the iodinated contrast medium generally used with CT. Iodinated contrast media make it necessary to delay the postoperative administration of radioactive iodine-131. The diagnosis of thyroid cancer must be confirmed by needle biopsy or open biopsy of the tumor. Further information for clinical staging may be obtained by biopsy of lymph nodes or other areas of suspected local or distant spread. All information available prior to first treatment should be used.

Pathologic Staging.   Pathologic staging requires the use of all information obtained in the clinical staging, as well as histologic study of the surgically resected specimen. The surgeon's description of gross unresected residual tumor must also be included.

DEFINITION OF TNM

Primary Tumor (T)

Note: All categories may be subdivided: (a) solitary tumor, (b) multifocal tumor (the largest determines the classification).

TX   Primary tumor cannot be assessed
T0   No evidence of primary tumor
T1   Tumor 2 cm or less in greatest dimension limited to the thyroid
T2   Tumor more than 2 cm but not more than 4 cm in greatest dimension limited to the thyroid
T3   Tumor more than 4 cm in greatest dimension limited to the thyroid or any tumor with minimal extrathyroid extension (e.g., extension to sternothyroid muscle or perithyroid soft tissues)
T4a Tumor of any size extending beyond the thyroid capsule to invade subcutaneous soft tissues, larynx, trachea, esophagus, or recurrent laryngeal nerve
T4b Tumor invades prevertebral fascia or encases carotid artery or mediastinal vessels

All anaplastic carcinomas are considered T4 tumors.

T4a Intrathyroidal anaplastic carcinoma—surgically resectable.
T4b Extrathyroidal anaplastic carcinoma—surgically unresectable

Regional Lymph Nodes (N)
Regional lymph nodes are the central compartment, lateral cervical, and upper mediastinal lymph nodes.
NX   Regional lymph nodes cannot be assessed.
N0   No regional lymph node metastasis
N1   Regional lymph node metastasis
N1a Metastasis to Level VI (pretracheal, paratracheal, and prelaryngeal/Delphian lymph nodes)
N1b Metastasis to unilateral, bilateral, or contralateral cervical or superior mediastinal lymph nodes

Distant Metastasis (M)
MX   Distant metastasis cannot be assessed
M0   No distant metastasis
M1   Distant metastasis

STAGE GROUPING

Separate stage groupings are recommended for papillary or follicular, medullary, and anaplastic (undifferentiated) carcinoma.

Papillary or Follicular
UNDER 45 YEARS

Stage I	Any T	Any N	M0
Stage II	Any T	Any N	M1

Papillary or Follicular
45 YEARS AND OLDER

Stage I	T1	N0	M0
Stage II	T2	N0	M0
Stage III	T3	N0	M0
	T1	N1a	M0
	T2	N1a	M0
	T3	N1a	M0
Stage IVA	T4a	N0	M0
	T4a	N1a	M0
	T1	N1b	M0
	T2	N1b	M0
	T3	N1b	M0
	T4a	N1b	M0
Stage IVB	T4b	Any N	M0
Stage IVC	Any T	Any N	M1

Medullary Carcinoma

Stage I	T1	N0	M0
Stage II	T2	N0	M0
Stage III	T3	N0	M0
	T1	N1a	M0
	T2	N1a	M0
	T3	N1a	M0
Stage IVA	T4a	N0	M0
	T4a	N1a	M0
	T1	N1b	M0
	T2	N1b	M0
	T3	N1b	M0
	T4a	N1b	M0
Stage IVB	T4b	Any N	M0
Stage IVC	Any T	Any N	M1

Anaplastic Carcinoma
All anaplastic carcinomas are considered Stage IV

Stage IVA	T4a	Any N	M0
Stage IVB	T4b	Any N	M0
Stage IVC	Any T	Any N	M1

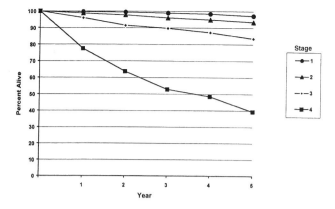

OBSERVED SURVIVAL BY STAGE	1	2	3	4	5	95% CIs*	CASES
1	99.4	98.9	98.4	97.9	97.2	96.7 – 97.7	4223
2	98.7	97.7	95.9	94.8	93.4	91.9 – 94.9	1225
3	95.9	91.4	89.7	87.2	83.5	80.9 – 86.1	928
4	77.5	63.7	52.8	48.5	39.3	31.9 – 46.7	200

FIG. 8.1A. Five-year, observed survival by "combined" AJCC stage for papillary adenocarcinoma of the thyroid gland, 1985–1991. (*95% confidence intervals correspond to year-5 survival rates.)

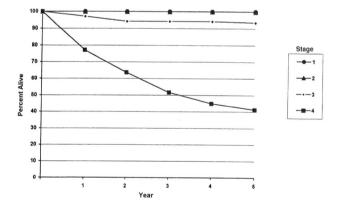

RELATIVE SURVIVAL BY STAGE	1	2	3	4	5	95% CIs*	CASES
1	100	100	100	100	100	100 – 100	4232
2	100	100	100	100	100	100 – 100	1227
3	98.1	96.2	96.2	96.2	95.8	92.8 – 98.8	930
4	78.6	66.1	57.0	53.2	45.3	36.9 – 53.8	201

FIG. 8.1B. Five-year, relative survival by "combined" AJCC stage for papillary adenocarcinoma of the thyroid gland, 1985–1991. (*95% confidence intervals correspond to year-5 survival rates.)

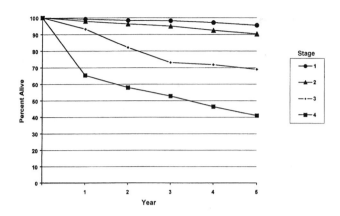

FIG. 8.2A. Five-year, observed survival by "combined" AJCC stage for follicular adenocarcinoma of the thyroid gland, 1985–1991. (*95% confidence intervals correspond to year-5 survival rates.)

OBSERVED SURVIVAL BY STAGE	1	2	3	4	5	95% CIs*	CASES
1	99.2	98.4	98.2	97.1	95.4	93.4 – 97.3	540
2	97.9	96.2	94.9	92.7	90.3	87.1 – 93.5	394
3	93.2	82.2	73.1	71.8	69.0	58.9 – 79.2	91
4	65.4	58.0	52.8	46.4	41.0	31.2 – 50.8	104

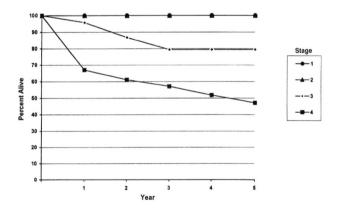

FIG. 8.2B. Five-year, relative survival by "combined" AJCC stage for follicular adenocarcinoma of the thyroid gland, 1985–1991. (*95% confidence intervals correspond to year-5 survival rates.)

RELATIVE SURVIVAL BY STAGE	1	2	3	4	5	95% CIs*	CASES
1	100	100	100	100	100	100 – 100	540
2	100	100	100	100	100	100 – 100	395
3	95.8	86.8	79.4	79.4	79.4	67.9 – 91.2	91
4	67.1	61.1	57.1	51.8	47.1	35.8 – 58.4	104

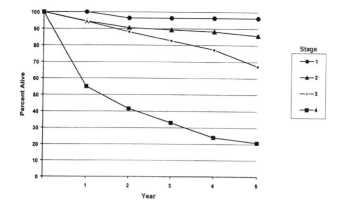

FIG. 8.3A. Five-year, observed survival by "combined" AJCC stage for medullary carcinoma of the thyroid gland, 1985–1991. (*95% confidence intervals correspond to year-5 survival rates.)

OBSERVED SURVIVAL BY STAGE	1	2	3	4	5	95% CIs*	CASES
1	100	96.2	96.2	96.2	96.2	91.0 – 100	55
2	94.4	90.4	89.3	88.2	85.8	78.8 – 92.7	110
3	94.2	88.0	82.7	77.3	67.2	57.7 – 76.8	107
4	55.0	41.6	33.0	24.0	20.8	7.3 – 34.2	41

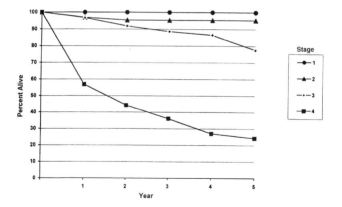

FIG. 8.3B. Five-year, relative survival by "combined" AJCC stage for medullary carcinoma of the thyroid gland, 1985–1991. (*95% confidence intervals correspond to year-5 survival rates.)

RELATIVE SURVIVAL BY STAGE	1	2	3	4	5	95% CIs*	CASES
1	100	100	100	100	100	100 – 100	57
2	96.9	95.3	96.8	96.8	96.8	90.3 – 100	110
3	96.7	91.8	88.6	86.5	77.6	66.7 – 88.4	107
4	56.9	44.2	36.1	27.0	24.3	8.83 – 39.9	41

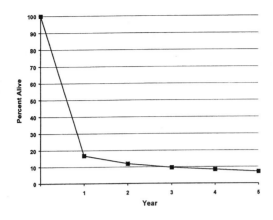

OBSERVED SURVIVAL FOR STAGE 4	1	2	3	4	5	95% CIs*	CASES
4	17.8	13.0	10.7	9.5	8.2	2.4 – 14.0	91

FIG. 8.4A. Five-year, observed survival by "combined" AJCC stage for Stage 4 anaplastic carcinoma of the thyroid gland, 1985–1991. (*95% confidence intervals correspond to year-5 survival rates.)

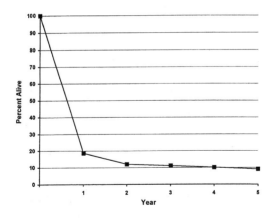

RELATIVE SURVIVAL FOR STAGE 4	1	2	3	4	5	95% CIs*	CASES
4	18.6	12.0	11.1	10.1	9.1	2.64 – 15.6	94

FIG. 8.4B. Five-year, relative survival by "combined" AJCC stage for Stage 4 anaplastic carcinoma of the thyroid gland, 1985–1991. (*95% confidence intervals correspond to year-5 survival rates.)

HISTOPATHOLOGIC TYPE

There are four major histopathologic types:

Papillary carcinoma (including follicular variant of papillary carcinoma)
Follicular carcinoma (including Hurthle cell carcinoma)
Medullary carcinoma
Undifferentiated (anaplastic) carcinoma

Figures 8.1A, 8.1B, 8.2A, 8.2B, 8.3A, 8.3B, 8.4A, 8.4B, show observed and relative survival rates for patients with papillary adenocarcinoma of the thyroid gland (8.1A,B), follicular adenocarcinoma of the thyroid gland (8.2A,B), medullar carcinoma of the thyroid gland (8.3A,B). Stage 4 anaplastic carcinoma of the thyroid gland (8.4A,B) and cancer of the thyroid gland.

BIBLIOGRAPHY

Ain KB: Papillary thyroid carcinoma: etiology, assessment, and therapy. Endocrinol Metab Clin North Am 24:711–760, 1995

Andersen PE, Kinsella J, Loree TR, Shaha AR, Shah JP: Differentiated carcinoma of the thyroid with extrathyroid extension—risks for failure and patterns of recurrence. Am J Surg 170:467–470, 1995

Antonacci A, Brierley G, Bacchi F, Consorti C, et al: Thyroid cancer. In Hermanek P, Gospodarowicz MK, Henson DE, et al (Eds.): Prognostic factors in cancer. Berlin: Springer-Verlag 28–36, 1995

Brierley JD, Panzarella T, Tsang RW, et al: Comparing staging classifications using thyroid cancer as an example. Cancer 79:2414–2413, 1997

Brierley J, Tsang R, Simpson WJ, et al: Medullary thyroid cancer—analyses of survival and prognostic factors and the role of radiation therapy in local control. Thyroid 6:305–310, 1996

Cady B, Rossi R, Silverman M, et al: Further evidence of the validity of risk group definition in differentiated thyroid carcinoma. Surgery 98:1171–1178, 1985

Cohn K, Blackdahl M, Forsslund G, et al: Prognostic value of nuclear DNA content in papillary thyroid carcinoma. World J Surg 8:474–480, 1984

Hay ID, Grant CS, Taylor WF, et al: Ipsilateral lobectomy versus bilateral lobar resection in papillary thyroid carcinoma: a retrospective analysis of surgical outcome using a novel prognostic scoring system. Surgery 102:1088–1095, 1987

Hedinger C. Histological typing of thyroid tumours: WHO international histological classification of tumours, 2nd ed. Berlin-Heidelberg-New York: Springer-Verlag, 1988

Hundahl SA, Cady B, Cunningham MP, Mazzaferri E, McKee R, Rosai J, Shah JP, Fremgen AM, Stewart AK, Holzer S (United States and German Thyroid Cancer Study Group): Initial results from a prospective cohort of 5,583 cases of thyroid carcinoma treated in the United States during 1996. Cancer 89:202–217, 2000

LiVolsi VA. Surgical pathology of the thyroid. Philadelphia: WB Saunders, 1990

Mazzaferri EL, Jhiang S: Long-term impact of initial surgical and medical therapy on papillary and follicular thyroid cancer. Am J Med 97:418–428, 1994

McConahey WM, Hay ID, Woolner LB, et al: Papillary thyroid cancer treated at the Mayo Clinic 1946–1970: initial manifestations, pathological findings, therapy and outcome. Mayo Clinic Proc 61:978–996, 1986

Rosai J, Carcangiu L, DeLellis RA: Tumors of the thyroid gland, 3rd series. Washington, DC: Armed Forces Institute of Pathology, 1992

Rossi R: Prognosis of undifferentiated carcinoma and lymphoma of the thyroid. Am J Surg 135:589–596, 1978

Saad MF, Ordonez NG, Rashid RK, et al: Medullary carcinoma of the thyroid: a study of the clinical features and prognostic factors in 161 patients. Medicine 63:319–342, 1984

Shah JP, Loree TR, Dharker D, et al: Prognostic factors in differentiated carcinoma of the thyroid gland. Am J Surg 1645:658–661, 1992

Shaha AR, Loree TR, Shah JP: Prognostic factors and risk group analysis in follicular carcinoma of the thyroid. Surgery 118:1131–1138, 1995

Shaha AR, Shah JP, Loree TR: Risk group stratification and prognostic factors in papillary carcinoma of the thyroid. Ann Surg Onc 3:534–538, 1996

Simpson WL, Panzarella T, Carruthers JS, et al: Papillary and follicular thyroid cancer: impact of treatment in 1,578 patients. Int J Radiation Oncol Biol Phys 14:1063–1075, 1988

Young RL, Mazzaferri EL, Rahea J, et al: Pure follicular thyroid carcinoma: impact of therapy in 214 patients. J Nucl Med 21:733–737, 1980

HISTOLOGIES—THYROID GLAND

8020/3	Carcinoma, undifferentiated, NOS
8021/3	Carcinoma, anaplastic, NOS
8050/3	Papillary carcinoma, NOS
8051/3	Verrucous carcinoma, NOS
8260/3	Papillary adenocarcinoma
8290/3	Hurthle cell adenocarcinoma
8330/3	Follicular adenocarcinoma
8331/3	Follicular adenocarcinoma, well differentiated
8335/3	Follicular carcinoma, minimally invasive
8337/3	Insular carcinoma
8340/3	Papillary carcinoma, follicular variant
8341/3	Papillary microcarcinoma
8342/3	Papillary carcinoma, oxyphilic cell
8343/3	Papillary carcinoma, encapsulated
8344/3	Papillary carcinoma, columnar cell
8345/3	Medullary carcinoma with amyloid stroma
8346/3	Mixed medullary-follicular carcinoma
8347/3	Mixed medullary-papillary carcinoma
8430/3	Mucoepidermoid carcinoma
8480/3	Mucinous adenocarcinoma
8481/3	Mucin-producing adenocarcinoma
8510/3	Medullary carcinoma, NOS

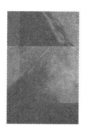

PART III
Digestive System

Esophagus

(Sarcomas are not included.)

C15.0 Cervical esophagus	C15.3 Upper third of esophagus	C15.8 Overlapping lesion of esophagus
C15.1 Thoracic esophagus	C15.4 Middle third of esophagus	C15.9 Esophagus, NOS
C15.2 Abdominal esophagus	C15.5 Lower third of esophagus	

SUMMARY OF CHANGES

- The definition of TNM and the Stage Grouping for this chapter have not changed from the Fifth Edition.

INTRODUCTION

Occurring more often in males, cancer of the esophagus accounts for 5.5% of all malignant tumors of the gastrointestinal tract and for less than 1% of all cancers in the United States. However, during the past 20 years, there has been a dramatic shift in the epidemiology of esophageal cancer in North America and most Western countries, characterized by a very rapid rise in the incidence of this disease and a marked shift from squamous cell carcinomas occurring predominantly in the middle third and distal esophagus to adenocarcinomas arising in the distal esophagus and the esophagogastric (EG) junction. Predisposing factors for squamous cell carcinomas include a high alcohol intake and heavy use of tobacco or nutritional deficiencies of vitamins and minerals. In contrast, EG junction carcinomas arise most frequently in Barrett's epithelium. The underlying causes for this marked epidemiologic change remain undefined.

Esophageal cancers, regardless of histologic type, may extend over wide areas of the mucosal surface. Squamous cell carcinomas often arise as multifocal tumors, presumably as a result of field carcinogenesis. Adenocarcinomas may have varying lengths of mucosal and submucosal disease, particularly in patients with long segments of Barrett's mucosa. However, only the depth of penetration into the esophageal wall and nodal status are considered in staging.

Many patients are asymptomatic during the early stages of disease. Early symptoms include those related to gastroesophageal reflux and associated Barrett's esophagus or odynophagia caused by esophageal ulceration. Unfortunately, the most common clinical symptom for all lesions is dysphagia, which occurs with large tumors that obstruct the lumen and deeply invade the esophageal wall. Therefore, most patients already have locally advanced or metastatic disease at diagnosis.

ANATOMY

Primary Site. Beginning at the hypopharynx, the esophagus lies posterior to the trachea and the heart, passing through the posterior mediastinum

---

and entering the stomach through an opening in the diaphragm called the hiatus.

Histologically, the esophagus has four layers: mucosa, submucosa, muscle coat or muscularis propria, and adventitia. There is no serosa.

For classification, staging, and reporting of cancer, the esophagus is divided into four regions. Because the behavior of esophageal cancer and its treatment vary with the anatomic divisions, these regions should be recorded and reported separately. The location of the esophageal cancer at the time of endoscopy is often measured from the incisors (front teeth).

Cervical esophagus. The cervical esophagus begins at the level of the lower border of the cricoid cartilage and ends at the thoracic inlet (the suprasternal notch), approximately 18 cm from the upper incisor teeth.

Intrathoracic and abdominal esophagus. This region is divided into two portions: The *upper thoracic portion* extends from the thoracic inlet to the level of the tracheal bifurcation, approximately 24 cm from the upper incisor teeth. The *midthoracic portion* of the esophagus lies between the tracheal bifurcation and the distal esophagus just above the esophagogastric junction. The lower level of this portion is approximately 32 cm from the upper incisor teeth.

Lower thoracic and abdominal portion. Approximately 3 cm in length, the lower esophagus also includes the intra-abdominal portion of the esophagus and the EG junction, which is located approximately 40 cm from the upper incisor teeth. Most adenocarcinomas arise from the EG junction and involve both the distal esophagus and the proximal stomach. Controversy exists over how to distinguish proximal gastric cancers involving the EG junction from distal esophageal and EG junction cancers extending inferiorly to involve the gastric cardia. In the absence of underlying Barrett's mucosa, making this distinction can be difficult. Siewert has proposed classifying EG junction cancers into types I, II and III depending on the relative extent of involvement of either the esophagus or the stomach. Further validation of this classification is needed to determine whether it is reliable for staging or for prognosis. In clinical practice, tumors arising within the EG junction and gastric cardia that have minimal (2 cm or less) involvement of the esophagus are considered primary gastric cancers.

Regional Lymph Nodes.   Specific regional lymph nodes are listed as follows:

Cervical esophagus
    Scalene
    Internal jugular
    Upper and lower cervical
    Periesophageal
    Supraclavicular
Intrathoracic esophagus—upper, middle, and lower
    Upper periesophageal (above the azygous vein)
    Subcarinal
    Lower periesophageal (below the azygous vein)

Gastroesophageal junction
>Lower esophageal (below the azygous vein)
>Diaphragmatic
>Pericardial
>Left gastric
>Celiac

Involvement of more distant lymph nodes (such as cervical or celiac axis nodes for intrathoracic tumors) is currently considered distant metastasis (M1a). However, recent analyses suggest that extensive nodal disease is associated with a better overall survival than visceral metastases and with an approximately 10% chance of cure at 5 years after surgical resection. On this basis, it has been suggested that the involvement of distant lymph nodes be classified as N2 disease rather than M1a, but such a change in classification requires further study.

The nomenclature used to indicate the location of involved lymph nodes has most frequently been that shown above, which provides a general anatomical description. More recently, a lymph node map that extends the nomenclature and numbering system used for the staging of non–small cell lung cancer has been developed and used in clinical trials. This map, which is shown in Figure 9.1, makes possible the more precise identification of involved lymph nodes.

Metastatic Sites. The liver, lungs, and pleura are the most common sites of distant metastases. Occasionally, the tumor may extend directly into mediastinal structures before distant metastasis is evident. This occurs most frequently with tumors of the intrathoracic esophagus, which may extend directly into the aorta, trachea, and pericardium.

RULES FOR CLASSIFICATION

Clinical Staging. Clinical staging depends on the anatomic extent of the primary tumor, which can be ascertained by examination before treatment. Such an examination includes some combination of medical history, physical examination, routine laboratory studies, esophagogastroscopy with biopsy, esophageal ultrasound (EUS), computed tomography (CT), and positron emission tomography (PET). EUS is considered the most accurate way to identify the depth of tumor invasion and may also reveal regional lymph node metastases. CT is more useful in identifying distant metastatic disease. Although the experience with PET is still limited, it appears to be more sensitive than CT in detecting distant metastases. The combined use of EUS, CT, and PET may prove to be the most accurate non-invasive means of staging esophageal carcinomas.

The anatomic location of the primary tumor (cervical, upper thoracic, midthoracic, or lower thoracic or gastroesophageal junction) should be recorded.

Pathologic Staging. Pathologic staging is based on surgical exploration and on the examination of the surgically resected esophagus and associated

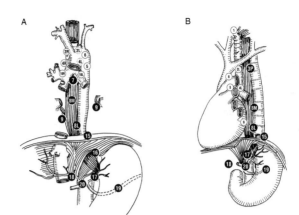

A

B

Regional lymph node stations for staging esophageal cancer, from front (A) and side (B).

1	Supraclavicular nodes	Above suprasternal notch and clavicles
2R	Right upper paratracheal nodes	Between intersection of caudal margin of innominate artery with trachea and the apex of the lung
2L	Left upper paratracheal nodes	Between top of aortic arch and apex of the lung
● 3P	Posterior mediastinal nodes	Upper paraesophageal nodes, above tracheal bifurcation
4R	Right lower paratracheal nodes	Between intersection of caudal margin of innominate artery with trachea and cephalic border of azygous vein
4L	Left lower paratracheal nodes	Between top of aortic arch and carina
5	Aortopulmonary nodes	Subaortic and para-aortic nodes lateral to the ligamentum arteriosum
6	Anterior mediastinal nodes	Anterior to ascending aorta or innominate artery
● 7	Subcarinal nodes	Caudal to the carina of the trachea
● 8M	Middle paraesophageal lymph nodes	From the tracheal bifurcation to the caudal margin of the inferior pulmonary vein
● 8L	Lower paraesophageal lymph nodes	From the caudal margin of the inferior pulmonary vein to the esophagogastric junction
● 9	Pulmonary ligament nodes	Within the inferior pulmonary ligament
10R	Right tracheobronchial nodes	From cephalic border of azygous vein to origin of RUL bronchus
10L	Left tracheobronchial nodes	Between carina and LUL bronchus
● 15	Diaphragmatic nodes	Lying on the dome of the diaphragm, and adjacent to or behind its crura
● 16	Paracardial nodes	Immediately adjacent to the gastroesophageal junction
● 17	Left gastric nodes	Along the course of the left gastric artery
● 18	Common hepatic nodes	Along the course of the common hepatic artery
● 19	Splenic nodes	Along the course of the splenic artery
● 20	Celiac nodes	At the base of the celiac artery

FIG. 9.1. Esophageal lymph node map indicating regional lymph node stations for staging esophageal cancer, from front (A) and side (B). (Reproduced with permission from Bristol-Myers Oncology Division.)

lymph nodes. Involvement of the adjacent structures depends on the location of the primary tumor. This extension and the presence of distant metastases should be specifically documented. A single classification serves all regions of the esophagus and the EG junction. It also serves both clinical and pathologic staging.

DEFINITION OF TNM

Primary Tumor (T)

TX   Primary tumor cannot be assessed
T0   No evidence of primary tumor
Tis   Carcinoma *in situ*
T1   Tumor invades lamina propria or submucosa
T2   Tumor invades muscularis propria
T3   Tumor invades adventitia
T4   Tumor invades adjacent structures

Regional Lymph Nodes (N)

NX   Regional lymph nodes cannot be assessed
N0   No regional lymph node metastasis
N1   Regional lymph node metastasis

Distant Metastasis (M)

MX   Distant metastasis cannot be assessed
M0   No distant metastasis
M1   Distant metastasis

Tumors of the lower thoracic esophagus:
M1a   Metastasis in celiac lymph nodes
M1b   Other distant metastasis

Tumors of the midthoracic esophagus:
M1a   Not applicable
M1b   Nonregional lymph nodes and/or other distant metastasis

Tumors of the upper thoracic esophagus:
M1a   Metastasis in cervical nodes
M1b   Other distant metastasis

STAGE GROUPING

Stage	T	N	M
Stage 0	Tis	N0	M0
Stage I	T1	N0	M0
Stage IIA	T2	N0	M0
	T3	N0	M0
Stage IIB	T1	N1	M0
	T2	N1	M0
Stage III	T3	N1	M0
	T4	Any N	M0
Stage IV	Any T	Any N	M1
Stage IVA	Any T	Any N	M1a
Stage IVB	Any T	Any N	M1b

HISTOPATHOLOGIC TYPE

The classification applies to all carcinomas. Sarcomas are not included. Worldwide, squamous cell carcinomas are the most common, but the incidence of adenocarcinoma is increasing. In North America and Europe, adenocarcinomas are more common than squamous cell carcinomas. Adenocarcinomas arising from Barrett's esophagus are included in the classification.

Barrett's esophagus (Barrett's mucosa) is a columnar metaplasia of the esophagus that is due to chronic gastroesophageal reflux. It is the only known precursor of esophageal adenocarcinoma, although the risk of Barrett's cancer varies greatly from one study to another. The diagnosis of Barrett's mucosa is made when two criteria are satisfied. First, there must be endoscopic or grossly abnormal columnar mucosa involving the distal esophagus, usually identified as tongues of pink mucosa extending above the normal squamocolumnar junction. This junction is the normal border between esophageal and gastric mucosa. Usually this junction coincides with the anatomic gastroesophageal junction, but sometimes it actually lies within the distal 2 cm of the tubular esophagus. Second, biopsies of the abnormal endoscopic areas must contain goblet cells in the columnar mucosa. Barrett's mucosa has been divided into two types based on length: short-segment disease that is less than 3 cm and long-segment disease that is 3 cm or longer. If all patients with short-segment and long-segment disease are compared, there is no significant difference in cancer risk, although there may be a gradual increase in risk with increasing length. The precursor lesion for carcinoma and the marker of very high cancer risk is high-grade dysplasia in the Barrett's mucosa. High-grade dysplasia includes all non-invasive neoplastic epithelium that was formally called carcinoma *in situ*, a diagnosis that is no longer used for columnar mucosae anywhere in the gastrointestinal tract.

HISTOLOGIC GRADE (G)

GX   Grade cannot be assessed
G1   Well differentiated
G2   Moderately differentiated
G3   Poorly differentiated
G4   Undifferentiated

PROGNOSTIC FACTORS

Anatomic location does not appear to be an important prognostic variable. However, upper thoracic and cervical esophageal lesions may be more difficult to manage surgically than more inferiorly located tumors because of their proximity to vital structures, including the trachea and great vessels. Depth of invasion (T) is an independent variable; tumor length is not. This has encouraged pretreatment endoscopic ultrasound for staging, particularly in patients who may be candidates for non-operative therapy. Lymphatic spread is a strong independent prognostic variable, as are distant metastases. In the latter category, distant organ metastasis appears to be associated with a worse prognosis than distant non-regional lymph node metastases. The histologic type (squamous cell carcinoma versus adenocarcinoma) is not a prognostic factor. Tumor differentiation, DNA ploidy status, and various oncogenes, growth factors, and other markers are being intensively studied as prognostic indicators, but data are still insufficient for a conclusive statement regarding these potential prognostic factors.

BIBLIOGRAPHY

Block MI, Patterson GA, Sundaresan RS, et al: Improvement in staging of esophageal cancer with the addition of positron emission tomography. Ann Thorac Surg 64:770–777, 1997

Casson AG, Rusch VW, Ginsberg RJ, Zankowicz N, Finley RJ: Lymph node mapping of esophageal cancer. Ann Thorac Surg 58:1569–1570, 1994

Ellis FH Jr, Heatley GJ, Krasna MJ, Williamson WA, Balogh K: Esophagogastrectomy for carcinoma of the esophagus and cardia: a comparison of findings and results after standard resection in three consecutive eight-year intervals with improved staging criteria. J Thorac Cardiovasc Surg 113:836–848, 1997

Kawahara K, Maekawa T, Okabayashi K, et al: The number of lymph node metastases influences survival in esophageal cancer. J Surg Oncol 67:160–163, 1998

Kelsen DP, Ginsberg R, Pajak TF, et al: Chemotherapy followed by surgery compared with surgery alone for localized esophageal cancer. N Engl J Med 339:1979–1984, 1998

Killinger WA, Jr., Rice TW, Adelstein DJ, et al: Stage II esophageal carcinoma: the significance of T and N. J Thorac Cardiovasc Surg 111:935–940, 1996

Lightdale CJ: Positron emission tomography: another useful test for staging esophageal cancer. J Clin Oncol 18:3199–3201, 2000

Nishimaki T, Tanaka O, Ando N, et al: Evaluation of the accuracy of preoperative staging in thoracic esophageal cancer. Ann Thorac Surg 68:2059–2064, 1999

Pera M, Cameron AJ, Trastek VF, Carpenter HA, Zinsmeister AR: Increasing incidence of adenocarcinoma of the esophagus and esophagogastric junction. Gastroenterol 104:510–513, 1993

Rudolph RE, Vaughan TL, Storer BE, et al: Effect of segment length on risk for neoplastic progression in patients with Barrett esophagus. Ann Int Med 132:612–620, 2000

Rusch VW, Levine DS, Haggitt R, Reid BJ: The management of high grade dysplasia and early cancer in Barrett's esophagus. Cancer 74:1225–1229, 1994

Sabik JF, Rice TW, Goldblum JR, et al: Superficial esophageal carcinoma. Ann Thorac Surg 60:896–902, 1995

Sampliner RE: Practice guidelines on the diagnosis, surveillance, and therapy of Barrett's esophagus: the Practice Parameters Committee of the American College of Gastroenterology. Am J Gastroenterol 93:1028–1032, 1998

Siewert JR, Feith M, Werner M, Stein HJ: Adenocarcinoma of the esophagogastric junction: results of surgical therapy based on anatomical/topographic classification in 1,002 consecutive patients. Trans Am Surg Assoc 118:67–75, 2000

Steup WH, De Leyn P, Deneffe G, Van Raemdonck D, Coosemans W, Lerut T: Tumors of the esophagogastric junction. Long term survival in relation to the pattern of lymph node metastasis and a critical analysis of the accuracy or inaccuracy of pTNM classification. J Thorac Cardiovasc Surg 111:85–95, 1996

Yang PC, Davis S: Incidence of cancer of the esophagus in the U.S. by histologic type. Cancer 61:612–617, 1988

8000/3	Neoplasm, malignant
8001/3	Tumor cells, malignant
8002/3	Malignant tumor, small cell type
8003/3	Malignant tumor, giant cell type
8004/3	Malignant tumor, spindle cell type
8005/3	Malignant tumor, clear cell type
8010/2	Carcinoma *in situ,* NOS
8010/3	Carcinoma, NOS
8011/3	Epithelioma, malignant
8012/3	Large cell carcinoma, NOS
8013/3	Large cell neuroendocrine carcinoma
8014/3	Large cell carcinoma with rhabdoid phenotype
8015/3	Glassy cell carcinoma
8020/3	Carcinoma, undifferentiated, NOS
8021/3	Carcinoma, anaplastic, NOS
8022/3	Pleomorphic carcinoma
8030/3	Giant cell and spindle cell carcinoma
8031/3	Giant cell carcinoma
8032/3	Spindle cell carcinoma, NOS
8033/3	Pseudosarcomatous carcinoma
8034/3	Polygonal cell carcinoma
8035/3	Carcinoma with osteoclast-like giant cells
8041/3	Small cell carcinoma, NOS
8042/3	Oat cell carcinoma
8043/3	Small cell carcinoma, fusiform cell
8044/3	Small cell carcinoma, intermediate cell
8045/3	Combined small cell carcinoma
8046/3	Non–small cell carcinoma
8050/3	Papillary carcinoma, NOS
8051/3	Verrucous carcinoma, NOS
8052/2	Papillary squamous cell carcinoma, non-invasive
8052/3	Papillary squamous cell carcinoma
8070/2	Squamous cell carcinoma *in situ,* NOS
8070/3	Squamous cell carcinoma, NOS
8071/3	Squamous cell carcinoma, keratinizing, NOS
8072/3	Squamous cell carcinoma, large cell, nonkeratinizing, NOS
8073/3	Squamous cell carcinoma, small cell, nonkeratinizing
8074/3	Squamous cell carcinoma, spindle cell
8075/3	Squamous cell carcinoma, adenoid
8076/2	Squamous cell carcinoma *in situ* with questionable stromal invasion
8076/3	Squamous cell carcinoma, microinvasive
8077/2	Squamous intraepithelial neoplasia, grade III
8082/3	Lymphoepithelial carcinoma
8083/3	Basaloid squamous cell carcinoma
8084/3	Squamous cell carcinoma, clear cell type
8090/3	Basal cell carcinoma, NOS
8091/3	Multifocal superficial basal cell carcinoma
8092/3	Infiltrating basal cell carcinoma, NOS
8093/3	Basal cell carcinoma, fibroepithelial
8094/3	Basosquamous carcinoma
8095/3	Metatypical carcinoma
8097/3	Basal cell carcinoma, nodular
8098/3	Adenoid basal carcinoma
8244/3	Composite carcinoid

8245/3	Adenocarcinoid tumor
8246/3	Neuroendocrine carcinoma, NOS
8247/3	Merkel cell carcinoma
8249/3	Atypical carcinoid tumor
8255/3	Adenocarcinoma with mixed subtypes
8260/3	Papillary adenocarcinoma, NOS
8430/3	Mucoepidermoid carcinoma
8440/3	Cystadenocarcinoma, NOS
8480/3	Mucinous adenocarcinoma
8481/3	Mucin-producing adenocarcinoma
8490/3	Signet ring cell carcinoma
8510/3	Medullary carcinoma, NOS
8560/3	Adenosquamous carcinoma
8570/3	Adenocarcinoma with squamous metaplasia
8571/3	Adenocarcinoma with cartilaginous and osseous metaplasia
8572/3	Adenocarcinoma with spindle cell metaplasia
8573/3	Adenocarcinoma with apocrine metaplasia
8574/3	Adenocarcinoma with neuroendocrine differentiation
8575/3	Metaplastic carcinoma, NOS
8830/3	Malignant fibrous histiocytoma
8933/3	Adenosarcoma
8940/3	Mixed tumor, malignant, NOS
8941/3	Carcinoma in pleomorphic adenoma

3

Stomach

(Lymphomas, sarcomas, and carcinoid tumors are not included.)

C16.0 Cardia, NOS
C16.1 Fundus of stomach
C16.2 Body of stomach
C16.3 Gastric antrum

C16.4 Pylorus
C16.5 Lesser curvature of
       stomach, NOS

C16.8 Greater curvature of
       stomach, NOS
C16.8 Overlapping lesion of
       stomach
C16.9 Stomach, NOS

SUMMARY OF CHANGES

- T2 lesions have been divided into T2a and T2b.
- T2a is defined as a tumor that invades the muscularis propria.
- T2b is defined as a tumor that invades into subserosa.

INTRODUCTION

Gastric adenocarcinoma has declined significantly in the United States over the past 70 years, but even so, during the early 21st century, an estimated 22,000 patients develop the disease each year. Of these patients, 13,000 will die, mainly because of nodal and metastatic disease present at the time of initial diagnosis. When worldwide figures are analyzed, the United States ranks 44th in both males and females dying from gastric adenocarcinoma. The highest rates of this disease continue to be in areas of Asia and Russia. Trends in survival rates from the 1970s to the 1990s have unfortunately shown very little improvement. During the 1990s, 20% of gastric carcinoma cases were diagnosed while localized to the gastric wall, whereas 30% had evidence of regional nodal disease. Disease resulting from metastasis to other solid organs within the abdomen, as well as to extra-abdominal sites, represents 35% of all cases. Although overall 5-year survival is approximately 15–20%, the 5-year survival is approximately 55% when disease is localized to the stomach (Fig. 10.1). The involvement of regional nodes reduces the 5-year survival to approximately 20%.

A notable shift in the site of gastric cancer reflects a proportionate increase in disease of the proximal stomach over the past several decades. Previously, there was a predominance of distal gastric cancers presenting as mass lesions or ulceration. Although other malignancies occur in the stomach, approximately 90% of all gastric neoplasms are adenocarcinomas. Tumors of the gastroesophageal (GE) junction may be difficult to stage as either a gastric or an esophageal primary, especially in view of the increased incidence of adenocarcinoma in the esophagus that presumably results from acid reflux disease. By convention, if more than 50% of the cancer involves the esophagus, the cancer is classified as esophageal. Similarly, if more than 50% of the tumor is below the GE junction, it is classified as gastric in origin. If the tumor is located equally above and below the GE junction, the histology determines the origin of the primary–

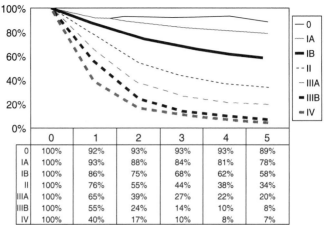

	0	1	2	3	4	5
0	100%	92%	93%	93%	93%	89%
IA	100%	93%	88%	84%	81%	78%
IB	100%	86%	75%	68%	62%	58%
II	100%	76%	55%	44%	38%	34%
IIIA	100%	65%	39%	27%	22%	20%
IIIB	100%	55%	24%	14%	10%	8%
IV	100%	40%	17%	10%	8%	7%

FIG. 10.1. One-year through 5-year survival rates of gastrectomy patients. Number of patients by stage group: Stage 0 (322), Stage IA (2,905), Stage IB (4,658), Stage II (6,541), Stage IIIA (7,481), Stage IIIB (2,330), and Stage IV (8,617). From Hundahl SA, Phillips JL, Menck HR: The National Cancer Data Base report on survival of U.S. gastric carcinoma patients treated with gastrectomy. Cancer 88:921–932, 2000. © 2000, American Cancer Society. Reprinted by permission of Wiley-Liss, Inc., a subsidiary of John Wiley & Sons, Inc.

squamous cell, small cell, and undifferentiated carcinomas are classified as esophageal, and adenocarcinoma and signet ring cell carcinomas are classified as gastric. When Barrett's esophagus (intestinal metaplasia) is present, adenocarcinoma in both the gastric cardia and lower esophagus is most likely to be esophageal in origin.

ANATOMY

Primary Site. The stomach is the first division of the abdominal portion of the alimentary tract, beginning at the gastroesophageal junction and extending to the pylorus. The proximal stomach is located immediately below the diaphragm and is termed the cardia. The remaining portions are the fundus (body) of the stomach and the distal portion of the stomach known as the antrum. The pylorus is a muscular ring that controls the flow of food content from the stomach into the first portion of the duodenum. The medial and lateral curvatures of the stomach are known as the lesser and greater curvatures, respectively. Histologically, the wall of the stomach has five layers: mucosal, submucosal, muscular, subserosal, and serosal.

Staging of primary gastric adenocarcinoma is dependent on the depth of penetration of the primary tumor. The T2 designation has been subdivided into T2a (invasion of the muscularis propria) and T2b (invasion of the subserosa) in order to discriminate between these intramural locations, even though there is no change in the designation in the stage grouping that involves T2a or T2b lesions.

Regional Lymph Nodes. Several groups of regional lymph nodes drain the wall of the stomach. These perigastric nodes are found along the lesser and greater curvatures. Other major nodal groups follow the main arterial and venous vessels from the aorta and the portal circulation. Adequate nodal dissection of these regional nodal areas is important to ensure appropriate designation of the pN determination. Although it is suggested that at least 15 regional nodes be assessed pathologically, a pN0 determination may be assigned on the basis of the actual number of nodes evaluated microscopically.

Involvement of other intra-abdominal lymph nodes, such as the hepatoduodenal, retropancreatic, mesenteric, and para-aortic, is classified as distant metastasis. The specific nodal areas are as follows:

Greater Curvature of Stomach:
Greater curvature, greater omental, gastroduodenal, gastroepiploic, pyloric, and pancreaticoduodenal

Pancreatic and Splenic Area:
Pancreaticolienal, peripancreatic, splenic

Lesser Curvature of Stomach:
Lesser curvature, lesser omental, left gastric, cardioesophageal, common hepatic, celiac, and hepatoduodenal

Distant Nodal Groups:
Retropancreatic, para-aortic, portal, retroperitoneal, mesenteric

Metastatic Sites. The most common metastatic distribution is to the liver, peritoneal surfaces, and nonregional or distant lymph nodes. Central nervous system and pulmonary metastases occur but are less frequent. With large, bulky lesions, direct extension may occur to the liver, transverse colon, pancreas, or undersurface of the diaphragm.

RULES FOR CLASSIFICATION

Clinical Staging. Designated as cTNM, clinical staging is based on evidence of extent of disease acquired before definitive treatment is instituted. It includes physical examination, radiologic imaging, endoscopy, biopsy, and laboratory findings. All cancers should be confirmed histologically.

Pathologic Staging. Pathologic staging depends on data acquired clinically, together with findings on subsequent surgical exploration and examination of the pathologic specimen if resection is accomplished. Pathologic assessment of the regional lymph nodes entails their removal and histologic examination to evaluate the total number, as well as the number that contain metastatic tumor. Metastatic nodules in the fat adjacent to a gastric carcinoma, without evidence of residual lymph node tissue, are considered regional lymph node metastases, but nodules implanted on peritoneal surfaces are considered distant metastasis. If there is uncertainty concerning the appropriate T, N, or M assignment, the lower (less advanced) category should be selected. This will also be reflected in the stage grouping.

DEFINITION OF TNM

Primary Tumor (T)

TX   Primary tumor cannot be assessed

T0   No evidence of primary tumor

Tis   Carcinoma *in situ:* intraepithelial tumor without invasion of the lamina propria

T1   Tumor invades lamina propria or submucosa

T2   Tumor invades muscularis propria or subserosa*

T2a   Tumor invades muscularis propria

T2b   Tumor invades subserosa

T3   Tumor penetrates serosa (visceral peritoneum) without invasion of adjacent structures**,***

T4   Tumor invades adjacent structures**,***

*Note: A tumor may penetrate the muscularis propria with extension into the gastrocolic or gastrohepatic ligaments, or into the greater or lesser omentum, without perforation of the visceral peritoneum covering these structures. In this case, the tumor is classified T2. If there is perforation of the visceral peritoneum covering the gastric ligaments or the omentum, the tumor should be classified T3.

**Note: The adjacent structures of the stomach include the spleen, transverse colon, liver, diaphragm, pancreas, abdominal wall, adrenal gland, kidney, small intestine, and retroperitoneum.

***Note: Intramural extension to the duodenum or esophagus is classified by the depth of the greatest invasion in any of these sites, including the stomach.

Regional Lymph Nodes (N)

NX   Regional lymph node(s) cannot be assessed

N0   No regional lymph node metastasis*

N1   Metastasis in 1 to 6 regional lymph nodes

N2   Metastasis in 7 to 15 regional lymph nodes

N3   Metastasis in more than 15 regional lymph nodes

*Note: A designation of pN0 should be used if all examined lymph nodes are negative, regardless of the total number removed and examined.

Distant Metastasis (M)

MX   Distant metastasis cannot be assessed

M0   No distant metastasis

M1   Distant metastasis

STAGE GROUPING

Stage 0	Tis	N0	M0
Stage IA	T1	N0	M0
Stage IB	T1	N1	M0
	T2a/b	N0	M0
Stage II	T1	N2	M0
	T2a/b	N1	M0
	T3	N0	M0
Stage IIIA	T2a/b	N2	M0
	T3	N1	M0
	T4	N0	M0
Stage IIIB	T3	N2	M0
Stage IV	T4	N1-3	M0
	T1-3	N3	M0
	Any T	Any N	M1

3

HISTOPATHOLOGIC TYPE

The staging recommendations apply only to carcinomas. Lymphomas, sarcomas, and carcinoid tumors are not included. Adenocarcinomas may be divided into the general subtypes listed below. In addition, the histologic terms intestinal, diffuse, and mixed may be applied.

The histologic subtypes are:

Adenocarcinoma
Papillary adenocarcinoma
Tubular adenocarcinoma
Mucinous adenocarcinoma
Signet ring cell carcinoma
Adenosquamous carcinoma
Squamous cell carcinoma
Small cell carcinoma
Undifferentiated carcinoma

HISTOLOGIC GRADE (G)

GX   Grade cannot be assessed
G1   Well differentiated
G2   Moderately differentiated
G3   Poorly differentiated
G4   Undifferentiated

PROGNOSTIC FACTORS

Treatment is a major prognostic factor for gastric cancer. Patients who are not resected have a poor prognosis, with survival ranging from 3 to 11 months. For those patients undergoing complete resection, the factors that affect prognosis include the location of the tumor in the stomach and the gross pathologic type, as well as the T and N classification. The prognosis for proximal gastric cancer is less favorable than for distal lesions, and the classic gross pathologic type, as described by Borrmann (I—polypoid, II—ulcerocancer, III—ulcerating and infiltrating, and IV—infiltrating), has prognostic impact. Polypoid and ulcerocancers (I and II) that are resected have a considerably better prognosis than Borrmann III and IV, independent of the presence or absence of regional lymph node involvement.

Depth of invasion into the gastric wall (T) correlates with reduced survival, but regional lymphatic spread is probably the most powerful prognostic factor. The histologic classification of Lauren has some impact on prognosis, but diffuse lesions are more often proximally located and larger than the intestinal-type lesions that generally tend to be distal. Histologic grade is an important prognostic factor. High preoperative serum levels for tumor markers CEA and CA 19–9 have been associated with a less favorable outcome.

BIBLIOGRAPHY

Alexander HR, Kelsen DG, Tepper JC: Cancer of the stomach. In DeVita VT, Hellman S, Rosenberg SA (Eds.): Cancer: principles and practice of oncology, 5th ed. Philadelphia: Lippincott-Raven, 1021–1054, 1997

Bonen Kamp JJ, Hermans J, Sasako M, et al: Extended lymph-node dissection for gastric cancer. Dutch Gastric Cancer Group. N Engl J Med 340:908–914, 1999

Bunt AM, Hermans J, Smith VT, et al: Surgical/pathologic-stage migration confounds comparisons of gastric cancer survival rates between Japan and Western countries. J Clin Oncol 13:19–25, 1995

Greenlee RT, Hill-Harmon M, Murray T, Thun M: Cancer statistics, 2001. Ca Cancer J Clin 51:15–36, 2001

Hermanek P. Prognostic factors in stomach cancer surgery. Eur J Surg Oncol 12:241–246, 1986

Hermanek P, Wittekind C. Residual tumor (R) classification and prognosis. Semin Surg Oncol 10:12–20, 1994

Hochwald SN, Kim S, Klimstra DS, et al: Analysis of 154 actual five-year survivors of gastric cancer. J Gastrointest Surg 4:520–525, 2000

Ichikura T, Tomimatsu S, Okusa Y, et al. Comparison of the prognostic significance between the number of metastatic lymph nodes and nodal stage based on their location in patients with gastric cancer. J Clin Oncol 11:1894–1900, 1993

Hundahl SA, Phillips JL, Menck HR. The National Cancer Data Base report on survival of U.S. gastric carcinoma patients treated with gastrectomy. Cancer 88:921–932, 2000

Kennedy BJ. Gastric cancer staging and natural history. In Wanebo HJ (Ed.): Surgery for gastrointestinal cancer: a multidisciplinary approach. Philadelphia: Lippincott-Raven, 299–303, 1977

Kodera Y, Yamamura Y, Shimizu Y, et al: The number of metastatic lymph nodes: a promising prognosis determinant for gastric carcinoma in the latest edition of the TNM classification. J Am Coll Surg 187:597–603, 1998

Lauren P. The two histological main types of gastric carcinoma: diffuse and so-called intestinal-type carcinoma. Acta Path Aicrobiol Scand 64:31–49, 1965

Lawrence W, Menck HR, Steele GD, et al: The National Cancer Data Base report on gastric cancer. Cancer 75:1734–1744, 1995

Wittekind C, Henson DE, Hutter RVP, Sobin LH: TNM supplement: a commentary on uniform use. 2nd ed. New York: Wiley-Liss, 2001

HISTOLOGIES—STOMACH

8010/2	Carcinoma *in situ*, NOS
8010/3	Carcinoma, NOS
8012/3	Large cell carcinoma, NOS
8013/3	Large cell neuroendocrine carcinoma
8014/3	Large cell carcinoma with rhabdoid phenotype
8020/3	Carcinoma, undifferentiated, NOS
8021/3	Carcinoma, anaplastic, NOS
8022/3	Pleomorphic carcinoma
8030/3	Giant cell and spindle cell carcinoma
8031/3	Giant cell carcinoma
8032/3	Spindle cell carcinoma, NOS
8033/3	Pseudosarcomatous carcinoma
8035/3	Carcinoma with osteoclast-like giant cells
8041/3	Small cell carcinoma, NOS
8042/3	Oat cell carcinoma
8043/3	Small cell carcinoma, fusiform cell
8044/3	Small cell carcinoma, intermediate cell
8045/3	Combined small cell carcinoma
8046/3	Non-small cell carcinoma
8070/2	Squamous cell carcinoma *in situ*, NOS
8070/3	Squamous cell carcinoma, NOS
8071/3	Squamous cell carcinoma, keratinizing, NOS
8072/3	Squamous cell carcinoma, large cell
8073/3	Squamous cell carcinoma, small cell, non-keratinizing
8074/3	Squamous cell carcinoma, spindle cell
8075/3	Squamous cell carcinoma, adenoid
8076/2	Squamous cell carcinoma *in situ* with questionable stromal invasion
8076/3	Squamous cell carcinoma, microinvasive
8082/3	Lymphoepithelial carcinoma
8083/3	Basaloid squamous cell carcinoma
8084/3	Squamous cell carcinoma, clear cell type
8140/2	Adenocarcinoma *in situ*, NOS
8140/3	Adenocarcinoma, NOS
8141/3	Scirrhous adenocarcinoma
8142/3	Linitis plastica
8143/3	Superficial spreading adenocarcinoma
8144/3	Adenocarcinoma, intestinal type
8145/3	Carcinoma, diffuse type
8147/3	Basal cell adenocarcinoma
8148/2	Glandular intraepithelial neoplasia, grade III
8210/2	Adenocarcinoma *in situ* in adenomatous polyp
8210/3	Adenocarcinoma in adenomatous polyp
8211/3	Tubular adenocarcinoma
8214/3	Parietal cell carcinoma
8221/3	Adenocarcinoma in multiple adenomatous polyps
8230/3	Solid carcinoma, NOS
8244/3	Composite carcinoid
8245/3	Adenocarcinoid tumor
8246/3	Neuroendocrine carcinoma, NOS
8255/3	Adenocarcinoma with mixed subtypes
8260/3	Papillary adenocarcinoma, NOS
8261/2	Adenocarcinoma *in situ* in villous adenoma
8261/3	Adenocarcinoma in villous adenoma
8262/3	Villous adenocarcinoma

3

8263/2	Adenocarcinoma *in situ* in tubulovillous adenoma
8263/3	Adenocarcinoma in tubulovillous adenoma
8310/3	Clear cell adenocarcinoma, NOS
8320/3	Granular cell carcinoma
8430/3	Mucoepidermoid carcinoma
8440/3	Cystadenocarcinoma, NOS
8441/3	Serous cystadenocarcinoma, NOS
8450/3	Papillary cystadenocarcinoma, NOS
8452/3	Solid pseudopapillary carcinoma
8453/2	Intraductal papillary-mucinous carcinoma, non-invasive
8453/3	Intraductal papillary-mucinous carcinoma, invasive
8460/3	Papillary serous cystadenocarcinoma
8461/3	Serous surface papillary carcinoma
8470/2	Mucinous cystadenocarcinoma, non-invasive
8470/3	Mucinous cystadenocarcinoma, NOS
8471/3	Papillary mucinous cystadenocarcinoma
8480/3	Mucinous adenocarcinoma
8481/3	Mucin-producing adenocarcinoma
8490/3	Signet ring cell carcinoma
8500/2	Intraductal carcinoma, non-infiltrating, NOS
8503/2	Non-infiltrating intraductal papillary adenocarcinoma
8503/3	Intraductal papillary adenocarcinoma with invasion
8550/3	Acinar cell carcinoma
8551/3	Acinar cell cystadenocarcinoma
8560/3	Adenosquamous carcinoma
8570/3	Adenocarcinoma with squamous metaplasia
8571/3	Adenocarcinoma with cartilaginous and osseous metaplasia
8572/3	Adenocarcinoma with spindle cell metaplasia

Small Intestine

(Lymphomas, carcinoid tumors, and visceral sarcomas are not included.)

C17.0 Duodenum
C17.1 Jejunum
C17.2 Ileum

C17.8 Overlapping lesion of small intestine

C17.9 Small intestine, NOS

SUMMARY OF CHANGES

• The definition of TNM and the Stage Grouping for this chapter have not changed from the Fifth Edition.

INTRODUCTION

Although the small intestine accounts for one of the largest surface areas in the human body, less than 2% of all malignant tumors of the gastrointestinal tract actually occur in the small bowel. Most cancers occur in the first or second portion of the duodenum and represent adenocarcinomas. A variety of tumors occur in the small intestine, approximately 50% of the primary malignant tumors being adenocarcinomas. An increased incidence of second malignancies has been noted in patients with primary small bowel adenocarcinoma. At the beginning of the 21st century, approximately 5,000 new cases of cancer involving the small intestine are seen annually in the United States. The 1,200 deaths predicted to occur from small intestinal cancer are divided equally between men and women. The patterns of local, regional, and metastatic spread for adenocarcinomas of the small intestine are comparable to those of similar histologic malignancies in other areas of the gastrointestinal tract. The classification and stage grouping described in this chapter are used for both clinical and pathologic staging of carcinomas of the small bowel and do not apply to other types of malignant small bowel tumors. Although small bowel carcinoid tumors are not traditionally staged using the TNM system, reports from the United States and throughout the world attempt to stage these neuroendocrine tumors using the TNM system.

ANATOMY

Primary Site. This classification applies to carcinomas arising in the duodenum, jejunum, and ileum. It does not apply to carcinomas arising in the ileocecal valve or to carcinomas that may arise in Meckel's diverticulum. Carcinomas arising in the ampulla of Vater are staged according to the system described in Chapter 17.

Duodenum. About 25 cm in length, the duodenum extends from the pyloric sphincter of the stomach to the jejunum. It is usually divided anatomically into four parts, with the common bile duct and pancreatic duct opening into the second part at the ampulla of Vater.

Jejunum and Ileum.   The jejunum (8 feet in length) and ileum (12 feet in length) extend from the junction with the duodenum proximally to the ileocecal valve distally. The division point between the jejunum and the ileum is arbitrary. As a general rule, the jejunum includes the proximal 40% and the ileum includes the distal 60% of the small intestine, exclusive of the duodenum.

General.   The jejunal and ileal portions of the small intestine are supported by a fold of the peritoneum containing the blood supply and the regional lymph nodes, the mesentery. The shortest segment, the duodenum, has no real mesentery and is covered only by peritoneum anteriorly. The wall of all parts of the small intestine has five layers: mucosal, submucosal, muscular, subserosal, and serosal. A very thin layer of smooth muscle cells, the muscularis mucosae, separates the mucosa from the submucosa. The small intestine is entirely ensheathed by peritoneum, except for a narrow strip of bowel that is attached to the mesentery and that part of the duodenum that is located retroperioneally.

Regional Lymph Nodes.   For pN, histologic examination of a regional lymphadenectomy specimen will ordinarily include a representative number of lymph nodes distributed along the mesenteric vessels extending to the base of the mesentery.

Duodenum:
Duodenal
Hepatic
Pancreaticoduodenal
Infrapyloric
Gastroduodenal
Pyloric
Superior mesenteric
Pericholedochal
Regional lymph nodes, NOS

Ileum and Jejunum:
Posterior cecal (terminal ileum only)
Ileocolic (terminal ileum only)
Superior mesenteric
Mesenteric, NOS
Regional lymph nodes, NOS

Metastatic Sites.   Cancers of the small intestine can metastasize to most organs, especially the liver, or to the peritoneal surfaces. Involvement of regional lymph nodes and invasion of adjacent structures are most common. Involvement of the celiac nodes is considered M1 disease for carcinomas of the duodenum, jejunum, and ileum. The presence of distant metastases and the presence of residual disease (R) have the most influence on survival.

RULES FOR CLASSIFICATION

Clinical Staging.   Imaging studies such as CT and MRI play a major role in clinical staging. Metastatic disease is assessed by routine chest films and chest CT. Intraoperative assessment plays a role in clinical evaluation, especially when tumor cannot be resected. Metastatic involvement of the liver may be evaluated by intraoperative ultrasonography.

Pathologic Staging.   The primary tumor is staged according to its depth of penetration and the involvement of adjacent structures or distant sites. Lateral spread within the duodenum, jejunum, or ileum is not considered in this classification. Only the depth of tumor penetration in the bowel wall defines the pT stage.

Although the two are similar, differences between this staging system and that of the colon should be noted. In the colon, pTis applies to intra-epithelial (*in situ*) as well as to intramucosal lesions. In the small intestine, intramucosal spread is listed as pT1 instead of pTis. In this regard, the pT1 definition for the small bowel is essentially the same as the pT1 defined for stomach lesions. Invasion through the wall is staged the same as for colon cancer. Discontinuous hematogenous metastases or peritoneal metastases are coded as M1. In addition, there is no subdivision within the N category based on the number of nodes involved with tumor.

DEFINITION OF TNM

Primary Tumor (T)
TX   Primary tumor cannot be assessed
T0   No evidence of primary tumor
Tis   Carcinoma *in situ*
T1   Tumor invades lamina propria or submucosa
T2   Tumor invades muscularis propria
T3   Tumor invades through the muscularis propria into the subserosa or into the nonperitonealized perimuscular tissue (mesentery or retroperitoneum) with extension 2 cm or less*
T4   Tumor perforates the visceral peritoneum or directly invades other organs or structures (includes other loops of small intestine, mesentery, or retroperitoneum more than 2 cm, and abdominal wall by way of serosa; for duodenum only, invasion of pancreas)

Note: The nonperitonealized perimuscular tissue is, for jejunum and ileum, part of the mesentery and, for duodenum in areas where serosa is lacking, part of the retroperitoneum.

Regional Lymph Nodes (N)
NX   Regional lymph nodes cannot be assessed
N0   No regional lymph node metastasis
N1   Regional lymph node metastasis

Distant Metastasis (M)

MX   Distant metastasis cannot be assessed
M0   No distant metastasis
M1   Distant metastasis

STAGE GROUPING			
Stage 0	Tis	N0	M0
Stage I	T1	N0	M0
	T2	N0	M0
Stage II	T3	N0	M0
	T4	N0	M0
Stage III	Any T	N1	M0
Stage IV	Any T	Any N	M1

HISTOPATHOLOGIC TYPE

This staging classification applies only to carcinomas arising in the small intestine. Lymphomas, carcinoid tumors, and visceral sarcomas are not included. The three major histopathologic types are carcinomas (such as adenocarcinoma), carcinoid tumors, and lymphomas (extranodal). Primary lymphomas are staged as extranodal lymphomas. Carcinoid tumors of the small intestine have no staging system, but size, depth of invasion, regional lymph node status, and distant metastasis are considered significant prognostic factors. Less common malignant tumors include leiomyosarcoma, although leiomyomas are plentiful. An increase in gastrointestinal stromal tumors (GIST) has occurred because of reclassification of stromal tumors of the gut wall into this category. The malignant GIST lesions are not classified using TNM nomenclature, but they should be denoted in registry data as localized or metastatic, which includes nodal or visceral metastases. Although carcinoid and GIST lesions are currently not staged in the TNM system, these lesions may be placed in appropriate TNM stage groupings in order to collect data sets that will enhance staging strategies according to outcomes.

HISTOLOGIC GRADE (G)

GX   Grade cannot be assessed
G1   Well differentiated
G2   Moderately differentiated
G3   Poorly differentiated
G4   Undifferentiated

PROGNOSTIC FACTORS

Small bowel carcinoma is rare, so various clinical prognostic factors such as age, gender, and ethnic origin are impossible to assess. The anatomic extent of the tumor is the strongest indicator of outcome when the tumor can be resected. Prognosis after incomplete removal is poor.

The pathologic extent of tumor, in terms of the depth of invasion through the bowel wall, is a significant prognostic factor, as is regional lymphatic spread. Prognosis is also influenced by histologic grade. There are insufficient data to assess the impact of other more sophisticated pathologic factors and serum tumor markers, but it is logical to believe that the effect of those factors would be similar to that observed with colorectal cancer.

BIBLIOGRAPHY

Brucher BL, Roder JD, Fink U, et al: Prognostic factors in resected primary small bowel tumors. Dig Surg 15:42–51, 1998

Coit D: Cancer of the small intestine. In DeVita VT, Hellman S, Rosenberg SA (Eds.): Cancer—principles and practice of oncology. Philadelphia: Lippincott-Raven, 1128–1143, 1997

Crosby JA, Catton CN, Davis A, et al: Malignant gastrointestinal stromal tumors of the small intestine: a review of 50 cases from a prospective database. Ann Surg Oncol 8:50–59, 2001

Greenlee RT, Hill-Harmon M, Murray T, Thun M: Cancer statistics, 2001. Ca Cancer J Clin 51:15–37, 2001

Ludwig DJ, Traverso LW: Gut stromal tumors and their clinical behavior. Am J Surg 173:390–394, 1997

Minardi AJ Jr, Zibari GB, Aultman DF, et al: Small-bowel tumors. J Am Coll Surg 186:664–668, 1998

Naef M, Buhlmann M, Baer HU. Small bowel tumors: diagnosis, therapy and prognostic factors. Lang Arch Surg 384:176–180, 1999

Negri E, Bosetti C, LaVecchia C, et al: Risk factors for adenocarcinoma of the small intestine. Int J Ca 82:171–174, 1999

Neugut AI, Jacobson JS, Suh S, et al: The epidemiology of cancer of the small bowel. Ca Epidemiol Bio Prev 7:243–51, 1998

Ripley D, Weinerman BH. Increased incidence of second malignancies associated with small bowel adenocarcinoma. Canad J Gastroenterol 11:65–68, 1997

HISTOLOGIES—SMALL INTESTINE

8010/2	Carcinoma *in situ*, NOS
8010/3	Carcinoma, NOS
8012/3	Large cell carcinoma, NOS
8013/3	Large cell neuroendocrine carcinoma
8014/3	Large cell carcinoma with rhabdoid phenotype
8020/3	Carcinoma, undifferentiated, NOS
8021/3	Carcinoma, anaplastic, NOS
8022/3	Pleomorphic carcinoma
8030/3	Giant cell and spindle cell carcinoma
8031/3	Giant cell carcinoma
8032/3	Spindle cell carcinoma, NOS
8033/3	Pseudosarcomatous carcinoma
8035/3	Carcinoma with osteoclast-like giant cells
8041/3	Small cell carcinoma, NOS
8042/3	Oat cell carcinoma
8043/3	Small cell carcinoma, fusiform cell
8044/3	Small cell carcinoma, intermediate cell
8045/3	Combined small cell carcinoma

8046/3	Non-small cell carcinoma
8070/2	Squamous cell carcinoma *in situ*, NOS
8070/3	Squamous cell carcinoma, NOS
8071/3	Squamous cell carcinoma, keratinizing, NOS
8072/3	Squamous cell carcinoma, large cell
8073/3	Squamous cell carcinoma, small cell, non-keratinizing
8074/3	Squamous cell carcinoma, spindle cell
8075/3	Squamous cell carcinoma, adenoid
8076/2	Squamous cell carcinoma *in situ* with questionable stromal invasion
8076/3	Squamous cell carcinoma, microinvasive
8082/3	Lymphoepithelial carcinoma
8083/3	Basaloid squamous cell carcinoma
8084/3	Squamous cell carcinoma, clear cell type
8140/2	Adenocarcinoma *in situ*, NOS
8140/3	Adenocarcinoma, NOS
8141/3	Scirrhous adenocarcinoma
8142/3	Linitis plastica
8143/3	Superficial spreading adenocarcinoma
8144/3	Adenocarcinoma, intestinal type
8145/3	Carcinoma, diffuse type
8147/3	Basal cell adenocarcinoma
8148/2	Glandular intraepithelial neoplasia, grade III
8210/2	Adenocarcinoma *in situ* in adenomatous polyp
8210/3	Adenocarcinoma in adenomatous polyp
8211/3	Tubular adenocarcinoma
8214/3	Parietal cell carcinoma
8221/3	Adenocarcinoma in multiple adenomatous polyps
8230/3	Solid carcinoma, NOS
8244/3	Composite carcinoid
8245/3	Adenocarcinoid tumor
8246/3	Neuroendocrine carcinoma, NOS
8255/3	Adenocarcinoma with mixed subtypes
8260/3	Papillary adenocarcinoma, NOS
8261/2	Adenocarcinoma *in situ* in villous adenoma
8261/3	Adenocarcinoma in villous adenoma
8262/3	Villous adenocarcinoma
8263/2	Adenocarcinoma *in situ* in tubulovillous adenoma
8263/3	Adenocarcinoma in tubulovillous adenoma
8310/3	Clear cell adenocarcinoma, NOS
8320/3	Granular cell carcinoma
8430/3	Mucoepidermoid carcinoma
8440/3	Cystadenocarcinoma, NOS
8441/3	Serous cystadenocarcinoma, NOS
8450/3	Papillary cystadenocarcinoma, NOS
8452/3	Solid pseudopapillary carcinoma
8453/2	Intraductal papillary-mucinous carcinoma, non-invasive
8453/3	Intraductal papillary-mucinous carcinoma, invasive
8460/3	Papillary serous cystadenocarcinoma
8461/3	Serous surface papillary carcinoma
8470/2	Mucinous cystadenocarcinoma, non-invasive
8470/3	Mucinous cystadenocarcinoma, NOS
8471/3	Papillary mucinous cystadenocarcinoma
8480/3	Mucinous adenocarcinoma
8481/3	Mucin-producing adenocarcinoma

8490/3	Signet ring cell carcinoma
8500/2	Intraductal carcinoma, non-infiltrating, NOS
8503/2	Non-infiltrating intraductal papillary adenocarcinoma
8503/3	Intraductal papillary adenocarcinoma with invasion
8550/3	Acinar cell carcinoma
8551/3	Acinar cell cystadenocarcinoma
8560/3	Adenosquamous carcinoma
8570/3	Adenocarcinoma with squamous metaplasia
8571/3	Adenocarcinoma with cartilaginous and osseous metaplasia
8572/3	Adenocarcinoma with spindle cell metaplasia

3

Colon and Rectum

(Sarcomas, lymphomas, and carcinoid tumors of the large intestine or appendix are not included.)

C18.0 Cecum	C18.4 Transverse colon	C18.8 Overlapping lesion of
C18.1 Appendix	C18.5 Splenic flexure of colon	colon
C18.2 Ascending colon	C18.6 Descending colon	C18.9 Colon, NOS
C18.3 Hepatic flexure of colon	C18.7 Sigmoid colon	C19.9 Rectosigmoid junction
		C20.9 Rectum, NOS

3

SUMMARY OF CHANGES

- A revised description of the anatomy of the colon and rectum better delineates the data concerning the boundaries between colon, rectum, and anal canal. Adenocarcinomas of the vermiform appendix are classified according to the TNM staging system but should be recorded separately, whereas cancers that occur in the anal canal are staged according to the classification used for the anus.

- Smooth metastatic nodules in the pericolic or perirectal fat are considered lymph node metastases and will be counted in the N staging. In contrast, irregularly contoured metastatic nodules in the peritumoral fat are considered vascular invasion and will be coded as an extension of the T category as either a V1 (microscopic vascular invasion) if only microscopically visible or a V2 (macroscopic vascular invasion) if grossly visible.

- Stage Group II is subdivided into IIA and IIB on the basis of whether the primary tumor is T3 or T4, respectively.

- Stage Group III is subdivided into IIIA (T1–2N1M0), IIIB (T3–4N1M0) or IIIC (any TN2M0).

The TNM classification for carcinomas of the colon and rectum provides more detail than other staging systems. Compatible with the Dukes' system, the TNM adds greater precision in the identification of prognostic subgroups. TNM staging is based on the depth of tumor invasion into the wall of the intestine (T), extension to adjacent structures (T), the number of regional lymph nodes involved (N), and the presence or absence of distant metastasis (M). The TNM classification applies to both clinical and pathologic staging. However, most cancers of the colon or rectum are staged after pathologic examination of the resected specimen. This staging system applies to all carcinomas arising in the colon or rectum. Adenocarcinomas of the vermiform appendix are classified according to the TNM staging system but should be recorded separately, whereas cancers that occur in the anal canal are staged according to the classification used for the anus (see Chapter 13).

ANATOMY

The divisions of the colon and rectum are as follows:

    Cecum
    Ascending colon
    Hepatic flexure
    Transverse colon
    Splenic flexure
    Descending colon
    Sigmoid colon
    Rectosigmoid junction
    Rectum

Primary Site. The large intestine (colorectum) extends from the terminal ileum to the anal canal. Excluding the rectum and vermiform appendix, the colon is divided into four parts: the right or ascending colon, the middle or transverse colon, the left or descending colon, and the sigmoid colon. The sigmoid is continuous with the rectum which terminates at the anal canal.

The cecum is a large, blind pouch that arises from the proximal segment of the right colon. It measures 6 cm by 9 cm and is covered with peritoneum. The ascending colon measures 15–20 cm in length. The posterior surface of the ascending (and descending) colon lacks peritoneum and thus is in direct contact with the retroperitoneum. In contrast, the anterior and lateral surfaces of the ascending (and descending) colon have serosa and are intraperitoneal. The hepatic flexure connects the ascending colon with the transverse colon, passing just inferior to the liver and anterior to the duodenum.

The transverse colon is entirely intraperitoneal, supported on a long mesentery that is attached to the pancreas. Anteriorly, its serosa is continuous with the gastrocolic ligament. The splenic flexure connects the transverse colon to the descending colon, passing inferior to the spleen and anterior to the tail of the pancreas. As noted above, the posterior aspect of the descending colon lacks serosa and is in direct contact with the retroperitoneum, whereas the lateral and anterior surfaces have serosa and are intraperitoneal. The descending colon measures 10–15 cm in length. The colon becomes completely intraperitoneal once again at the sigmoid colon, where the mesentery develops at the medial border of the left posterior major psoas muscle and extends to the rectum. The transition from sigmoid colon to rectum is marked by the fusion of the tenia of the sigmoid colon to the circumferential longitudinal muscle of the rectum. This occurs roughly 12–15 cm from the dentate line.

Approximately 12 cm in length, the rectum extends from the fusion of the tenia to the puborectalis ring. The rectum is covered by peritoneum in front and on both sides in its upper third and only on the anterior wall in its middle third. The peritoneum is reflected laterally from the rectum to form the perirectal fossa and, anteriorly, the uterine or rectovesical fold. There is no peritoneal covering in the lower third, which is often known as the rectal ampulla. The anal canal, which measures 3 to 5 cm in length, extends from the puborectalis sling to the anal verge.

Regional Lymph Nodes.   Regional nodes are located (1) along the course of the major vessels supplying the colon and rectum, (2) along the vascular arcades of the marginal artery, and (3) adjacent to the colon—that is, located along the mesocolic border of the colon. Specifically, the regional lymph nodes are the pericolic and perirectal nodes and those found along the ileocolic, right colic, middle colic, left colic, inferior mesenteric artery, superior rectal (hemorrhoidal), and internal iliac arteries.

For pN, the number of lymph nodes sampled should be recorded. The number of nodes examined from an operative specimen has been reported to be associated with improved survival, possibly because of increased accuracy in staging. It is important to obtain at least 7–14 lymph nodes in radical colon and rectum resections; however, in cases in which tumor is resected for palliation or in patients who have received preoperative radiation, only a few lymph nodes may be present. A pN0 determination may be assessed when these nodes are histologically negative, even though fewer than the recommended number of nodes have been analyzed.

The regional lymph nodes for each segment of the large bowel are designated as follows:

Segment	*Regional Lymph Nodes*
Cecum	Pericolic, anterior cecal, posterior cecal, ileocolic, right colic
Ascending colon	Pericolic, ileocolic, right colic, middle colic
Hepatic flexure	Pericolic, middle colic, right colic
Transverse colon	Pericolic, middle colic
Splenic flexure	Pericolic, middle colic, left colic, inferior mesenteric
Descending colon	Pericolic, left colic, inferior mesenteric, sigmoid
Sigmoid colon	Pericolic, inferior mesenteric, superior rectal (hemorrhoidal), sigmoidal, sigmoid mesenteric
Rectosigmoid	Pericolic, perirectal, left colic, sigmoid mesenteric, sigmoidal, inferior mesenteric, superior rectal (hemorrhoidal), middle rectal (hemorrhoidal)
Rectum	Perirectal, sigmoid mesenteric, inferior mesenteric, lateral sacral presacral, internal iliac, sacral promontory (Gerota's), internal iliac, superior rectal (hemorrhoidal), middle rectal (hemorrhoidal), inferior rectal (hemorrhoidal)

Metastatic Sites.   Although carcinomas of the colon and rectum can metastasize to almost any organ, the liver and lungs are the most common sites. Seeding of other segments of the colon, small intestine, or peritoneum can also occur.

RULES FOR CLASSIFICATION

Clinical Staging.   Clinical assessment is based on medical history, physical examination, sigmoidoscopy, and colonoscopy with biopsy. Special examinations designed to demonstrate the presence of extracolonic metastasis, such as chest films, computerized tomography, and PET scans, may be performed.

Pathologic Staging.   Colorectal cancers are usually staged after surgical exploration of the abdomen and pathologic examination of the resected specimen. The definition of *in situ* carcinoma—pTis—includes cancer cells confined within the glandular basement membrane (intraepithelial) or lamina propria (intramucosal) with no extension through the muscularis mucosae into the submucosa. Neither intraepithelial nor intramucosal carcinomas of the large intestine have a significant potential for metastasis.

Tumor that invades the stalk of a polyp is classified according to the pT definitions adopted for colorectal carcinomas. For instance, tumor that is limited to the lamina propria is listed as pTis, whereas tumor that has invaded the muscularis mucosae and entered the submucosa of the stalk is classified pT1.

Lymph nodes are classified N1 or N2 according to the number involved with metastatic tumor. Involvement of 1 to 3 nodes is pN1, and the presence of 4 or more nodes involved with tumor metastasis is considered pN2.

Patients with tumor located on the serosal surface as a result of direct extension through the wall of the colon or proximal rectum are assigned T4, as are those with lesions that directly invade other organs or structures. Seeding of abdominal organs—for instance, the distal ileum from a carcinoma of the transverse colon—is considered discontinuous metastasis and should be recorded as M1. Metastatic nodules or foci found in the pericolic or perirectal fat or in adjacent mesentery (mesocolic fat) without evidence of residual lymph node tissue are considered equivalent to regional lymph node metastasis if the nodule has the form and smooth contour of a lymph node. If the nodule has an irregular contour, it should be classified in the T category and also coded as V1 (microscopic venous invasion) or V2 (if it was grossly evident), because of the likelihood that it represents venous invasion. Multiple metastatic foci seen microscopically only in the pericolic fat should be considered lymph node metastases for classification.

Metastasis in the external iliac or common iliac lymph nodes is classified M1.

If the tumor recurs at the site of surgery, it is anatomically assigned to the proximal segment of the anastomosis and restaged by the TNM classification, using the r prefix for the recurrent tumor stage (rTNM).

Radial Margins.   It is important that accurate pathologic evaluation of the radial margin be performed. The radial margin is that surgically dissected surface adjacent to the deepest point of tumor invasion beyond the wall of the large bowel. The surgeon is encouraged to mark the area of deepest tumor penetration so that the pathologist may most directly evaluate the radial margin. This margin may reflect invasion either through the peritoneum covering the intraabdominal colon in which the lesion was adherent to an unresected structure or organ, or into retroperitoneal or infraperitoneal fat. The completeness of resection is dependent in large part on this radial margin, and the resection (R) codes should be given for each procedure: R0—complete tumor resection with all margins negative; R1—incomplete tumor resection with microscopic involvement of a margin (gross total marginal resection), and R2—incomplete tumor resection with gross residual tumor that was not resected.

DEFINITION OF TNM

The same classification is used for both clinical and pathologic staging.

Primary Tumor (T)

TX	Primary tumor cannot be assessed
T0	No evidence of primary tumor
Tis	Carcinoma *in situ:* intraepithelial or invasion of lamina propria*
T1	Tumor invades submucosa
T2	Tumor invades muscularis propria
T3	Tumor invades through the muscularis propria into the subserosa, or into non-peritonealized pericolic or perirectal tissues
T4	Tumor directly invades other organs or structures, and/or perforates visceral peritoneum**,***

*Note: Tis includes cancer cells confined within the glandular basement membrane (intraepithelial) or lamina propria (intramucosal) with no extension through the muscularis mucosae into the submucosa.

**Note: Direct invasion in T4 includes invasion of other segments of the colorectum by way of the serosa; for example, invasion of the sigmoid colon by a carcinoma of the cecum.

***Tumor that is adherent to other organs or structures, macroscopically, is classified T4. However, if no tumor is present in the adhesion, microscopically, the classification should be pT3. The V and L substaging should be used to identify the presence or absence of vascular or lymphatic invasion.

Regional Lymph Nodes (N)

NX	Regional lymph nodes cannot be assessed
N0	No regional lymph node metastasis
N1	Metastasis in 1 to 3 regional lymph nodes
N2	Metastasis in 4 or more regional lymph nodes

Note: A tumor nodule in the pericolorectal adipose tissue of a primary carcinoma without histologic evidence of residual lymph node in the nodule is classified in the pN category as a regional lymph node metastasis if the nodule has the form and smooth contour of a lymph node. If the nodule has an irregular contour, it should be classified in the T category and also coded as V1 (microscopic venous invasion) or as V2 (if it was grossly evident), because there is a strong likelihood that it represents venous invasion.

Distant Metastasis (M)

MX   Distant metastasis cannot be assessed
M0   No distant metastasis
M1   Distant metastasis

STAGE GROUPING

Stage	T	N	M	Dukes*	MAC*
0	Tis	N0	M0	-	-
I	T1	N0	M0	A	A
	T2	N0	M0	A	B1
IIA	T3	N0	M0	B	B2
IIB	T4	N0	M0	B	B3
IIIA	T1-T2	N1	M0	C	C1
IIIB	T3-T4	N1	M0	C	C2/C3
IIIC	Any T	N2	M0	C	C1/C2/C3
IV	Any T	Any N	M1	-	D

*Dukes B is a composite of better (T3 N0 M0) and worse (T4 N0 M0) prognostic groups, as is Dukes C (Any TN1 M0 and Any T N2 M0). MAC is the modified Astler-Coller classification.

Note: The y prefix is to be used for those cancers that are classified after pretreatment, whereas the r prefix is to be used for those cancers that have recurred.

HISTOPATHOLOGIC TYPE

This staging classification applies to carcinomas that arise in the colon or rectum. The classification does not apply to sarcomas, to lymphomas, or to carcinoid tumors of the large intestine or appendix. The histologic types include:

Adenocarcinoma *in situ**
Adenocarcinoma
Medullary carcinoma
Mucinous carcinoma (colloid type) (greater than 50% mucinous carcinoma)
Signet ring cell carcinoma (greater than 50% signet ring cell)
Squamous cell (epidermoid) carcinoma
Adenosquamous carcinoma
Small cell carcinoma
Undifferentiated carcinoma
Carcinoma, NOS

*The terms "high grade dysplasia" and "severe dysplasia" may be used as synonyms for *in situ* adenocarcinoma and *in situ* carcinoma. These cases should be assigned pTis.

HISTOLOGIC GRADE (G)

GX Grade cannot be assessed
G1 Well differentiated
G2 Moderately differentiated
G3 Poorly differentiated
G4 Undifferentiated

It is recommended that the terms "low-grade" (G1–G2) and "high-grade" (G3–G4) be applied, because data indicate that low and high grade may be associated with outcome independently of TNM stage group for both colon and rectum adenocarcinoma. Some authors suggest that G4 lesions be identified separately because they may represent a small subgroup of carcinomas that are very aggressive.

RESIDUAL TUMOR (R)

R0 Complete resection, margins histologically negative, no residual tumor left after resection
R1 Incomplete resection, margins histologically involved, microscopic tumor remains after resection of gross disease
R2 Incomplete resection, margins involved or gross disease remains after resection

PROGNOSTIC FACTORS

In addition to the TNM, independent prognostic factors that are generally used in patient management and are well supported in the literature include residual disease, histologic type, histologic grade, serum carcinoembryonic antigen and cytokine levels, extramural venous invasion, and submucosal vascular invasion by carcinomas arising in adenomas. Small cell carcinomas, signet ring cell carcinomas, and undifferentiated carcinomas have a less favorable outcome than other histologic types. Submucosal vascular invasion by carcinomas arising in adenomas is associated with a greater risk of regional lymph node involvement. In the future, the intratumoral expression of specific molecules (e.g., Deleted in Colorectal Cancer (DCC), p27^{Kip1}, DNA microsatellite instability, thymidylate synthase) may be proven to be associated either with prognosis or response to therapy and yet be independent of TNM stage group or histologic grade. These molecular markers are currently not part of the staging system, but it is recommended that they be recorded if available and studied within the context of a clinical trial.

BIBLIOGRAPHY

Adam IJ, Mohamdee MO, Martin IG, et al: Role of circumferential margin involvement in the local recurrence of rectal cancer. Lancet 344:707–711, 1994

Astler VB, Coller FA: The prognostic significance of direct extension of carcinoma of the colon and rectum. Ann Surg 139:846–852, 1954

Bast RC, Desch CE, Ravdin P, et al: Clinical practice guidelines for the use of tumor markers in breast and colorectal cancer: report of the American

Society of Clinical Oncology Expert Panel. J Clin Oncol 14:2843–2877, 1996

Bauer K, Bagwell C, Giaretti W, et al: Consensus review of the clinical utility of DNA flow cytometry in colorectal cancer. Cytometry 14:486–491, 1993

Belluco C, Esposito G, Bertorelle R, et al: Absence of the cell cycle inhibitor p27Kip1 protein predicts poor outcome in patients with stage I–III colorectal cancer. Ann Surg Oncol 6:19–25, 1999

Belluco C, Frantz M, Carnio S, et al: IL-6 blood level is associated with circulating CEA and prognosis in patients with colorectal cancer. Ann Surg Oncol 7:133–138, 2000

Butch RJ, Stark DD, Wittenberg J, et al: Staging rectal cancer by MR and CT. Am J Roentgenol 146:1155–1160, 1986

Caplin S, Cerottini JP, Bosman FT, et al: For patients with Dukes' B (TNM Stage II) colorectal carcinoma, examination of six or fewer lymph nodes is related to poor prognosis. Cancer 83:666–672, 1998

Chapuis PH, Fisher R, Dent DF, et al: The relationship between different staging methods and survival in colorectal carcinoma. Dis Colon Rectum 28:158–161, 1985

Coia LR, Gunderson LL, Haller D, et al: Outcomes of patients receiving radiation for carcinoma of the rectum. Results of the 1988–1989 patterns of care study. Cancer 86:1952–1958, 1999

Compton CC: Updated protocol for the examination of specimens removed from patients with colorectal carcinoma. Arch Pathol Lab Med 124:1016–1025, 2000

Compton CC, Fenoglio-Prieser CM, Pettigrew N, Fielding LP: American Joint Committee on Cancer Prognostic Factors Consensus Conference: Colorectal Working Group. Cancer 88:1739–1757, 2000

Compton CC, Fielding LP, Burgart LJ, et al: Prognostic factors in colorectal cancer: College of American Pathologists Consensus Statement 1999. Arch Pathol Lab Med 124:979–994, 2000

Copeland EM, Miller LD, Jones RS: Prognostic factors in carcinoma of the colon and rectum. Am J Surg 116:875–881, 1968

Dukes CE: Cancer of the rectum: an analysis of 1000 cases. J Pathol Bacteriol 50:527–539, 1940

Fenoglio-Prieser CM, Hutter RVP: Colorectal polyps: pathologic diagnosis and clinical significance. Cancer J Clin 35:322–344, 1985

Fielding LP, Arsenault PA, Chapuis PH, et al: Clinicopathological staging for colorectal cancer: an International Documentation System (IDS) and an International Comprehensive Anatomical Terminology (ICAT). Gastroenterol Hepatol 6:325–344, 1991

Fielding LP, Pettigrew N: College of American Pathologists Conference XXVI on clinical relevance of prognostic markers in solid tumors: report of the Colorectal Working Group. Arch Pathol Lab Med 119:1115–1121, 1995

Fielding LP, Phillips RK, Frey JS, et al: The prediction of outcome after curative resection for large bowel cancer. Lancet 2:904–907, 1986

Fielding LP, Phillips RK, Hittinger R: Factors influencing mortality after curative resection for large bowel cancer in elderly patients. Lancet 1:595–597, 1989

Gilbert SG. Symptomatic local tumor failure following abdomino-perineal resection. Int J Radiat Oncol Biol Phys. 4:801–807, 1978

Goldstein NS, Turner JR. Pericolonic tumor deposits in patients with T3N + M0 colon adenocarcinomas: a marker for reduced disease-free survival and intra-abdominal metastasis. Cancer 88:2228–2238, 2000

Griffin MR, Bergstralh EJ, Coffey RJ, et al: Predictors of survival after curative resection of carcinoma of the colon and rectum. Cancer 60:2318–2324, 1987

Gunderson LL, Sosin H: Areas of failure found at reoperation (second or symptomatic look) following "curative surgery" for adenocarcinoma of the rectum. Clinicopathologic correlation and implications for adjuvant therapy. Cancer. 34:1278–1292, 1974

Hall NR, Finan PJ, al-Jaberi T, et al: Circumferential margin involvement after mesorectal excision of rectal cancer with curative intent: predictor of survival but not local recurrence? Dis Colon Rectum 41:979–983, 1998

Halling KC, French AJ, McDonnell SK, et al: Microsatellite imbalance in stage B2 and C colorectal cancers. J Natl Cancer Inst 91:1295–1303, 1999

Harrison JC, Dean PJ, El-Zeky F, Vander Zwaag R: From Dukes through Jass. Pathological prognostic indicators in rectal cancer. Hum Pathol 25:498–505, 1994

Harrison JC, Dean PJ, El-Zeky F, Vander Zwaag R: Impact of the Crohn's-like lymphoid reaction on staging of right-sided colon cancer: results of a multivariate analysis. Hum Pathol 26:31–38, 1995

Hermanek P: Colorectal carcinoma. Histopathological diagnosis and staging. Baillieres Clin Gastroenterol 3:511–529, 1989

Hermanek P: Problems of pTNM classification of carcinoma of the stomach, colorectum and anal margin. Pathol Res Pract 181:296–300, 1986

Hermanek P, Gall FP: Early (microinvasive) colorectal carcinoma: pathology, diagnosis, surgical treatment. Int J Colorectal Dis 1:79–84, 1986

Hermanek P, Giedl J, Dworak O: Two programs for examination of regional lymph nodes in colorectal carcinoma with regard to the new pN classification. Pathol Res Pract 185:867–873, 1989

Hermanek P, Guggenmoos-Holzmann I, Gall FP: Prognostic factors in rectal carcinoma: a contribution to the further development of tumor classification. Dis Colon Rectum 32:593–599, 1989

Hermanek P, Henson DE, Hutter RVP, Sobin LH: TNM Supplement 1993: a commentary on uniform use. Berlin: Springer-Verlag, 1993

Hermanek P, Sobin LH: Colorectal carcinoma. In Hermanek P, Gospodarowicz MK, Henson DE, et al (Eds.): Prognostic factors in cancer. Berlin: Springer-Verlag, 1995

Herrera-Ornelas L, Justiniano J, Castillo N, et al: Metastases in small lymph nodes from colon cancer. Arch Surg 122:1253–1256, 1987

Hoskins RB, Gunderson LL, Dosoretz DE, et al: Adjuvant postoperative radiotherapy in carcinoma of the rectum and rectosigmoid. Cancer 55:61–71, 1985

Jass JR, Atkin WS, Cuzick J, et al: The grading of rectal cancer: historical perspectives and a multivariate analysis of 447 cases. Histopathology 10:437–459, 1986

Jass JR, Love SB, Northover JMA: A new prognostic classification of rectal cancer. Lancet 1:1303–1306, 1987

Jass JR, Mukawa K, Goh HS, et al: Clinical importance of DNA content in rectal cancer measured by flow cytometry. J Clin Pathol 42:254–259, 1989

Jass JR, Sobin LH: Histological typing of intestinal tumours. In WHO international histological classification of tumours, 2nd ed. Berlin-New York: Springer-Verlag, 1989

Jen J, Kim H, Piantidosi S, et al: Allelic loss of chromosome 18q and prognosis in colorectal cancer. N Eng J Med 331:213–221, 1994

Kokal W, Sheibani K, Terz J, et al: Tumor DNA content in the prognosis of colorectal carcinoma. JAMA 255:3123–3127, 1986

Kotanagi H, Fukuoka T, Shibata Y, et al: Blood vessel invasions in metastatic nodes for development of liver metastasis in colorectal cancer. Hepato-Gastroenterol 42:771–774, 1995

Lindmark G, Gerdin B, Sundberg C, et al: Prognostic significance of the microvascular count in colorectal cancer. J Clin Oncol 14:461–466, 1996

Lipper S, Kahn LB, Ackerman LV: The significance of microscopic invasive cancer in endoscopically removed polyps of the large bowel: a clinico-pathologic study of 51 cases. Cancer 52:1691, 1983

Loda M, Cukor B, Tam SW, et al: Increased proteasome-dependent degradation of the cyclin-dependent kinase inhibitor p27 in aggressive colorectal carcinomas. Nature Medicine 3:231–234, 1997

Minsky BD, Mies C, Rich TA, et al: Lymphatic vessel invasion is an independent prognostic factor for survival in colorectal cancer. Int J Radiat Oncol 17:311–318, 1989

Newland RC, Chapuis PH, Pheils MT, et al: The relationship of survival to staging and grading of colorectal carcinoma: a prospective study of 503 cases. Cancer 47:1424–1429, 1981

Ondero H, Maetani S, Nishikawa T, et al: The reappraisal of prognostic classifications for colorectal cancer. Dis Colon Rectum 32:609–614, 1989

Phillips RKS, Hittinger R, Blesovsky L, et al: Large bowel cancer: surgical pathology and its relationship to survival. Br J Surg 71:604–610, 1984

Pocard M, Panis Y, Malassagne B, et al: Assessing the effectiveness of mesorectal excision in rectal cancer: prognostic value of the number of lymph nodes found in resected specimens. Dis Colon Rectum 41:839–845, 1998

Qizilbash AH: Pathologic studies in colorectal cancer: a guide to the surgical pathology examination of colorectal specimens and review of features of prognostic significance. Pathol Annu 17(l):1–46, 1982

Ratto C, Sofo L, Ippoliti M, et al: Accurate lymph-node detection in colorectal specimens resected for cancer is of prognostic significance. Dis Colon Rectum 42:143–154, 1999

Rich T, Gunderson LL, Lew R, et al: Patterns of recurrence of rectal cancer after potentially curative surgery. Cancer 52:1317–1329, 1983

Schild SE, Martenson JA Jr, Gunderson LL, et al: Postoperative adjuvant therapy of rectal cancer: an analysis of disease control, survival, and prognostic factors. Int J Radiat Oncol Biol Phys. 17:55–62, 1989

Scott KWM, Grace RH: Detection of lymph node metastases in colorectal carcinoma before and after fat clearance. Br J Surg 76:1165–1167, 1989

Scott NA, Rainwater LM, Wieland HS, et al: The relative prognostic value of flow cytometric DNA analysis and conventional clinicopathologic criteria in patients with operative rectal carcinoma. Dis Colon Rectum 30:513–520, 1987

Shepherd NA, Saraga EP, Love SB, et al: Prognostic factors in colonic cancer. Histopathology 14:613–620, 1989

Shibata D, Reale MA, Lavin P, et al: The DCC protein and prognosis in colorectal cancer. N Engl J Med 335:1727–1732, 1996

Steinberg SM, Barkin JS, Kaplan RS, et al: Prognostic indicators of colon tumors: the gastrointestinal tumor study group experience. Cancer 57:1866–1870, 1986

Talbot IC, Ritchie S, Leighton MH, et al: The clinical significance of invasion of veins by rectal cancer. Br J Surg 67:439–442, 1980

Talbot IC, Ritchie S, Leighton MH, et al: Spread of rectal cancer within veins: histologic features and clinical significance. Am J Surg 141:15–17, 1981

Tepper JE, Cohen AM, Wood WC, et al: Postoperative radiation therapy of rectal cancer. Int J Radiat Oncol Biol Phys 13:5–10, 1987

Tepper JE, O'Connell MJ, Niedzwiecki D, et al: Impact of number of nodes retrieved on outcome in patients with rectal cancer. J Clin Oncol 19:157–163, 2001

Willett CG, Tepper JE, Kaufman DS, et al: Adjuvant postoperative radiation therapy for rectal adenocarcinoma. Am J Clin Oncol 15:371–375, 1992

Williams NS, Durdey P, Qwihe P, et al: Pre-operative staging of rectal neoplasm and its impact on clinical management. Br J Surg 72:868–874, 1985

Wolmark N, Fisher B, Wieand HS: The prognostic value of the modifications of the Dukes C class of colorectal cancer: an analysis of the NSABP clinical trials. Ann Surg 203:115–122, 1986

Wolmark N, Fisher ER, Wieand HS, et al: The relationship of depth of penetration and tumor size to the number of positive nodes in Dukes C colorectal cancer. Cancer 53:2707–2712, 1984

Wong JH, Severino R, Honnebier MB, et al: Number of nodes examined and staging accuracy in colorectal carcinoma. J Clin Oncol 17:2896–2900, 1999

Wright CM, Dent OF, Barker M, et al: Prognostic significance of extensive microsatellite instabilty in sporadic clinicopathological stage C colorectal cancer. Brit J Surg 87:1197–1202, 2000

3

HISTOLOGIES—COLON AND RECTUM

8000/3	Neoplasm, malignant
8001/3	Tumor cells, malignant
8002/3	Malignant tumor, small cell type
8004/3	Malignant tumor, spindle cell type
8005/3	Malignant tumor, clear cell type
8010/2	Carcinoma *in situ,* NOS
8010/3	Carcinoma, NOS
8012/3	Large cell carcinoma, NOS
8013/3	Large cell neuroendocrine carcinoma
8020/3	Carcinoma, undifferentiated, NOS
8021/3	Carcinoma, anaplastic, NOS
8032/3	Spindle cell carcinoma, NOS
8041/3	Small cell carcinoma, NOS
8042/3	Oat cell carcinoma
8043/3	Small cell carcinoma, fusiform cell
8044/3	Small cell carcinoma, intermediate cell
8045/3	Combined small cell carcinoma
8050/3	Papillary carcinoma
8070/3	Squamous cell carcinoma, NOS
8140/2	Adenocarcinoma *in situ,* NOS
8140/3	Adenocarcinoma, NOS
8141/3	Scirrhous adenocarcinoma
8210/2	Adenocarcinoma *in situ* in adenomatous polyp
8210/3	Adenocarcinoma in adenomatous polyp
8211/3	Tubular adenocarcinoma
8214/3	Parietal cell carcinoma
8215/3	Adenocarcinoma of anal glands
8220/3	Adenocarcinoma in adenomatous polyposis coli
8221/3	Adenocarcinoma in multiple adenomatous polyps
8230/2	Ductal carcinoma *in situ,* solid type
8230/3	Solid carcinoma, NOS
8240/3	Carcinoid tumor, NOS
8244/3	Composite carcinoid
8245/3	Adenocarcinoid tumor
8246/3	Neuroendocrine carcinoma, NOS
8249/3	Atypical carcinoid tumor
8261/2	Adenocarcinoma *in situ* in villous adenoma
8261/3	Adenocarcinoma in villous adenoma
8262/3	Villous adenocarcinoma
8263/2	Adenocarcinoma *in situ* in tubulovillous adenoma
8263/3	Adenocarcinoma in tubulovillous adenoma

8480/3	Mucinous adenocarcinoma
8481/3	Mucin-producing adenocarcinoma
8490/3	Signet ring cell carcinoma
8510/3	Medullary carcinoma, NOS
8560/3	Adenosquamous carcinoma
8570/3	Adenocarcinoma with squamous metaplasia
8571/3	Adenocarcinoma with cartilaginous and osseous metaplasia
8935/3	Stromal sarcoma, NOS
8936/3	Gastrointestinal stromal sarcoma

13

Anal Canal

(The classification applies to carcinomas only; melanomas, carcinoid tumors, and sarcomas are not included.)

C21.0 Anus, NOS	C21.2 Cloacogenic zone	C21.8 Overlapping lesion of rectum, anus, and anal canal
C21.1 Anal canal		

INTRODUCTION

The proximal region of the anus encompasses true mucosa of three different histologic types: glandular, transitional, and squamous (proximal to distal, respectively). Distally, the squamous mucosa merges with the perianal skin (true epidermis). This mucocutaneous junction historically has been called the anal verge or margin. Thus, two distinct categories of tumors arise in the anal region. Tumors that develop from mucosa (of any of the three types) are termed anal canal cancers, whereas those that arise within skin at or distal to the squamous mucocutaneous junction are termed anal margin tumors. The proximal boundary of the anal margin is indistinct on macroscopic examination and, anatomically, may vary with the patient's body habitus. A proximal boundary located 5–6 cm from the squamous mucocutaneous junction applies in the majority of adults.

Anal canal tumors are staged using the classification system described herein. Anal margin tumors are biologically comparable to other skin tumors and therefore are classified by the schema presented in Chapter 23. However, the regional nodal drainage (relevant to the N category) of the skin of the anal margin is uniquely specific to this anatomic site, as outlined in this section.

Because the primary management of carcinomas of the anal canal has shifted from surgical resection to non-surgical treatment, they are typically staged clinically according to the size and extent of the primary tumor. Thus, patients with cancer of the anal canal may be staged at the time of presentation by inspection, palpation and biopsy of the mass, palpation (and biopsy as needed) of regional lymph nodes, and radiologic imaging of chest, abdomen, and pelvis.

ANATOMY

Primary site. The anal canal begins where the rectum enters the puborectalis sling at the apex of the anal sphincter complex (palpable as the anorectal ring on digital exam) and ends at the squamous mucocutaneous junction with the perianal skin. The most proximal aspect of the anal canal is lined by colorectal mucosa, and at the dentate line, a narrow zone of transitional mucosa that is similar to urothelium is variably present. This proximal zone (from the top of the puborectalis to the dentate line, including the transitional zone) measures approximately 1–2 cm. In the region of the dentate line, anal glands may be found subjacent to the mucosa, often extending across the internal sphincter to the intersphincteric plane. A proximal boundary located distal to the dentate line and extending to the mucocutaneous junction is a non-keratinizing squamous epithelium devoid of skin appendages (hair follicles, apocrine glands, and sweat glands).

Carcinomas that overlap the anorectal junction may be problematic. They should be staged as rectal tumors if their epicenter is located more than 2 cm proximal to the dentate line and as anal tumors if their epicenter is 2 cm or less from the dentate line. However, extension of low rectal tumors beyond the dentate line implies risk of metastatic spread to the superficial inguinal lymph nodes.

Regional Lymph Nodes.   Lymphatic drainage and nodal involvement of anal cancers depend on the location of the primary tumor. Tumors above the dentate line spread primarily to the anorectal, perirectal, and paravertebral nodes, whereas tumors below the dentate line spread to the superficial inguinal nodes.

The regional lymph nodes are as follows:

Perirectal
   Anorectal
   Perirectal
   Lateral sacral
Internal iliac (hypogastric)
Inguinal
   Superficial
   Deep femoral

All other nodal groups represent sites of distant metastasis.

Metastatic Sites.   Cancers of the anus may metastasize to any organs, but the liver and lungs are the distal organs that are most frequently involved. Involvement of the abdominal cavity is not unusual.

RULES FOR CLASSIFICATION

Clinical Staging.   The TNM classification for tumors of the anal canal depends largely on clinical observations. The primary tumor is staged according to its greatest dimension and local extent as determined by clinical and/or pathologic examination. Palpation and radiologic imaging assess extension to the anorectal, perirectal, and superficial inguinal or femoral nodes, as well as to adjacent structures. Metastasis to other nodal groups, such as the inferior mesenteric, may also be assessed radiologically. Tumor may extend to the rectal mucosa or submucosa, subcutaneous perianal tissue, perianal skin, ischiorectal fat, and/or local skeletal muscles, such as the external anal sphincter, levator ani, and coccygeus muscles. Local extension of tumor may also include the perineum, vulva, prostate gland, urinary bladder, urethra, vagina, cervix uteri, corpus uteri, pelvic peritoneum, and broad ligaments. Organs invaded by tumor should be specified.

Pathologic Staging.   Surgical excision is infrequently performed for anal carcinoma, so few tumors are staged pathologically. The size of the tumor is assessed by macroscopic examination and confirmed microscopically. Accurate assessment of the involvement of local structures or organs may require specific orientation of the specimen or other identification by the surgeon. Perirectal lymph nodes may be identified within the surgical specimen on pathologic examination, but specific identification of internal iliac and inguinal lymph nodes by the surgeon is required.

DEFINITION OF TNM

Primary Tumor (T)

TX   Primary tumor cannot be assessed
T0   No evidence of primary tumor
Tis   Carcinoma *in situ*
T1   Tumor 2 cm or less in greatest dimension
T2   Tumor more than 2 cm but not more than 5 cm in greatest dimension
T3   Tumor more than 5 cm in greatest dimension
T4   Tumor of any size invades adjacent organ(s), e.g., vagina, urethra, bladder*

*Note: Direct invasion of the rectal wall, perirectal skin, subcutaneous tissue, or the sphincter muscle(s) is not classified as T4.

Regional Lymph Nodes (N)

NX   Regional lymph nodes cannot be assessed
N0   No regional lymph node metastasis
N1   Metastasis in perirectal lymph node(s)
N2   Metastasis in unilateral internal iliac and/or inguinal lymph node(s)
N3   Metastasis in perirectal and inguinal lymph nodes and/or bilateral internal iliac and/or inguinal lymph nodes

Distant Metastasis (M)

MX   Distant metastasis cannot be assessed
M0   No distant metastasis
M1   Distant metastasis

Stage 0	Tis	N0	M0
Stage I	T1	N0	M0
Stage II	T2	N0	M0
	T3	N0	M0
Stage IIIA	T1	N1	M0
	T2	N1	M0
	T3	N1	M0
	T4	N0	M0
Stage IIIB	T4	N1	M0
	Any T	N2	M0
	Any T	N3	M0
Stage IV	Any T	Any N	M1

HISTOPATHOLOGIC TYPE

The staging system applies to all carcinomas arising in the anal canal, including carcinomas that arise within anorectal fistulas. Melanomas, carcinoid tumors, and sarcomas are excluded from this staging system. Most carcinomas of the anal canal are squamous cell carcinomas. The WHO classification of the types and subtypes of carcinomas of the anal canal is shown below. The terms *transitional cell* and *cloacogenic carcinoma* have been abandoned, because these tumors are now recognized as non-keratinizing types of squamous cell carcinoma.

WHO Classification of Carcinoma of the Anal Canal*
Squamous cell carcinoma
Adenocarcinoma
   Rectal type
   Of anal glands
   Within anorectal fistula
Mucinous adenocarcinoma
Small cell carcinoma
Undifferentiated carcinoma

*Note: The term *carcinoma, NOS* (not otherwise specified) is not part of the WHO classification.

Perianal skin and anal margin (junction of squamous mucosa and skin) tumor types include squamous cell carcinoma, giant condyloma (verrucous carcinoma), basal cell carcinoma, Bowen's disease, and Paget's disease. These tumors are staged as skin cancers according to the system outlined in Chapter 23.

HISTOLOGIC GRADE (G)

GX   Grade cannot be assessed
G1   Well differentiated
G2   Moderately differentiated

G3   Poorly differentiated
G4   Undifferentiated

PROGNOSTIC FACTORS

Because of the infrequent occurrence of carcinomas of the anal canal, the definitive identification of prognostic factors is problematic. However, poor histologic grade or histologic types that are categorized by convention as high-grade, such as small cell carcinoma, have been shown to be adverse prognostic factors.

3

BIBLIOGRAPHY

Boman BM, Moertel CG, O'Connell MJ, et al: Carcinoma of the anal canal: a clinical and pathologic study of 188 cases. Cancer 54:114–125, 1984

Cummings BJ: Anal canal carcinoma. In Hermanek P, Gospodarowicz MK, Henson DE, et al (Eds.): Prognostic factors in cancer. Berlin: Springer-Verlag, 1995

Dean GT, McAleer JJA, Spence RAJ: Malignant anal tumors. Br J Surg 81:500–508, 1994

Fenger C, Frisch M, Marti MC, Parc R: Tumors of the anal canal. In Hamilton SR, Aaltonen LA (Eds): World Health Organization classification of tumors: pathology and genetics of tumors of the digestive system. Lyon: IARC Press, 146, 2000

Flam MS, John M, Lovalvo LJ, et al: Definitive nonsurgical therapy of epithelial malignancies of the anal canal. Cancer 51:1378–1387, 1983

Longo WE, Vernava AM III, Wade TP, et al: Recurrent squamous cell carcinoma of the anal canal: predictors of initial treatment failure and results of salvage therapy. Ann Surg 220:40–49, 1994

Nigro ND: An evaluation of combined therapy for squamous cell cancer of the anal canal. Dis Colon Rectum 27:763–766, 1984

Nigro ND, Vaitkeviceus VK, Herskovic AM: Preservation of function in the treatment of cancer of the anus. Important Adv Oncol 161–177, 1989

Paradis P, Douglass HO Jr, Holyoke ED: The clinical implications of a staging system for carcinoma of the anus. Surg Gynecol Obstet 141:411–416, 1975

Pintor MP, Northover JM, Nicholls RJ: Squamous cell carcinoma of the anus at one hospital from 1948. Br J Surg 76:806–810, 1989

Roseau G, Palazzo L, Colardelle P, et al: Endoscopic ultrasonography in the staging and follow-up of epidermoid carcinoma of the anal canal. Gastrointest Endosc 40:447–450, 1994

Ryan DP, Compton CC, Mayer RJ: Carcinoma of the anal canal. NEJM 342(11):792–800, 2000

Shepherd NA, Scholefield JH, Love SB, et al: Prognostic factors in anal squamous carcinoma: a multivariate analysis of clinical, pathological and flow cytometric parameters in 235 cases. Histopathology 16:545–555, 1990

HISTOLOGIES—ANAL CANAL

8000/3	Neoplasm, malignant
8001/3	Tumor cells, malignant
8002/3	Malignant tumor, small cell type
8004/3	Malignant tumor, spindle cell type
8005/3	Malignant tumor, clear cell type
8010/2	Carcinoma *in situ*, NOS

8010/3	Carcinoma, NOS
8020/3	Carcinoma, undifferentiated, NOS
8021/3	Carcinoma, anaplastic, NOS
8032/3	Spindle cell carcinoma, NOS
8033/3	Pseudosarcomatous carcinoma
8041/3	Small cell carcinoma, NOS
8042/3	Oat cell carcinoma
8045/3	Combined small cell carcinoma
8051/3	Verrucous carcinoma, NOS
8070/2	Squamous cell carcinoma *in situ*, NOS
8070/3	Squamous cell carcinoma, NOS
8071/3	Squamous cell carcinoma, keratinizing, NOS
8072/3	Squamous cell carcinoma, large cell, non-keratinizing, NOS
8073/3	Squamous cell carcinoma, small cell, non-keratinizing
8074/3	Squamous cell carcinoma, spindle cell
8076/2	Squamous cell carcinoma *in situ* with questionable stromal invasion
8076/3	Squamous cell carcinoma, microinvasive
8083/3	Basaloid squamous cell carcinoma
8084/3	Squamous cell carcinoma, clear cell type
8123/3	Basaloid carcinoma
8124/3	Cloacogenic carcinoma
8140/2	Adenocarcinoma *in situ*, NOS
8140/3	Adenocarcinoma, NOS
8141/3	Scirrhous adenocarcinoma
8210/2	Adenocarcinoma *in situ* in adenomatous polyp
8210/3	Adenocarcinoma in adenomatous polyp
8215/3	Adenocarcinoma of anal glands
8244/3	Composite carcinoid
8245/3	Adenocarcinoid tumor
8246/3	Neuroendocrine carcinoma, NOS
8249/3	Atypical carcinoid tumor
8255/3	Adenocarcinoma with mixed subtypes
8310/3	Clear cell adenocarcinoma, NOS
8480/3	Mucinous adenocarcinoma
8481/3	Mucin-producing adenocarcinoma
8490/3	Signet ring cell carcinoma
8510/3	Medullary carcinoma, NOS
8560/3	Adenosquamous carcinoma
8933/3	Adenosarcoma

14

Liver (Including Intrahepatic Bile Ducts)

(Sarcomas and tumors metastatic to the liver are not included.)

C22.0 Liver   C22.1 Intrahepatic bile duct

SUMMARY OF CHANGES

- The T categories in this edition have been redefined and simplified.

- All solitary tumors without vascular invasion, regardless of size, are classified as T1 because of similar prognosis.

- All solitary tumors with vascular invasion (again regardless of size) are combined with multiple tumors ≤ 5 cm and classified as T2 because of similar prognosis.

- Multiple tumors > 5 cm and tumors with evidence of major vascular invasion are combined and classified as T3 because of similarly poor prognosis.

- Tumor(s) with direct invasion of adjacent organs other than the gallbladder or with perforation of visceral peritoneum are classified separately as T4.

- The separate subcategory for multiple bilobar tumors has been eliminated because of a lack of distinct prognostic value.

- T3 N0 tumors and tumors with lymph node involvement are combined into Stage III because of similar prognosis.

- Stage IV defines metastatic disease only. The subcategories IVA and IVB have been eliminated.

INTRODUCTION

Primary malignancies of the liver include tumors arising from the hepatocytes (hepatocellular carcinoma), intrahepatic bile ducts (intrahepatic cholangiocarcinoma and cystadenocarcinoma), and mesenchymal elements (primary sarcomas, not covered in this chapter). Hepatocellular carcinoma is the most common primary cancer of the liver and is a leading cause of death from cancer worldwide. Although it is uncommon in the United States, its incidence is rising. The majority of hepatocellular carcinomas arise in a background of chronic liver disease due to viral hepatitis (B or C) or ethanol abuse. Cirrhosis may dominate the clinical picture and determine the prognosis. Other important indicators of the outcome of hepatocellular carcinoma are resectability for cure and the extent of vascular invasion.

ANATOMY

Primary Site.   The liver has a dual blood supply: the hepatic artery, which branches from the celiac artery, and the portal vein, which drains the intestine. Blood from the liver passes through the hepatic vein and enters

---

the inferior vena cava. The liver is divided into right and left lobes by a plane (Cantlie's line) projecting between the gallbladder fossa and the vena cava and defined by the middle hepatic vein. Couinaud refined knowledge about the functional anatomy of the liver and proposed division of the liver into four sectors (formerly called segments) and eight segments. In this nomenclature, the liver is divided by vertical and oblique planes or scissurae defined by the three main hepatic veins and a transverse plane or scissura that follows a line drawn through the right and left portal branches. Thus, the four traditional segments (right anterior, right posterior, left medial, and left lateral) are replaced by sectors (right anterior, right posterior, left anterior, and left posterior), and these sectors are divided into segments by the transverse scissura (Fig. 14.1). The eight segments are numbered clockwise in a frontal plane. Recent advances in hepatic surgery have made possible anatomic (also called typical) resections along these planes.

Histologically, the liver is divided into lobules with central veins draining each lobule. The portal spaces between the lobules contain the intrahepatic bile ducts and the blood supply, which consists of small branches of the hepatic artery and portal vein (portal triads).

Regional Lymph Nodes. The regional lymph nodes are the hilar, hepatoduodenal ligament lymph nodes, and caval lymph nodes, among which the most prominent are the hepatic artery and portal vein lymph nodes. Histologic examination of a regional lymphadenectomy specimen will ordinarily include a minimum of three lymph nodes.

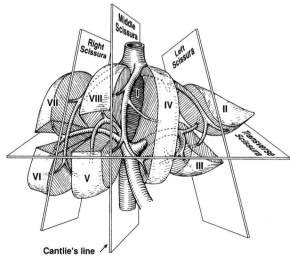

Fig. 14.1. Anatomy of the liver. (Reproduced with permission from JN Vauthey. Liver imaging. Radiol Clin North Am 1998; 36(2):445.)

Nodal involvement beyond these lymph nodes is considered distant metastasis and should be coded as M1. Involvement of the inferior phrenic lymph nodes should also be considered M1.

Metastatic Sites. The main mode of dissemination of liver carcinomas is via the portal veins (intrahepatic) and hepatic veins. Intrahepatic venous dissemination cannot be differentiated from satellitosis or multifocal tumors and is classified as multiple tumors. The most common sites of extrahepatic dissemination are the lungs and bones. Tumors may extend through the liver capsule to adjacent organs (adrenal, diaphragm, and colon) or may rupture, causing acute hemorrhage and peritoneal carcinomatosis.

RULES FOR CLASSIFICATION

The T classification is based on the results of multivariate analyses of factors affecting prognosis after resection of liver carcinomas. The classification considers the presence or absence of vascular invasion (as assessed radiographically or pathologically), the number of tumor nodules (single versus multiple), and the size of the largest tumor ($\leq$ 5 cm versus > 5 cm). For pathologic classification, vascular invasion includes gross as well as microscopic involvement of vessels. Major vascular invasion (T3) is defined as invasion of the branches of the main portal vein (right or left portal vein, this does not include sectoral or segmental branches) or as invasion of one or more of the three hepatic veins (right, middle, or left). Multiple tumors include satellitosis, multifocal tumors, and intrahepatic metastases. Invasion of adjacent organs other than the gallbladder or with perforation of the visceral peritoneum is considered T4.

Clinical Staging. Clinical staging depends on imaging procedures designed to demonstrate the size of the primary tumor and vascular invasion. Surgical exploration is not carried out if imaging shows that complete resection is not possible or if the hepatic reserve is deemed insufficient for safe resection. In the presence of cirrhosis, the Child-Pugh class should be recorded using a point system. When advanced underlying liver disease (cirrhosis) dominates the prognosis, primary tumor factors (T stage) may become irrelevant in terms of prognosis. In these instances, another clinical staging system (Okuda staging, Cancer of the Liver Italian Program [CLIP] score, or Barcelona Clinic Liver Cancer [BCLC] staging) that combines the evaluation of liver disease and hepatocellular carcinoma may be helpful.

Pathologic Staging. Complete pathologic staging consists of evaluation of the primary tumor, including histologic grade; regional lymph nodes; and underlying liver disease. Regional lymph node involvement is rare (5%) except in the fibrolamellar variant of hepatocellular carcinoma. Tumors with positive lymph nodes are classified as Stage III because they carry the same prognosis as multiple tumors > 5 cm and tumors with evidence of major vascular invasion. The grade is based on the cytopathologic study of nuclear pleiomorphism as described by Edmonson and

Steiner. Because of the prognostic significance of underlying liver disease in hepatocellular carcinoma, it is recommended that the results of the histopathologic analysis of the adjacent (non-tumorous) liver be reported. Severe fibrosis/cirrhosis (F1; Ishak score of 5–6) is associated with a worse prognosis than is no or moderate fibrosis (F0; Ishak score of 0–4). Although grade and underlying liver disease have prognostic significance, they are not included in the current staging system.

DEFINITION OF TNM

Primary Tumor (T)

TX Primary tumor cannot be assessed

T0 No evidence of primary tumor

T1 Solitary tumor without vascular invasion

T2 Solitary tumor with vascular invasion or multiple tumors none more than 5 cm

T3 Multiple tumors more than 5 cm or tumor involving a major branch of the portal or hepatic vein(s)

T4 Tumor(s) with direct invasion of adjacent organs other than the gallbladder or with perforation of visceral peritoneum.

Regional Lymph Nodes (N)

NX Regional lymph nodes cannot be assessed

N0 No regional lymph node metastasis

N1 Regional lymph node metastasis

Distant Metastasis (M)

MX Distant metastasis cannot be assessed

M0 No distant metastasis

M1 Distant metastasis

STAGE GROUPING

Stage	T	N	M
Stage I	T1	N0	M0
Stage II	T2	N0	M0
Stage IIIA	T3	N0	M0
IIIB	T4	N0	M0
IIIC	Any T	N1	M0
Stage IV	Any T	Any N	M1

Validation. Validation of T1, T2, and T3 categories of this staging system is based on multivariate analyses of outcome and survival data of single-institution and multi-institution studies of hepatic resection of hepatocellular carcinoma worldwide (totaling 741 patients at seven institutions worldwide). The survival curves obtained from analysis of the database of the International Cooperative Study Group for Hepatocellular Carcinoma are presented in Figures 14.2, 14.3 and 14.4.

HISTOPATHOLOGIC TYPE

The staging system applies only to primary carcinomas of the liver. These include

> Hepatocellular carcinoma
> Intrahepatic bile duct carcinoma
> Mixed types

Hepatocellular carcinoma is by far the most common. The classification does not apply to primary sarcomas or metastatic tumors. The histologic type and subtype should be recorded, since they may provide prognostic information.

HISTOLOGIC GRADE (G)

The grading scheme of Edmondson and Steiner is recommended. The system employs four grades as follows:

G1 Well differentiated
G2 Moderately differentiated
G3 Poorly differentiated
G4 Undifferentiated

FIBROSIS SCORE (F)

The fibrosis score as defined by Ishak is recommended because of its prognostic value in overall survival. This scoring system uses a 0–6 scale.

F0 Fibrosis score 0–4 (none to moderate fibrosis)
F1 Fibrosis score 5–6 (severe fibrosis or cirrhosis)

PROGNOSTIC FACTORS

Clinical factors predictive of decreased survival duration include an elevated serum alpha-fetoprotein level and Child-Pugh class B and C liver disease. For patients who undergo tumor resection, the main predictor of poor outcome is a positive surgical margin (grossly or microscopically incomplete resection). The effect of margin size (< 10 mm versus ≥ 10 mm) remains controversial. Other prognostic factors associated with decreased survival include major vascular invasion and tumor size > 5 cm in patients with multiple tumors.

Intrahepatic bile duct cancer (cholangiocarcinoma) is currently staged similarly to hepatocellular carcinoma because of limited data regarding the factors that affect prognosis; we anticipate including a separate chapter for the staging of intrahepatic cholangiocarcinoma in the seventh edition of this manual.

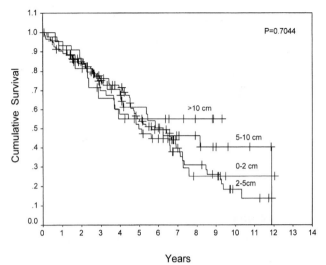

Fig. 14.2. Survival of patients with T1 tumors (solitary tumor without vascular invasion) stratified by size. Size does not affect prognosis for this category. (Reproduced with permission from Vauthey JN, Lauwers GY, Esnaola N, et al: A simplified staging for hepatocellular carcinoma. J Clin Oncol [in press].)

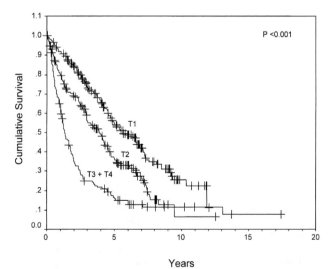

Fig. 14.3. Survival stratified according to T classification. (Reproduced with permission from Vauthey JN, Lauwers GY, Esnaola N, et al: A simplified staging for hepatocellular carcinoma. J Clin Oncol [in press].)

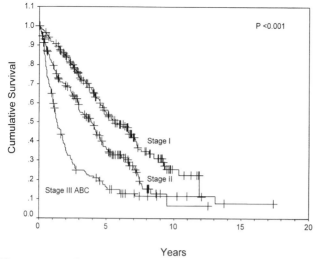

Fig. 14.4. Survival stratified according to stage grouping. (Reproduced with permission from Vauthey JN, Lauwers GY, Esnaola N, et al: A simplified staging for hepatocellular carcinoma. J Clin Oncol [in press].)

BIBLIOGRAPHY

Bilimoria MM, Lauwers GY, Nagorney DM, et al: Underlying liver disease but not tumor factors predict long-term survival after hepatic resection of hepatocellular carcinoma. Arch Surg 136:528–535, 2001

Cance WG, Stewart AK, Menck HR: The National Cancer Data Base report on treatment patterns for hepatocellular carcinomas: improved survival of surgically resected patients, 1985–1996. Cancer 88:912–920, 2000

The Cancer of the Liver Italian Program (CLIP) investigators: Prospective validation of the CLIP score: a new prognostic system for patients with cirrhosis and hepatocellular carcinoma. Hepatology 31:840–845, 2000

Cantlie J: On a new arrangement of the right and left lobes of the liver. J Anat Physiol 32:iv–ix, 1897

Couinaud C: Basic knowledge of interest: the paracaval segments of the liver. J Hep Bil Pancr Surg 2:145–151, 1994

Edmondson HA, Steiner PE: Primary carcinoma of the liver: a study of 100 cases among 48,900 necropsies. Cancer 7:462–503, 1954

El-Serag HB, Mason AC: Rising incidence of hepatocellular carcinoma in the United States. N Engl J Med 340:745–750, 1999

Fong Y, Sun RL, Jarnagin W, et al: An analysis of 412 cases of hepatocellular carcinoma at a western center. Ann Surg 229:790–800, 1998

Ikai I, Yamaoka Y, Yamamoto Y, et al: Surgical intervention for patients with stage IV-A hepatocellular carcinoma without lymph node metastasis: proposal as a standard therapy. Ann Surg 227:433–439, 1998

Ishak K, Baptista A, Bianchi L, et al: Histological grading and staging of chronic hepatitis. J Hepatol 22:696–699, 1995

Izumi R, Shimizu K, Ii T, Yagi M, et al: Prognostic factors of hepatocellular carcinoma in patients undergoing hepatic resection. Gastroenterology 106:720–727, 1994

Jeng KS, Chen BF, Lin HJ: En bloc resection for extensive hepatocellular carcinoma: is it advisable? World J Surg 18:834–839, 1994

Kosuge T, Makuuchi M, Takayama T, et al: Long-term results after resection of hepatocellular carcinoma: experience of 480 cases. Hepatogastroenterology 40:328–332, 1993

Lau WY, Leung KL, Leung TW, et al: Resection of hepatocellular carcinoma with diaphragmatic invasion. Br J Surg 82:264–266, 1995

Lauwers GY, Vauthey JN: Pathological aspects of hepatocellular carcinoma: a critical review of prognostic factors. Hepatogastroenterology 45 (Suppl 3):1197–1202, 1998

Llovet JM, Bru C, Bruix J: Prognosis of hepatocellular carcinoma: the BCLC staging classification. Semin Liver Dis 19:329–338, 1999

Nzeako UC, Goodman ZD, Ishak KG: Hepatocellular carcinoma in cirrhotic and noncirrhotic livers. A clinico-histopathologic study of 804 North American patients. Am J Clin Pathol 105:65–75, 1996

Okuda K, Ohtsuki T, Obata H, et al: Natural history of hepatocellular carcinoma and prognosis in relation to treatment. Study of 850 patients. Cancer 56:918–928, 1985

Poon RT, Fan ST, Ng IO, et al: Significance of resection margin in hepatectomy for hepatocellular carcinoma: a critical reappraisal. Ann Surg 231:544–551, 2000

Pugh RN, Murray-Lyon IM, Dawson JL, et al: Transection of the oesophagus for bleeding oesophageal varices. Br J Surg 60:646–649, 1973

Satoh, S, Ikai, I, Honda, G, et al: Clinicopathologic evaluation of hepatocellular carcinoma with bile duct thrombi. Surgery 128:779–783, 2000

Staudacher C, Chiappa A, Biella F, et al: Validation of the modified TNM-Izumi classification for hepatocellular carcinoma. Tumori 86:8–11, 2000

Tsai TJ, Chau GY, Lui WY, et al: Clinical significance of microscopic tumor venous invasion in patients with resectable hepatocellular carcinoma. Surgery 127:603–608, 2000

Tung WY, Chau GY, Loong CC, et al: Surgical resection of primary hepatocellular carcinoma extending to adjacent organ(s). Eur J Surg Oncol 22:516–520, 1996

Vauthey JN, Klimstra D, Franceschi D, et al: Factors affecting long-term outcome after hepatic resection for hepatocellular carcinoma. Am J Surg 169:28–35, 1995

Vauthey JN, Lauwers GY, Esnaola N, et al: A simplified staging for hepatocellular carcinoma. J Clin Oncol (in press)

Weimann A, Varnholt H, Schlitt HJ, et al: Retrospective analysis of prognostic factors after liver resection and transplantation for cholangiocellular carcinoma. Br J Surg 87:1182–1187, 2000

Wu CC, Ho WL, Lin MC, et al: Hepatic resection for bilobar multicentric hepatocellular carcinoma: is it justified? Surgery 123:270–277, 1998

Zhu LX, Wang GS, Fan, ST: Spontaneous rupture of hepatocellular carcinoma. Br J Surg 83:602–607, 2000

HISTOLOGIES—LIVER

8010/3	Carcinoma, NOS
8012/3	Large cell carcinoma, NOS
8013/3	Large cell neuroendocrine carcinoma
8014/3	Large cell carcinoma with rhabdoid phenotype
8020/3	Carcinoma, undifferentiated, NOS
8021/3	Carcinoma, anaplastic, NOS

8022/3	Pleomorphic carcinoma
8030/3	Giant cell and spindle cell carcinoma
8031/3	Giant cell carcinoma
8032/3	Spindle cell carcinoma, NOS
8033/3	Pseudosarcomatous carcinoma
8035/3	Carcinoma with osteoclast-like giant cells
8140/2	Adenocarcinoma *in situ*, NOS
8140/3	Adenocarcinoma, NOS
8141/3	Scirrhous adenocarcinoma
8142/3	Linitis plastica
8143/3	Superficial spreading adenocarcinoma
8144/3	Adenocarcinoma, intestinal type
8145/3	Carcinoma, diffuse type
8147/3	Basal cell adenocarcinoma
8148/2	Glandular intraepithelial neoplasia, grade III
8160/3	Cholangiocarcinoma
8161/3	Bile duct cystadenocarcinoma
8162/3	Klatskin tumor
8170/3	Hepatocellular carcinoma
8171/3	Hepatocellular carcinoma, fibrolamellar
8172/3	Hepatocellular carcinoma, scirrhous
8173/3	Hepatocellular carcinoma, spindle cell variant
8174/3	Hepatocellular carcinoma, clear cell type
8175/3	Hepatocellular carcinoma, pleomorphic type
8180/3	Combined hepatocellular carcinoma and cholangiocarcinoma
8214/3	Parietal cell carcinoma
8230/3	Solid carcinoma, NOS
8244/3	Composite carcinoid
8245/3	Adenocarcinoid tumor
8246/3	Neuroendocrine carcinoma, NOS
8255/3	Adenocarcinoma with mixed subtypes
8260/3	Papillary adenocarcinoma, NOS
8310/3	Clear cell adenocarcinoma, NOS
8320/3	Granular cell carcinoma
8430/3	Mucoepidermoid carcinoma
8440/3	Cystadenocarcinoma, NOS
8452/3	Solid pseudopapillary carcinoma
8460/3	Papillary serous cystadenocarcinoma
8461/3	Serous surface papillary carcinoma
8470/2	Mucinous cystadenocarcinoma, non-invasive
8470/3	Mucinous cystadenocarcinoma, NOS
8471/3	Papillary mucinous cystadenocarcinoma
8480/3	Mucinous adenocarcinoma
8481/3	Mucin-producing adenocarcinoma
8490/3	Signet ring cell carcinoma
8500/2	Intraductal carcinoma, noninfiltrating, NOS
8503/2	Noninfiltrating intraductal papillary adenocarcinoma
8503/3	Intraductal papillary adenocarcinoma with invasion
8550/3	Acinar cell carcinoma
8551/3	Acinar cell cystadenocarcinoma

3

15

Gallbladder

(Carcinoid tumors and sarcomas are not included.)

C23.9 Gallbladder

SUMMARY OF CHANGES

- The T and N classifications have been simplified in an effort to separate locally invasive tumors into potentially resectable (T3) and unresectable (T4).

- There is no longer a distinction between T3 and T4 based on the depth of liver invasion.

- Lymph node metastasis is now classified as Stage IIB, and Stage IIA is reserved for large, invasive tumors (resectable), without lymph node metastasis.

- Stage grouping has been changed to allow Stage III to signify locally un-resectable disease and Stage IV to indicate metastatic disease.

INTRODUCTION

Cancers of the gallbladder are staged according to their depth of penetration and extent of spread. These cancers frequently spread to the liver, which is involved in 70% of patients at the time of surgical evaluation. Malignant tumors of the gallbladder can also directly invade other adjacent organs, particularly the common bile duct, the duodenum, and the transverse colon. Gallbladder cancers are insidious in their growth, often metastasizing early, before a diagnosis is made. Tumors can also perforate the wall of the gallbladder, eventually causing intra-abdominal metastases, carcinomatosis, and ascites. Because gallbladder cancer is uncommon and is usually diagnosed late, physicians have tended to ignore anatomic staging, even though its importance for survival, management, and prognosis has been emphasized. Many cases are not suspected clinically and are first discovered at laparotomy or incidentally by the pathologist. More than 75% of carcinomas of the gallbladder are associated with cholelithiasis. Survival correlates with the stage of disease.

ANATOMY

Primary Site.   The gallbladder is a pear-shaped saccular organ located under the liver in the gallbladder fossa. It has three parts: a fundus, a body, and a neck that tapers into the cystic duct. The wall of the gallbladder is much thinner than that of the intestine and lacks a circular and transverse muscle layer. The wall has a mucosa (that is, an epithelial lining and lamina propria), a smooth muscle layer analogous to the muscularis propria of the small intestine, perimuscular connective tissue, and serosa. In contrast

---

to the intestine, there is no submucosa. Along the attachment to the liver, no serosa exists, and the perimuscular connective tissue is continuous with the interlobular connective tissue of the liver. Tumors that arise in the cystic duct are classified according to the scheme for the extrahepatic bile ducts.

Regional Lymph Nodes. Accurate tumor staging requires that all lymph nodes that are removed be analyzed. Optimal histologic examination of a regional lymphadenectomy specimen should include analysis of a minimum of three lymph nodes. The regional lymph nodes include the following: hilar, celiac, periduodenal, peripancreatic, and superior mesenteric. The hilar nodes include the lymph nodes along the common bile duct, hepatic artery, portal vein, and cystic duct.

Metastatic disease in peripancreatic nodes located along the body and tail of the pancreas are considered sites of distant metastasis.

Metastatic Sites. Cancers of the gallbladder usually metastasize to the peritoneum and liver and occasionally to the lungs and pleura.

RULES FOR CLASSIFICATION

Gallbladder cancers are staged primarily on the basis of surgical exploration or resection. However, because not all patients with gallbladder cancer undergo surgical resection, a single TNM classification must apply to both clinical and pathologic staging. Therefore, in this edition of the *AJCC Cancer Staging Manual*, we have attempted to combine clinical and pathologic staging.

Many *in situ* and early-stage carcinomas are not recognized grossly. They are usually staged pathologically after histologic examination of the resected specimen. The T classification depends on the depth of tumor penetration into the wall of the gallbladder, on the presence or absence of tumor invasion into the liver, hepatic artery, or portal vein, and on the presence or absence of adjacent organ involvement. Direct tumor extension into the liver is not considered a metastatic (M) site. Direct invasion of other adjacent organs, including colon, duodenum, stomach, common bile duct, abdominal wall, and diaphragm, is also not considered a metastasis. Tumor confined to the gallbladder is classified as either T1 or T2, depending on the depth of invasion. It must be noted that because there is no serosa on the gallbladder on the side attached to the liver, a simple cholecystectomy may not completely remove a T2 tumor, even though such tumors are considered to be confined to the gallbladder.

Clinical Staging. Clinical evaluation usually depends on the results of ultrasonography and computed tomography. In recent years, magnetic resonance cholangiopancreatography has also proved to be a useful diagnostic and staging modality. Clinical staging may also be based on findings from surgical exploration when the main tumor mass is not resected.

Pathologic Staging. Pathologic staging is based on examination of the resected specimen.

Note: The extent of resection (R0, complete resection with grossly and microscopically negative margins of resection; R1, grossly negative but microscopically positive margins of resection; R2, grossly and microscopically positive margins of resection) is not part of the TNM staging system but is prognostically of great significance.

DEFINITION OF TNM

Primary Tumor (T)

TX   Primary tumor cannot be assessed
T0   No evidence of primary tumor
Tis   Carcinoma *in situ*
T1   Tumor invades lamina propria or muscle layer (Fig. 15.1)
T1a   Tumor invades lamina propria
T1b   Tumor invades muscle layer
T2   Tumor invades perimuscular connective tissue; no extension beyond serosa or into liver (Fig. 15.2)
T3   Tumor perforates the serosa (visceral peritoneum) and/or directly invades the liver and/or one other adjacent organ or structure, such as the stomach, duodenum, colon, or pancreas, omentum or extrahepatic bile ducts
T4   Tumor invades main portal vein or hepatic artery or invades multiple extrahepatic organs or structures

Regional Lymph Nodes (N)

NX   Regional lymph nodes cannot be assessed
N0   No regional lymph node metastasis
N1   Regional lymph node metastasis

Distant Metastasis (M)

MX   Distant metastasis cannot be assessed
M0   No distant metastasis
M1   Distant metastasis

STAGE GROUPING			
Stage 0	Tis	N0	M0
Stage IA	T1	N0	M0
Stage IB	T2	N0	M0
Stage IIA	T3	N0	M0
Stage IIB	T1	N1	M0
	T2	N1	M0
	T3	N1	M0
Stage III	T4	Any N	M0
Stage IV	Any T	Any N	M1

HISTOPATHOLOGIC TYPE

The staging system applies only to primary carcinomas of the gallbladder. It does not apply to carcinoid tumors or to sarcomas. Adenocarcinomas are the most common histologic type. More that 98% of gallbladder cancers are carcinomas. The carcinomas are listed below.

Carcinoma *in situ*
Adenocarcinoma, NOS
Papillary carcinoma
Adenocarcinoma, intestinal type
Clear cell adenocarcinoma
Mucinous carcinoma
Signet ring cell carcinoma
Squamous carcinoma
Adenosquamous carcinoma
Small cell carcinoma*
Undifferentiated carcinoma*
   Spindle and giant cell types
   Small cell types
Carcinoma, NOS
Carcinosarcoma
Other (specify)

*Grade 4 by definition

HISTOLOGIC GRADE (G)

GX   Grade cannot be assessed
G1   Well differentiated
G2   Moderately differentiated
G3   Poorly differentiated
G4   Undifferentiated

PROGNOSTIC FACTORS

Many patients' gallbladder malignancies are discovered at pathologic analysis after simple cholecystectomy for presumed gallstone disease. Five-year survival is 85–100% for patients with T1 stage tumors. Patients with T2 tumors have a 5-year survival rate of approximately 30–40%, which appears to be improved (to a 5-year survival rate as high as 80–90%) with more radical resection. Patients with lymph node metastases or locally advanced tumors (Stages IIB and III) rarely experience long-term survival. The prognostic factors include histologic type, histologic grade, and vascular invasion. Papillary carcinomas have the most favorable prognosis. Unfavorable histologic types include small cell carcinomas and undifferentiated carcinomas. Lymphatic and/or blood vessel invasion indicates a less favorable outcome. Histologic grade also correlates with outcome.

Patients with T2–3 cancers discovered at pathologic analysis are usually offered a repeat operation for radical resection of residual tumor. There are indications that patients who require such repeat surgery for

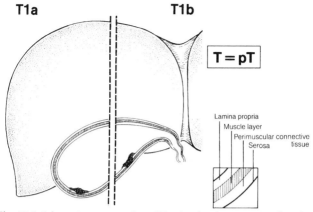

Fig. 15.1. Schematic representation of T1, showing the tumor invading the lamina propria or muscle layer of the gallbladder.

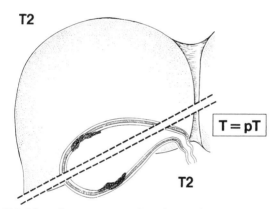

Fig. 15.2. Schematic representation of T2, showing the tumor invading perimuscular connective tissue of the gallbladder with no extension of tumor beyond serosa or into the liver.

definitive treatment of gallbladder cancer do worse than patients who undergo only a single radical procedure for tumor resection; the former have higher incidences of peritoneal dissemination and local tumor recurrence. For patients who undergo two operations for treatment of gallbladder cancer, a classification to indicate reoperative therapy should be reported so that comparisons can be made with patients who had a single operation.

BIBLIOGRAPHY

Albores-Saavedra J, Henson DE: Tumors of the gallbladder and extrahepatic bile ducts. In Atlas of tumor pathology, 2nd series, fascicle 22. Washington, DC: Armed Forces Institute of Pathology, 1986

Albores-Saavedra J, Henson DE, Sobin LH: Histological typing of tumours of the gallbladder and extrahepatic bile ducts. In WHO international histological classification of tumours. Berlin: Springer-Verlag, 1991

Bergdahl L: Gallbladder carcinoma first diagnosed at microscopic examination of gallbladders removed for presumed benign disease. Ann Surg 191:19–22, 1980

Bivins BA, Meeker MR, Griffen WO Jr: Importance of histologic classification of carcinoma of the gallbladder. Am Surg 41:121–124, 1975

de Arexabala X, Roa IS, Burgos LA, et al: Curative resection in potentially resectable tumours of the gallbladder. Euro J Surg 163:419–426, 1997

Donohue JH, Nagorney DM, Grant CS, et al: Carcinoma of the gallbladder: does radical resection improve outcome? Arch Surg 125:237–241, 1990

Donohue JH, Stewart AK, Menck HR: The National Cancer Data Base report on carcinoma of the gallbladder, 1989–1995. Cancer 83:2618–2628, 1998

Fahim RB, McDonald JR, Richards JC, et al: Carcinoma of the gallbladder: a study of its modes of spread. Ann Surg 156:114–124, 1962

Fong Y, Brennan MF, Turnbull A, et al: Gallbladder cancers discovered during laparoscopic surgery: potential for iatrogenic tumor dissemination. Arch Surg 128:1054–1056, 1993

Fong Y, Jarnagin W, Blumgart LH: Gallbladder cancer: comparison of patients presenting initially for definitive operation with those presenting after prior noncurative intervention. Ann Surg 232:557–569, 2000

Guo K J, Yamaguchi K, Enjoji M: Undifferentiated carcinoma of the gallbladder. A clinicopathologic, histochemical, and immunohistochemical study of 21 patients with a poor prognosis. Cancer 61:1872–1879, 1988

Henson DE, Albores-Saavedra J, Corle D: Carcinoma of the gallbladder. Histologic types, stage of disease, grade, and survival rates. Cancer 70:1493–1497, 1992

Hisatomi K, Haratake J, Horie A, et al: Relation of histopathological features to prognosis of gallbladder cancer. Am J Gastroenterol 85:567–572, 1990

Jones RS: Carcinoma of the gallbladder [review]. Surg Clin North Am 70:1419–1428, 1990

Nevin JE, Moran TJ, Kay S, et al: Carcinoma of the gallbladder: staging, treatment, and prognosis. Cancer 37:141–148, 1976

Ogura Y, Mizumoto R, Isaji S, et al: Radical operations for carcinoma of the gallbladder: present status in Japan. World J Surg 15:337–343, 1991

Ohtani T, Shirai Y, Tsukada K, et al: Carcinoma of the gallbladder: CT evaluation of lymphatic spread. Radiology 189:875–880, 1993

Ouchi K, Owada Y, Matsuno S, et al: Prognostic factors in the surgical treatment of gallbladder carcinoma. Surgery 101:731–737, 1987

Perpetuo MD, Valdivieso M, Heilbrun LK, et al: Natural history of gallbladder cancer. Cancer 42:330–335, 1978

Shirai Y, Ohtani T, Hatakeyama K: Laparoscopic cholecystectomy may disseminate gallbladder carcinoma. Hepatogastroenterology 45:81–82, 1998

Shirai Y, Tsukada K, Ohtani T, et al: Hepatic metastases from carcinoma of the gallbladder. Cancer 75:2063–2068, 1995

Shirai Y, Yoshida K, Tsukada K, et al: Identification of the regional lymphatic system of the gallbladder by vital staining. Br J Surg 79:659–662, 1992

Todoroki T, Kawamoto T, Takahashi H, et al: Treatment of gallbladder cancer by radical resection. Br J Surg 86:622–627, 1999

Yamamoto M, Nakajo S, Tahara E: Carcinoma of the gallbladder: the correlation between histogenesis and prognosis. Virchows Archiv A, Pathological Anatomy and Histopathology 414:83–90, 1989

HISTOLOGIES—GALLBLADDER

8010/2	Carcinoma *in situ*, NOS
8010/3	Carcinoma, NOS
8020/3	Undifferentiated carcinoma
8041/3	Small cell carcinoma, NOS
8070/3	Squamous cell carcinoma, NOS
8082/3	Lymphoepithelial carcinoma
8083/3	Basaloid squamous cell carcinoma
8084/3	Squamous cell carcinoma, clear cell type
8140/2	Adenocarcinoma *in situ*, NOS
8140/3	Adenocarcinoma, NOS
8144/3	Adenocarcinoma, intestinal type
8255/3	Adenocarcinoma with mixed subtypes
8260/3	Papillary adenocarcinoma, NOS
8310/3	Clear cell adenocarcinoma
8480/3	Mucinous adenocarcinoma
8490/3	Signet ring cell carcinoma
8560/3	Adenosquamous carcinoma
8980/3	Carcinosarcoma

3

16

Extrahepatic Bile Ducts

(Sarcomas and carcinoid tumors are not included.)

C24.0 Extrahapetic bile duct   C24.8 Overlapping lesion of   C24.9 Biliary tract, NOS
                                            biliary tract

SUMMARY OF CHANGES

- The T and N classifications have been redefined and simplified.

- Invasion of the subepithelial fibro (muscular) connective tissue is classified as T1 irrespective of muscular invasion, which cannot always be noted because of the scarcity of muscle fibers in some bile duct segments.

- T2 is defined as invasion beyond the wall of the bile duct.

- The T classification allows one to separate locally invasive tumors into resectable (T3) and unresectable (T4).

- Invasion of branches of the portal vein (right or left), hepatic artery, or liver is classified as T3.

- Invasion of the main portal vein, common hepatic artery, and/or regional organs is classified as T4.

- The stage grouping has been changed to allow Stage III to signify locally unresectable disease and Stage IV to indicate metastatic disease.

INTRODUCTION

Malignant tumors can develop anywhere along the extrahepatic bile ducts (Fig. 16.1). Of these tumors, 70–80% involve the confluence of the right and left hepatic ducts (hilar carcinomas), and about 20–30% arise more distally. Diffuse involvement of the ducts is rare, occurring in only about 2% of cases. All malignant tumors of the extrahepatic bile ducts inevitably cause partial or complete ductal obstruction. Because the bile ducts have a small diameter, the signs and symptoms of obstruction usually occur while tumors are relatively small. Because of their invasion of major vascular structures and direct extension to the liver, hilar carcinomas are more difficult to resect than those that arise distally and are associated with a worse prognosis (because of the low rate of resectability).

This TNM classification applies only to cancers arising in the extrahepatic bile ducts above the ampulla of Vater. This includes malignant tumors that develop in congenital choledochal cysts and tumors that arise in the intrapancreatic portion of the common bile duct. Patients with advanced (metastatic) disease and a primary tumor in the intrapancreatic portion of the common bile duct may be misclassified as having pancreatic cancer if surgical resection is not performed. In such cases, it is often impossible to determine (from radiographic images or endoscopy) whether a tumor arises from the intrapancreatic portion of the bile duct, the ampulla of Vater, or the pancreas. Tumors of the pancreas and ampulla of Vater are classified separately.

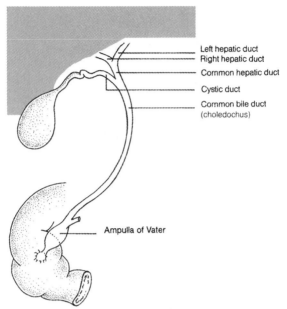

Fig. 16.1. Anatomy of the extrahepatic bile ducts.

ANATOMY

Primary Site. Emerging from the transverse scissura of the liver are the right and left hepatic bile ducts, which join to form the common hepatic duct. The cystic duct, which connects to the gallbladder, joins the common hepatic duct to form the common bile duct, which passes posterior to the first part of the duodenum, traverses the head of the pancreas, and then enters the second part of the duodenum through the ampulla of Vater. Histologically, the bile ducts are lined by a single layer of tall, uniform columnar cells. The mucosa usually forms irregular pleats or small longitudinal folds. The walls of the bile ducts have a layer of subepithelial connective tissue and muscle fibers. It should be noted that the muscle fibers are most prominent in the distal segment of the common bile duct. More proximally, the muscle fibers are sparse or absent, and the walls of the bile ducts consist largely of fibrous tissue.

Regional Lymph Nodes. Accurate tumor staging requires that all lymph nodes that are removed be analyzed. Optimal histologic examination of a regional lymphadenectomy specimen should include analysis of a minimum of three lymph nodes. The regional lymph nodes are the same as those listed for the gallbladder cancer and include the following: hilar, celiac, periduodenal, peripancreatic, and superior mesenteric. The hilar nodes include the lymph nodes along the common bile duct, hepatic artery, portal vein, and cystic duct.

Metastatic Sites.   Extrahepatic bile duct carcinomas can extend to the liver, pancreas, ampulla of Vater, duodenum, colon, omentum, stomach, or gallbladder. Tumors arising in the right or left hepatic ducts usually extend proximally into the liver or distally to the common hepatic duct. Neoplasms from the cystic duct invade the gallbladder, common bile duct, or both. Carcinomas that arise in the distal segment of the common bile duct can spread to the pancreas, duodenum, stomach, colon, or omentum. Distant metastases usually occur late in the course of the disease and are most often found in the liver, lungs, and peritoneum.

RULES FOR CLASSIFICATION

Although for most malignancies, patients are staged following surgery and pathologic examination, this is often not true of patients with carcinoma of the extrahepatic bile ducts. In a third to a half of cases, surgical resection is not attempted because of local/regional extension, and patients are treated without pathologic staging. A single TNM classification must apply to both clinical and pathologic staging. In this edition of the *AJCC Cancer Staging Manual*, we have attempted to combine clinical and pathologic staging. With advances in imaging, integrated radiologic and pathologic staging of patients can be satisfactorily achieved.

Clinical Staging.   Clinical evaluation usually depends on the results of ultrasonography, computed tomography, and magnetic resonance cholangiopancreatography. Clinical staging may also be based on findings from surgical exploration when the main tumor mass is not resected.

Pathologic Staging.   Pathologic staging is based on examination of the resected specimen.

Note: The extent of resection (R0, complete resection with grossly and microscopically negative margins of resection; R1, grossly negative but microscopically positive margins of resection; R2, grossly and microscopically positive margins of resection) is not part of the TNM staging system but is prognostically of great significance.

DEFINITION OF TNM

Primary Tumor (T)
TX   Primary tumor cannot be assessed
T0   No evidence of primary tumor
Tis   Carcinoma *in situ*
T1   Tumor confined to the bile duct histologically
T2   Tumor invades beyond the wall of the bile duct
T3   Tumor invades the liver, gallbladder, pancreas, and/or unilateral branches of the portal vein (right or left) or hepatic artery (right or left)

T4   Tumor invades any of the following: main portal vein or its branches bilaterally, common hepatic artery, or other adjacent structures, such as the colon, stomach, duodenum, or abdominal wall

Regional Lymph Nodes (N)
NX   Regional lymph nodes cannot be assessed
N0   No regional lymph node metastasis
N1   Regional lymph node metastasis

Distant Metastasis (M)
MX   Distant metastasis cannot be assessed
M0   No distant metastasis
M1   Distant metastasis

STAGE GROUPING			
Stage 0	Tis	N0	M0
Stage IA	T1	N0	M0
Stage IB	T2	N0	M0
Stage IIA	T3	N0	M0
Stage IIB	T1	N1	M0
	T2	N1	M0
	T3	N1	M0
Stage III	T4	Any N	M0
Stage IV	Any T	Any N	M1

HISTOPATHOLOGIC TYPE

The staging system applies to all carcinomas that arise in the extrahepatic bile ducts or in the cystic duct. Sarcomas and carcinoid tumors are excluded. "Adenocarcinoma, NOS" is the most common histologic type. Carcinomas account for more than 98% of cancers of the extrahepatic bile ducts. The histologic types include:

Carcinomas *in situ*
Adenocarcinoma, NOS
Adenocarcinoma, intestinal type
Clear cell adenocarcinoma
Mucinous carcinoma
Signet ring cell carcinoma
Squamous cell carcinoma
Adenosquamous carcinoma
Small cell carcinoma*
Undifferentiated carcinoma*
    Spindle and giant cell types
    Small cell types
Papillomatosis
Papillary carcinoma, non-invasive
Papillary carcinoma, invasive

Carcinoma, NOS
Other (specify)

*Grade 4 by definition

HISTOLOGIC GRADE (G)

GX   Grade cannot be assessed
G1   Well differentiated
G2   Moderately differentiated
G3   Poorly differentiated
G4   Undifferentiated

PROGNOSTIC FACTORS

Patients who undergo surgical resection for localized bile duct adenocarcinoma have a median survival of approximately 2 years and a 5-year survival of 20–40% based on extent of disease at the time of surgery. Several prognostic factors based on the pathologic characteristics of the primary tumor have been reported for carcinomas of the extrahepatic bile ducts. These include histologic type, histologic grade, and vascular, lymphatic, and perineural invasion. Papillary carcinomas have a more favorable outcome than other types of carcinoma. High-grade tumors (grades 3–4) have a less favorable outcome than low-grade tumors (grades 1–2). Positive surgical margins have emerged as a very important prognostic factor. Residual tumor classification (R0, R1, R2) should be reported if the margins are involved.

BIBLIOGRAPHY

Albores-Saavedra J, Henson DE: Tumors of the gallbladder and extrahepatic bile ducts. In Atlas of tumor pathology, 2nd series, fascicle 22, Washington, DC: Armed Forces Institute of Pathology, 1986

Albores-Saavedra J, Henson DE, Sobin LH: Histological typing of tumours of the gallbladder and extrahepatic bile ducts. In WHO international histological classification of tumors. Berlin: Springer-Verlag, 1991

Bhuiya MMR, Nimura Y, Kamiya J, et al: Clinicopathologic factors influencing survival of patients with bile duct carcinoma: multivariate statistical analysis. World J Surg 17:653, 1993

Bhuiya MMR, Nimura Y, Kamiya J, et al: Clinicopathologic studies on perineural invasion of bile duct carcinoma. Ann Surg 215:344–349, 1992

Braasch JW, Warren KW, Kune GA: Malignant neoplasms of the bile ducts. Surg Clin North Am 47:627–638, 1967

Burke EC, Jarnagin WR, Hochwald SN, et al: Hilar cholangiocarcinoma: patterns of spread, the importance of hepatic resection for curative operation, and a presurgical clinical staging system. Ann Surg 228:385–394, 1998

Hayashi S, Miyazaki M, Kondo Y, et al: Invasive growth patterns of hepatic hilar ductal carcinoma: a histologic analysis of 18 surgical cases. Cancer 73:2922–2929, 1994

Henson DE, Albores-Saavedra J, Corle D: Carcinoma of the extrahepatic bile ducts: histologic types, stage of disease, grade and survival. Cancer 70:1498–1501, 1992

Hong SM, Kang GH, Lee HY: Smooth muscle distribution in the extrahepatic bile duct: histologic and immunohistochemical studies of 122 cases. Am J Surg Pathol 24:660–667, 2000

Kayahara M, Nagakawa T, Tsukioka Y, et al: Neural invasion and nodal involvement in distal bile duct cancer. Hepatogastroenterology 41:190–194, 1994

Kayahara M, Nagakawa T, Ueno K, et al: Lymphatic flow in carcinoma of the distal bile duct based on a clinicopathologic study. Cancer 72:2112–2117, 1993

Kosuge T, Yamamoto J, Shimada K, et al: Improved surgical results for hilar cholangiocarcinoma with procedures including major hepatic resection. Ann Surg 230:663–671, 1999

Longmire WP Jr, McArthur MS, Bastounis EA, et al: Carcinoma of the extrahepatic biliary tract. Ann Surg 178:333–345, 1973

Nakeeb A, Pitt HA, Sohn TA, et al: Cholangiocarcinoma. A spectrum of intrahepatic, perihilar, and distal tumors. Ann Surg 224:463–475, 1996

Ogura Y, Takahashi K, Tabata M, et al: Clinicopathological study on carcinoma of the extrahepatic bile duct with special focus on cancer invasion on the surgical margins. World J Surg 18:778–784, 1994

Ouchi K, Suzuki M, Hashimoto L, et al: Histologic findings and prognostic factors in carcinoma of the upper bile duct. Am J Surg 157:552–556, 1989

Suzuki M, Takahashi T, Ouchi K, et al: The development and extension of hepatohilar bile duct carcinoma: a three-dimensional tumor mapping in the intrahepatic biliary tree visualized with the aid of a graphics computer system. Cancer 64:658–666, 1989

Tamada K, Ido K, Ueno N, et al: Preoperative staging of extrahepatic bile duct cancer: comparison with pathological staging. Gastroenterology 100(pt 1):1351–1361, 1991

Tio TL, Wijers OB, Sars PR, et al: Preoperative TNM classification of proximal extrahepatic bile duct carcinoma by endosonography. Semin Liver Dis 10:114–120, 1990

Tompkins RK, Saunders K, Roslyn JJ, et al: Changing patterns in diagnosis and management of bile duct cancer. Ann Surg 211:613–620, 1990

Tompkins RK, Thomas D, Wile A, et al: Prognostic factors in bile duct carcinoma. Ann Surg 194:447–455, 1981

Tsunodo T, Eto T, Koga M, et al: Early carcinoma of the extrahepatic bile duct. Jpn J Surg 19:691–698, 1989

Yamaguchi K: Early bile duct carcinoma. Aust N Z J Surg 62:525–529, 1992

HISTOLOGIES—EXTRAHEPATIC BILE DUCTS

8002/3	Malignant tumor, small cell type
8003/3	Malignant tumor, giant cell type
8005/3	Malignant tumor, clear cell type
8010/2	Carcinoma *in situ*, NOS
8010/3	Carcinoma, NOS
8020/3	Carcinoma, undifferentiated, NOS
8021/3	Carcinoma, anaplastic, NOS
8022/3	Pleomorphic carcinoma
8030/3	Giant cell and spindle cell carcinoma
8031/3	Giant cell carcinoma
8032/3	Spindle cell carcinoma, NOS
8041/3	Small cell carcinoma, NOS
8042/3	Oat cell carcinoma
8043/3	Small cell carcinoma, fusiform cell

8044/3	Small cell carcinoma, intermediate cell
8045/3	Combined small cell carcinoma
8070/3	Squamous cell carcinoma, NOS
8140/2	Adenocarcinoma *in situ*, NOS
8140/3	Adenocarcinoma, NOS
8144/3	Adenocarcinoma, intestinal type
8160/3	Cholangiocarcinoma
8161/3	Bile duct cystadenocarcinoma
8162/3	Klatskin tumor
8180/3	Combined hepatocellular carcinoma and cholangiocarcinoma
8260/3	Papillary adenocarcinoma, NOS
8310/3	Clear cell adenocarcinoma
8480/3	Mucinous adenocarcinoma
8490/3	Signet ring cell carcinoma
8560/3	Adenosquamous carcinoma

3

17

Ampulla of Vater

(Carcinoid tumors and other neuroendocrine tumors are not included.)

C24.1 Ampulla of Vater

SUMMARY OF CHANGES

- There is no longer a distinction between T3 and T4 on the basis of the depth of pancreatic invasion.

- The stage grouping has been revised.

- Stage I has been replaced with Stage IA and Stage IB.

- Stage II has been replaced with Stage IIA and Stage IIB.

- Node positive disease has been moved to Stage IIB to retain consistency with the staging of tumors of the bile duct and of the pancreas.

INTRODUCTION

The ampulla of Vater is strategically located at the confluence of the pancreatic and common bile ducts (Fig. 17.1). Most tumors that arise in this small structure will obstruct the common bile duct, causing jaundice, abdominal pain, and occasionally pancreatitis. Clinically and pathologically, carcinomas of the ampulla may be difficult to differentiate from those

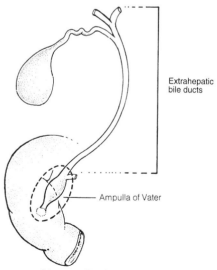

Fig. 17.1. Anatomy of the ampulla of Vater, strategically located at the confluence of the pancreatic and common bile ducts.

arising in the head of the pancreas or in the distal segment of the common bile duct. Primary cancers of the ampulla are not common, although they constitute a high proportion of malignant tumors occurring in the duodenum. Tumors of the ampulla must be differentiated from those arising in the second part of the duodenum and invading the ampulla. Carcinomas of the ampulla and periampullary region are often associated with the adenomatous polyposis coli syndrome.

ANATOMY

Primary Site. The ampulla is a small dilated duct less than 1.5 cm long, formed in most individuals by the union of the terminal segments of the pancreatic and common bile ducts. In 42% of individuals, however, the ampulla is the termination of the common duct only, the pancreatic duct having its own entrance into the duodenum adjacent to the ampulla. In these individuals, the ampulla may be difficult to locate or even nonexistent. The ampulla opens into the duodenum, usually on the posterior-medial wall, through a small mucosal elevation, the duodenal papilla, which is also called the papilla of Vater. Although carcinomas can arise either in the ampulla or on the papilla, they most commonly arise near the junction of the mucosa of the ampulla with that of the papilla. Nearly all cancers that arise in this area are well-differentiated adenocarcinomas. They have a variety of designations, including carcinoma of the ampulla of Vater, carcinoma of the periampullary portion of the duodenum, and carcinoma of the peripapillary portion of the duodenum. It may not be possible to determine the exact site of origin for large tumors.

Regional Lymph Nodes. A rich lymphatic network surrounds the pancreas and periampullary region, and accurate tumor staging requires that all lymph nodes that are removed be analyzed. Optimal histologic examination of a pancreaticoduodenectomy specimen should include analysis of a minimum of 10 lymph nodes. The regional lymph nodes are the peripancreatic lymph nodes, which also include the lymph nodes along the hepatic artery, celiac axis, and pyloric regions. Anatomic division of regional lymph nodes is not necessary; however, separately submitted lymph nodes should be reported as submitted.

Metastatic Sites. Tumors of the ampulla may infiltrate adjacent structures, such as the wall of the duodenum, the head of the pancreas, and extrahepatic bile ducts. Metastatic disease is most commonly found in the liver and peritoneum and is less commonly seen in the lungs and pleura.

RULES FOR CLASSIFICATION

Most patients are staged pathologically after examination of the resected specimen. Classification is based primarily on local extension. The T classification depends on extension of the primary tumor through the ampulla of Vater or the sphincter of Oddi into the duodenal wall or beyond into the head of the pancreas or contiguous soft tissue. The designation T4 most commonly refers to local soft tissue invasion. Unlike the case with other solid tumors, even T4 tumors are usually locally resectable.

Clinical Staging.   Endoscopic ultrasonography and computed tomography are effective in preoperative staging and in evaluating resectability of ampullary carcinomas. Laparoscopy is occasionally performed on patients who are believed to have localized, potentially resectable tumors to exclude peritoneal metastases and small metastases on the surface of the liver.

Pathologic Staging.   Pathologic staging depends on surgical resection and pathologic examination of the specimen and associated lymph nodes.

Note: The extent of resection (R0, complete resection with grossly and microscopically negative margins of resection; R1, grossly negative but microscopically positive margins of resection; R2, grossly and microscopically positive margins of resection) is not part of the TNM staging system but is prognostically of great significance.

DEFINITION OF TNM

Primary Tumor (T)
TX	Primary tumor cannot be assessed
T0	No evidence of primary tumor
Tis	Carcinoma *in situ*
T1	Tumor limited to ampulla of Vater or sphincter of Oddi
T2	Tumor invades duodenal wall
T3	Tumor invades pancreas
T4	Tumor invades peripancreatic soft tissues or other adjacent organs or structures

Regional Lymph Nodes (N)
NX	Regional lymph nodes cannot be assessed
N0	No regional lymph node metastasis
N1	Regional lymph node metastasis

Distant Metastasis (M)
MX	Distant metastasis cannot be assessed
M0	No distant metastasis
M1	Distant metastasis

STAGE GROUPING

Stage 0	Tis	N0	M0
Stage IA	T1	N0	M0
Stage IB	T2	N0	M0
Stage IIA	T3	N0	M0
Stage IIB	T1	N1	M0
	T2	N1	M0
	T3	N1	M0
Stage III	T4	Any N	M0
Stage IV	Any T	Any N	M1

HISTOPATHOLOGIC TYPE

The staging system applies to all primary carcinomas that arise in the ampulla or on the duodenal papilla. Adenocarcinomas are the most common histologic type. The classification does not apply to carcinoid tumors or to other neuroendocrine tumors. The following histologic types are included:

Carcinoma *in situ*
Adenocarcinoma, NOS
Adenocarcinoma, intestinal type
Clear cell adenocarcinoma
Mucinous carcinoma
Signet ring cell carcinoma
Squamous cell carcinoma
Adenosquamous carcinoma
Small cell carcinoma*
Undifferentiated carcinoma*
   Spindle and giant cell types
   Small cell types
Papillomatosis
Papillary carcinoma, non-invasive
Papillary carcinoma, invasive
Carcinoma, NOS
Other (specify)

*Grade 4 by definition

HISTOLOGIC GRADE (G)

GX   Grade cannot be assessed
G1   Well differentiated
G2   Moderately differentiated
G3   Poorly differentiated
G4   Undifferentiated

PROGNOSTIC FACTORS

Patients who undergo pancreaticoduodenectomy for localized periampullary adenocarcinoma of non-pancreatic origin have a superior survival duration compared with similarly treated patients who have adenocarcinoma of pancreatic origin (median survival 3–4 years compared to 18–24 months; 5-year survival 35–45% compared to 10–20%). However, as is true of the natural history of pancreatic adenocarcinoma, extent of disease and the histologic characteristics of the primary tumor predict survival duration. Even in patients who undergo a potentially curative resection, the presence of lymph node metastases, poorly differentiated histology, positive margins of resection, and tumor invasion into the pancreas are associated with a less favorable outcome. Histologic evidence of tumor extension from the ampulla into the pancreatic parenchyma appears to reflect the extent of both local and regional disease. Perineural invasion, ulceration, and high histopathologic grade are also adverse prognostic factors.

Although tumor size is not part of the TNM classification, it has prognostic significance. Tumor involvement (positivity) of resection margins has consistently been demonstrated to be an adverse prognostic factor. The residual tumor classification (R0, R1, or R2) should be reported if the margins are involved.

In contrast to the natural history of adenocarcinoma of pancreatic origin, lymph node metastasis in patients with adenocarcinoma of the ampulla of Vater are not as powerful a predictor of disease recurrence or short survival duration. The actuarial 5-year survival following potentially curative surgery in node-positive patients with pancreatic adenocarcinoma is 0–5%; in those with ampullary adenocarcinoma it is 15–30%. Tumors with papillary histology have a better outcome than non-papillary tumors.

BIBLIOGRAPHY

Allema JH, Reinders ME, van Gulik TM, et al: Prognostic factors for survival after pancreaticoduodenectomy for patients with carcinoma of the pancreatic head region. Cancer 75:2069–2076, 1995

Bakkevold KE, Kambestad B: Long-term survival following radical and palliative treatment of patients with carcinoma of the pancreas and papilla of Vater—the prognostic factors influencing the long-term results: a prospective multicentre study. Eur J Surg Oncol 19:147–161, 1993

Bakkevold KE, Kambestad B: Staging of carcinoma of the pancreas and ampulla of Vater: tumor (T), lymph node (N), and distant metastasis (M) as prognostic factors. Int J Pancreatol 17:249–259, 1995

Beger HG, Treitschke F, Gansauge F, et al: Tumor of the ampulla of Vater. Arch Surg 134:526–532, 1999

Bottger TC, Boddin J, Heintz A, et al: Clinicopathologic study for the assessment of resection for ampullary carcinoma. World J Surg 21:379–383, 1997

Compton CC: Protocol for the examination of specimens from patients with carcinoma of the ampulla of Vater. Arch Pathol Lab Med. 121:673–677, 1997

Cubilla AL, Fitzgerald PJ: Tumors of the exocrine pancreas. In Atlas of tumor pathology, 2nd series, fascicle 19, Washington, DC: Armed Forces Institute of Pathology, 1984

Delcore R Jr, Connor CS, Thomas JH, et al: Significance of tumor spread in adenocarcinoma of the ampulla of Vater. Am J Surg 158:593–596, 1989

Dorandeau A, Raoul J-L, Sisiser F, Leclercq-Rioux N, et al: Carcinoma of the ampulla of Vater: prognostic factors after curative surgery: a series of 45 cases. Gut 40:350–355, 1997

Griffanti-Bartoli F, Arnone GB, Ceppa P, et al: Malignant tumors in the head of the pancreas and the periampullary region: diagnostic and prognostic aspects. Anticancer Res 14:657–666, 1994

Harada N, Treitschke F, Imaizumi T, Beger HG. Pancreatic invasion is a prognostic indicator after radical resection for carcinoma of the ampulla of Vater. J Hep Bil Pancr Surg 4:215–219, 1997

Howe JR, Klimstra DS, Moccia RD, et al: Factors predictive of survival in ampullary carcinoma. Ann Surg 228:87–94, 1998

Kayahara M, Nagakawa T, Ohta T, Kitagawa H, Miyazaki I. Surgical strategy for carcinoma of the papilla of Vater on the basis of lymphatic spread and mode of recurrence. Surgery 121:611–617, 1997

Klempnauer J, Ridder GH, Bektas H, et al: Surgery for exocrine pancreatic cancer—who are the 5- and 10-year survivors? Oncology 52:353–359, 1995

Knox RA, Kingston RD: Carcinoma of the ampulla of Vater. Br J Surg 73:72–73, 1976

Lee JH, Whittington R, Williams NN, et al: Outcome of pancreaticoduodenectomy and impact of adjuvant therapy for ampullary carcinomas. Int J Radiat Oncol Biol Phys 47:945–953, 2000

Makipour H, Cooperman A, Danzi JT, et al: Carcinoma of the ampulla of Vater. Ann Surg 183:341–344, 1976

Martin MF, Rossi RL, Dorucci V, et al: Clinical and pathologic correlations in patients with periampullary tumors. Arch Surg 125:723–726, 1990

Monson JRT, Donohue JH, McEntee GP, et al: Radical resection for carcinoma of the ampulla of Vater. Arch Surg 126:353–357, 1991

Mori K, Ikei S, Yamane T, et al: Pathological factors influencing survival of carcinoma of the ampulla of Vater. Eur J Surg Oncol 16:183–188, 1990

Nelptolemos JP, Talbot IC, Shaw DC, et al: Long-term survival after resection of ampullary carcinoma is associated independently with tumor grade and a new staging classification that assesses local invasiveness. Cancer 61:1403–1407, 1988

Roberts RH, Krige JE, Bornman PC, Terblanche J. Pancreaticoduodenectomy of ampullary carcinoma. Am Surg 65:1043–1048, 1999

Shirai Y, Tsukada K, Ohtani T, et al: Carcinoma of the ampulla of Vater: histopathologic analysis of tumor spread in Whipple pancreatoduodenectomy specimens. World J Surg 19:102–107, 1995

Talamini MA, Moesinger RC, Pitt HA, et al: Adenocarcinoma of the ampulla of Vater: a 28-year experience. Ann Surg 225:590–600, 1997

Willett CG, Warshaw AL, Convery K, et al: Patterns of failure after pancreaticoduodenectomy for ampullary carcinoma. Surg Gynecol Obstet 176:33–38, 1993

Wise L, Pizzimbono C, Dehner IP: Periampullary cancer. Am J Surg 131:141–148, 1976

Yamaguchi K, Enjoji M: Carcinoma of the ampulla of Vater: a clinicopathologic study and pathologic staging of 109 cases of carcinoma and 5 cases of adenoma. Cancer 59:506–515, 1987

Yasuda K, Mukai H, Cho E, et al: The use of endoscopic ultrasonography in the diagnosis and staging of carcinoma of the papilla of Vater. Endoscopy 20(Suppl):218–222, 1988

HISTOLOGIES—AMPULLA OF VATER

8010/2	Carcinoma *in situ*, NOS
8010/3	Carcinoma, NOS
8020/3	Undifferentiated carcinoma
8032/3	Spindle cell carcinoma, NOS
8041/3	Small cell carcinoma, NOS
8042/3	Oat cell carcinoma
8070/3	Squamous cell carcinoma, NOS
8140/2	Adenocarcinoma *in situ*, NOS
8140/3	Adenocarcinoma, NOS
8144/3	Adenocarcinoma, intestinal type
8210/2	Adenocarcinoma *in situ* in adenomatous polyp
8210/3	Adenocarcinoma in adenomatous polyp
8255/3	Adenocarcinoma with mixed subtypes
8260/3	Papillary adenocarcinoma, NOS
8261/3	Adenocarcinoma in villous adenoma

8310/3   Clear cell adenocarcinoma, NOS
8480/3   Mucinous adenocarcinoma
8481/3   Mucin-producing adenocarcinoma
8490/3   Signet ring cell carcinoma
8560/3   Adenosquamous carcinoma

3

18

Exocrine Pancreas

(Endocrine tumors arising from the islets of Langerhans and carcinoid tumors are not included.)

C25.0 Head of pancreas	C25.3 Pancreatic duct	C25.8 Overlapping lesion of
C25.1 Body of pancreas	C25.7 Other specified parts of	pancreas
C25.2 Tail of pancreas	pancreas	C25.9 Pancreas, NOS

SUMMARY OF CHANGES

- The T classification reflects the distinction between potentially resectable (T3) and locally advanced (T4) primary pancreatic tumors.

- Stage grouping has been changed to allow Stage III to signify unresectable, locally advanced pancreatic cancer, while Stage IV is reserved for patients with metastatic disease.

INTRODUCTION

In the United States, pancreatic cancer is the second most common malignant tumor of the gastrointestinal tract and the fifth leading cause of cancer-related death in adults. The disease is difficult to diagnose, especially in its early stages. Most pancreatic cancers arise in the head of the pancreas, often causing bile duct obstruction that results in clinically evident jaundice. Cancers that arise in either the body or the tail of the pancreas are insidious in their development and often far advanced when first detected. Most pancreatic cancers are adenocarcinomas, which usually originate from the pancreatic duct cells. Surgical resection remains the only potentially curative approach, although multimodality therapy that includes innovative systemic agents and often radiation therapy is available.

Staging of exocrine pancreatic cancers depends on the size and extent of the primary tumor. This TNM classification does not apply to endocrine tumors.

ANATOMY

Primary Site. The pancreas is a long, coarsely lobulated gland that lies transversely across the posterior abdomen and extends from the duodenum to the splenic hilum. The organ is divided into a head with a small uncinate process, a neck, a body, and a tail. The anterior aspect of the body of the pancreas is in direct contact with the posterior wall of the stomach; posteriorly, the pancreas extends to the aorta, splenic vein, and left kidney.

Regional Lymph Nodes. A rich lymphatic network surrounds the pancreas, and accurate tumor staging requires that all lymph nodes that are removed be analyzed. Optimal histologic examination of a

---

pancreaticoduodenectomy specimen should include analysis of a minimum of 10 lymph nodes, although pathologic analysis of at least 10 lymph nodes may still result in a pN0 designation. The regional lymph nodes are the peripancreatic lymph nodes, which also include the lymph nodes along the hepatic artery, the celiac axis, and the pyloric and splenic regions. Anatomic division of regional lymph nodes is not necessary; however, separately submitted lymph nodes should be reported as submitted.

Metastatic Sites. Distant spread occurs commonly to the liver, peritoneal cavity, and lungs. Metastases to other sites are uncommon (or rarely detected), possibly because of the short interval from diagnosis of distant metastases to death.

DEFINITION OF LOCATION

Tumors of the head of the pancreas are those arising to the right of the superior mesenteric–portal vein confluence (Fig. 18.1). The uncinate process is part of the pancreatic head. Tumors of the body of the pancreas are roughly defined as those arising between the superior mesenteric–portal vein confluence and the aorta. Tumors of the tail of the pancreas are those arising between the aorta and the hilum of the spleen.

RULES FOR CLASSIFICATION

Because only a minority of patients with pancreatic cancer undergo surgical resection of the pancreas (and adjacent lymph nodes), a single TNM classification must apply to both clinical and pathologic staging.

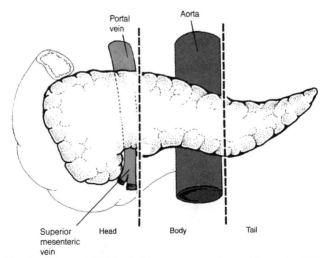

Fig. 18.1. Tumors of the head of the pancreas are those arising to the right of the superior mesenteric–portal vein confluence.

RULES FOR CLASSIFICATION AND CHANGES FROM THE FIFTH EDITION

Since only a minority of patients with pancreatic cancer undergo surgical resection of the pancreas (and adjacent lymph nodes), a single TNM classification must apply to both clinical and pathologic staging. In this edition of the *AJCC Cancer Staging Manual*, the editorial consultants have attempted to combine clinical and pathologic staging to address the following problems presented by previous editions:

1. We have changed the T classification to a more clinically relevant system, based upon both preoperative CT-assessment of resectability and final pathologic evaluation of the resected specimen. It is important to distinguish between resectable (T1, T2, and T3) and locally advanced (T4) primary tumors. Pancreatic tumors are judged unresectable when they cannot be separated (on high-quality CT images) from the adjacent large arterial structures (celiac axis or superior mesenteric artery). It would be unusual for an exocrine pancreatic cancer to exhibit local tumor extension to the retroperitoneum or adjacent structures, which would preclude surgical resection, in the absence of arterial involvement. Tumor involvement of the superior mesenteric or portal veins is classified as T3 in the current AJCC T classification; such tumors are considered resectable in some centers and there are few data on the prognostic value of venous invasion. The distinction between T3 and T4 in this chapter reflects the distinction between potentially resectable (T3) and locally advanced (T4) primary pancreatic tumors, both of which demonstrate radiographic or pathologic evidence of extrapancreatic tumor extension.

2. In the fifth edition, patients with unresectable T3 primary tumors were considered to have stage II disease (the lymph node status was unknown since no surgical resection was performed); in contrast, a patient with a 1-cm primary tumor and 1 positive regional lymph node who had undergone pancreaticoduodenectomy would be classified as having stage III disease. We acknowledge the prognostic importance of positive lymph nodes, but in general, patients with completely resected (R0 or R1; see below) N1 pancreatic cancer have a superior survival duration compared to patients with locally advanced (unresectable) or metastatic disease. Therefore, in the current edition, we reserve stage III for patients with unresectable, locally advanced pancreatic cancer.

It is important to note that the extent of resection (R0, complete resection with grossly and microscopically negative margins of resection; R1, grossly negative but positive microscopically margins of resection; R2, grossly and microscopically positive margins of resection) is not part of the TNM staging system but is prognostically of great significance.

Clinical Staging. Information necessary for the clinical staging of exocrine pancreatic cancer can be obtained from a physical examination and high-quality computed tomography (CT) images. The standard imaging procedure for pancreatic neoplasms is contrast-enhanced multislice CT (arterial and venous phases of contrast enhancement). On the basis of the interpretation of CT images and chest radiographs, patients can be classified as having localized resectable (Stage I or II), locally advanced (Stage III), or metastatic (Stage IV) pancreatic cancer. Endoscopic ultrasonography (when done by experienced gastroenterologists) also provides information helpful for clinical staging and is the procedure of choice for performing fine-needle aspiration biopsy of the pancreas. Laparoscopy is commonly performed on patients believed to have localized, potentially resectable tumors to exclude peritoneal metastases and small metastases on the surface of the liver. Laparoscopy will reveal tiny (<1 cm) peritoneal or liver metastases and up-stage (to Stage IV) approximately 10% of patients with tumors in the pancreatic head, and up to 40% of patients with tumors in the body and tail, who had been believed to have Stage I or Stage II disease on the basis of CT alone. Endoscopic retrograde cholangiopancreatography and placement of an endobiliary stent are commonly performed in patients with biliary obstruction.

Pathologic Staging.   Partial resection (pancreaticoduodenectomy or distal pancreatectomy) or complete resection of the pancreas, including the tumor and associated regional lymph nodes, provides the information necessary for pathologic staging.

In pancreaticoduodenectomy specimens, the bile duct, pancreatic duct, and retroperitoneal margins should be evaluated grossly and microscopically. In total pancreatectomy specimens, the bile duct and retroperitoneal margins should be assessed. Duodenal (with pylorus-preserving pancreaticoduodenectomy) and gastric (with standard pancreaticoduodenectomy) margins are rarely involved, but their status should be included in the surgical pathology report. Reporting of margins may be facilitated by use of the following checklist:

Surgical Margin	*Status*
Common bile (hepatic) duct	
Pancreatic neck	
Retroperitoneal margin	
Other soft tissue margins (such as posterior pancreatic)	
Duodenum	
Stomach	

Particular attention should be paid to the retroperitoneal (also referred to as the mesenteric or uncinate) pancreatic margin (soft tissue that often contains perineural tissue adjacent to the superior mesenteric artery; see Fig. 18.2) because most local recurrences arise in the pancreatic bed along

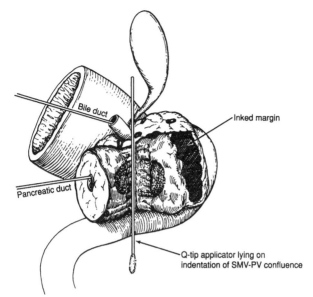

Bile duct

Inked margin

Pancreatic duct

Q-tip applicator lying on
indentation of SMV-PV confluence

Fig. 18.2. The retroperitoneal (also referred to as the mesenteric or uncinate) pancreatic margin (soft tissue that often contains perineural tissue adjacent to the superior mesenteric artery).

this critical margin. The soft tissue between the anterior surface of the inferior vena cava and the posterior aspect of the pancreatic head and duodenum is best referred to as the posterior pancreatic margin (not the retroperitoneal margin). The retroperitoneal margin should be inked as part of the gross evaluation of the specimen; the specimen is then cut perpendicular to the inked margin for histologic analysis. The closest microscopic approach of the tumor to the margin should be recorded in millimeters.

Seeding of the peritoneum (even if limited to the lesser sac region) is considered M1. Similarly, peritoneal fluid that contains cytologic (microscopic) evidence of carcinoma is considered M1. In patients without ascites, the implications of positive peritoneal cytology are not clear at this time, although the available data suggest that this finding predicts a short survival. Therefore, positive peritoneal cytology is also considered M1.

Note: The extent of resection (R0, complete resection with grossly and microscopically negative margins of resection; R1, grossly negative but microscopically positive margins of resection; R2, grossly and microscopically positive margins of resection) is not part of the TNM staging system but is prognostically of great significance.

DEFINITION OF TNM

Primary Tumor (T)

TX   Primary tumor cannot be assessed
T0   No evidence of primary tumor
Tis   Carcinoma *in situ**
T1   Tumor limited to the pancreas, 2 cm or less in greatest dimension
T2   Tumor limited to the pancreas, more than 2 cm in greatest dimension
T3   Tumor extends beyond the pancreas but without involvement of the celiac axis or the superior mesenteric artery
T4   Tumor involves the celiac axis or the superior mesenteric artery (unresectable primary tumor)

Regional Lymph Nodes (N)

NX   Regional lymph nodes cannot be assessed
N0   No regional lymph node metastasis
N1   Regional lymph node metastasis

Distant Metastasis (M)

MX   Distant metastasis cannot be assessed
M0   No distant metastasis
M1   Distant metastasis

*This also includes the "PanInIII" classification

STAGE GROUPING

Stage 0	Tis	N0	M0
Stage IA	T1	N0	M0
Stage IB	T2	N0	M0
Stage IIA	T3	N0	M0
Stage IIB	T1	N1	M0
	T2	N1	M0
	T3	N1	M0
Stage III	T4	Any N	M0
Stage IV	Any T	Any N	M1

HISTOPATHOLOGIC TYPE

The staging system applies to all exocrine carcinomas that arise in the pancreas. It does not apply to endocrine tumors, which usually arise from the islets of Langerhans. Carcinoid tumors are also excluded. More than 90% of malignant tumors of the pancreas are exocrine carcinomas. The following carcinomas are included:

Severe ductal dysplasia/carcinoma *in situ* (PanIn III; pancreatic intraepithelial neoplasia)
Ductal adenocarcinoma
Mucinous noncystic carcinoma

Signet ring cell carcinoma
Adenosquamous carcinoma
Undifferentiated carcinoma
   Spindle and giant cell types
   Small cell types
Mixed ductal-endocrine carcinoma
Osteoclast-like giant cell tumor
Serous cystadenocarcinoma
Mucinous cystadenocarcinoma
Intraductal papillary mucinous carcinoma with or without invasion
   (IPMN)
Acinar cell carcinoma
Acinar cell cystadenocarcinoma
Mixed acinar-endocrine carcinoma
Pancreaticoblastoma
Solid pseudopapillary carcinoma
Borderline (uncertain malignant potential) tumors
   Mucinous cystic tumor with moderate dysplasia
   Intraductal papillary-mucinous tumor with moderate
      dysplasia
   Solid pseudopapillary tumor
Other

HISTOLOGIC GRADE (G)

GX   Grade cannot be assessed
G1   Well differentiated
G2   Moderately differentiated
G3   Poorly differentiated
G4   Undifferentiated

PROGNOSTIC FACTORS

Patients who undergo surgical resection for localized non-metastatic adenocarcinoma of the pancreas have a long-term survival rate of approximately 20% and a median survival of 12–20 months. Patients with locally advanced, non-metastatic disease have a median survival of 6–10 months. Patients with metastatic disease have a short survival (3–6 months), the length of which depends on the extent of disease and performance status.

A number of investigators have examined pathologic factors of the resected tumor (in patients with apparently localized, resectable pancreatic cancer) in an effort to establish reliable prognostic variables associated with decreased survival duration. Metastatic disease in regional lymph nodes, poorly differentiated histology, and increased size of the primary tumor have been associated with decreased survival duration. The prognostic factor of greatest significance for decreased survival duration in patients who undergo pancreaticoduodenectomy is incomplete resection. Therefore, margin assessment is of major importance in the gross and microscopic evaluation of the pancreaticoduodenectomy specimen. Retrospective pathologic analysis of archival material does not allow accurate assessment of the margins of resection or of the number of lymph nodes retrieved; this information must be obtained when the specimen is removed and examined in the surgical pathology laboratory. The margin of resection most likely to be positive is the retroperitoneal (or mesenteric) margin along the right lateral border of the superior mesenteric artery. This margin is defined as the soft tissue margin directly adjacent to the proximal 3–4 cm of the superior mesenteric artery and is inked for evaluation of margin status on permanent-section histologic evaluation (see the "Pathologic Staging" section). Incomplete resection resulting in a grossly positive retroperitoneal margin provides no survival advantage from surgical resection (compared to those who receive chemoradiation and no surgery).

BIBLIOGRAPHY

Albores-Saavedra J, Heffess C, Hruban RH, et al: Recommendations for the reporting of pancreatic specimens containing malignant tumors. Am J Clin Pathol 111:304–307, 1999

Association of Directors of Anatomic and Surgical Pathology: Recommendations for the reporting of pancreatic specimens containing malignant tumors. Hum Pathol 29:893–895, 1998

Birkmeyer JD, Finlayson SR, Tosteson AN, et al: Effect of hospital volume on in-hospital mortality with pancreaticoduodenectomy. Surgery 125:250–256, 1999

Birkmeyer JD, Warshaw AL, Finlayson SR, et al: Relationship between hospital volume and late survival after pancreaticoduodenectomy. Surgery 126:178–183, 1999

Bold RJ, Charnsangavej C, Cleary KR, et al: Major vascular resection as part of pancreaticoduodenectomy for cancer: radiologic, intraoperative, and pathologic analysis. J Gastrointest Surg 3:233–243, 1999

Compton CC, Henson DE: Protocol for the examination of specimens removed from patients with carcinoma of the exocrine pancreas: a basis for checklists. Arch Pathol Lab Med 121:1129–1136, 1997

Conlon KC, Klimstra DS, Brennan MF: Long-term survival after curative resection for pancreatic ductal adenocarcinoma: clinicopathologic analysis of 5-year survivors. Ann Surg 223:273–279, 1996

Cubilla AL, Fitzgerald PJ: Tumors of the exocrine pancreas. In Atlas of tumor pathology, 2nd series, facicle 19, Washington DC: Armed Forces Institute of Pathology, 1984

Cubilla AL, Fortner J, Fitzgerald PJ. Lymph node involvement in carcinoma of the head of the pancreas area. Cancer 41:880–887, 1978

Evans DB, Abbruzzese JL, Willett CG. Cancer of the pancreas. In DeVita VT, Hellman S, Rosenberg SA (Eds): Cancer, principles and practice of oncology, 6th ed. Philadelphia: J.B. Lippincott, 2002

Evans DB, Lee JE, Pisters PWT: Pancreaticoduodenectomy (Whipple operation) and total pancreatectomy for cancer. In Nyhus LM, Baker RJ, Fischer JF (Eds.): Mastery of surgery, 3rd ed. Boston: Little, Brown, 1233–1249, 1997

Fuhrman GM, Charnsangavej C, Abbruzzese JL, et al: Thin-section contrast-enhanced computed tomography accurately predicts resectability of malignant pancreatic neoplasms. Am J Surg 167:104–111, 1994

Geer RJ, Brennan MF: Prognostic indicators for survival after resection of pancreatic adenocarcinoma. Am J Surg 165:68–72, 1993

Gold EB, Goldin SB: Epidemiology of and risk factors for pancreatic cancer. Surg Oncol Clin N Am 7:67–91, 1998

Greenlee RT, Murray T, Bolden S, et al: Cancer statistics, 2000. CA Cancer J Clin 50:7–13, 2000

Griffin JF, Smalley SR, Jewell W: Patterns of failure after curative resection of pancreatic carcinoma. Cancer 66:56–61, 1990

Kloppel G, Hruban RH, Longnecker DS, Adler G, Kern SE, Partanen TJ. Ductal adenocarcinoma of the pancreas. In Hamilton SR, Aaltonen LA, eds. World Health Organization Classification of Tumors: Pathology and Genetics, Tumors of the Digestive System. Lyon, IARC Press, 2000, pp 221–230.

Leach SD, Lee JE, Charnsangavej C, et al: Survival following pancreaticoduodenectomy with resection of the superior mesenteric–portal vein confluence for adenocarcinoma of the pancreatic head. Br J Surg 85:611–617, 1998

Millikan KW, Deziel DJ, Silverstein JC, et al: Prognostic factors associated with resectable adenocarcinoma of the head of the pancreas. Am Surg 65:618–624, 1999

Nitecki SS, Sarr MG, Colby TV, et al: Long-term survival after resection for ductal adenocarcinoma of the pancreas: is it really improving? Ann Surg 221:59–66, 1995

Pedrazzoli S, Bger HG, Obertop H, et al: A surgical and pathological based classification of resective treatment of pancreatic cancer. Dig Surg 16:337–345, 1999

Sohn TA, Yeo CJ, Cameron JL, et al. Resected adenocarcinoma of the pancreas–616 patients: results, outcomes, and prognostic indicators. J Gastrointest Surg. 4:567–579, 2000.

Staley C, Cleary K, Abbruzzese J, et al: Need for standardized pathologic staging of pancreaticoduodenectomy specimens. Pancreas 12:373–380, 1996

Suits J, Frazee R, Erickson RA: Endoscopic ultrasound and fine-needle aspiration for the valuation of pancreatic masses. Arch Surg 134:639–643, 1999

Traverso LW, Longmire WP Jr: Preservation of the pylorus in pancreaticoduodenectomy. Surg Gynecol Obstet 146:959–962, 1978

Tyler DS, Evans DB: Reoperative pancreaticoduodenectomy. Ann Surg 219:211–221, 1994

Westerdahl J, Andrén-Sandeberg Å, Ihse I: Recurrence of exocrine pancreatic cancer—local or hepatic? Hepatogastroenterology 40:384–387, 1993

Whipple AO, Parsons WW, Mullin CR: Treatment of carcinoma of the ampulla of Vater. Ann Surg 102:763–269, 1935

Willett CG, Lewandrowski K, Warshaw AL, et al: Resection margins in carcinoma of the head of the pancreas: implications for radiation therapy. Ann Surg 217:144–148, 1993

Yeo CJ, Cameron JL, Sohn TA, et al: Six hundred fifty consecutive pancreaticoduodenectomies in the 1990s: pathology, complications, and outcomes. Ann Surg 226:248–257, 1997

HISTOLOGIES—EXOCRINE PANCREAS

8010/2	Carcinoma *in situ*, NOS
8010/3	Carcinoma, NOS
8012/3	Large cell carcinoma, NOS
8013/3	Large cell neuroendocrine carcinoma
8014/3	Large cell carcinoma with rhabdoid phenotype
8020/3	Carcinoma, undifferentiated, NOS
8020/3	Undifferentiated carcinoma
8021/3	Carcinoma, anaplastic, NOS
8022/3	Pleomorphic carcinoma

8030/3	Giant cell and spindle cell carcinoma
8031/3	Giant cell carcinoma
8032/3	Spindle cell carcinoma, NOS
8035/3	Osteoclast-like giant cell tumor
8041/3	Small cell carcinoma, NOS
8042/3	Oat cell carcinoma
8043/3	Small cell carcinoma, fusiform cell
8044/3	Small cell carcinoma, intermediate cell
8045/3	Combined small cell carcinoma
8046/3	Non–small cell carcinoma
8070/2	Squamous cell carcinoma *in situ*, NOS
8070/3	Squamous cell carcinoma, NOS
8140/3	Adenocarcinoma, NOS
8141/3	Scirrhous adenocarcinoma
8144/3	Adenocarcinoma, intestinal type
8145/3	Carcinoma, diffuse type
8148/2	Glandular intraepithelial neoplasia, grade III
8154/3	Mixed acinar-endocrine carcinoma
8154/3	Mixed ductal-endocrine carcinoma
8214/3	Parietal cell carcinoma
8246/3	Neuroendocrine carcinoma, NOS
8255/3	Adenocarcinoma with mixed subtypes
8260/3	Papillary adenocarcinoma, NOS
8310/3	Clear cell adenocarcinoma, NOS
8320/3	Granular cell carcinoma
8430/3	Mucoepidermoid carcinoma
8441/3	Serous cystadenocarcinoma
8452/3	Solid pseudopapillary carcinoma
8453/2	Intraductal papillary-mucinous carcinoma, non-invasive
8453/3	Intraductal papillary-mucinous carcinoma, invasive
8470/3	Mucinous cystadenocarcinoma
8480/3	Mucinous adenocarcinoma
8481/3	Mucin-producing adenocarcinoma
8490/3	Signet ring cell carcinoma
8500/3	Ductal adenocarcinoma
8550/3	Acinar cell carcinoma
8551/3	Acinar cell cystadenocarcinoma
8560/3	Adenosquamous carcinoma
8971/3	Pancreaticoblastoma

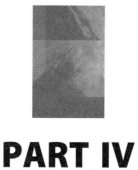

PART IV
Thorax

19

Lung

(Sarcomas and other rare tumors are not included.)

C34.0 Main bronchus
C34.1 Upper lobe, lung
C34.2 Middle lobe, lung
C34.3 Lower lobe, lung
C34.8 Overlapping lesion of lung
C34.9 Lung, NOS

SUMMARY OF CHANGES

- The definition of TNM and the Stage Grouping for this chapter have not changed from the Fifth Edition.

4

INTRODUCTION

Lung cancer is among the most common malignancies in the Western world and is the leading cause of cancer deaths in both men and women. It is one of the few tumors with a known carcinogen, namely tobacco, contributing to its etiology. In recent years we have come to appreciate that the initiation of lung cancer is a complex process that also involves certain biologic factors, such as the body's ability to process carcinogens. This disease is usually not diagnosed early, and therefore the overall 5-year survival rate is approximately 15%. The treatment of lung cancer depends on the extent of disease, the location of the primary tumor, and the presence or absence of medical comorbidities. The assessment of extrapulmonary intrathoracic and extrathoracic metastasis is important for staging and patient evaluation.

ANATOMY

Primary Site. Carcinomas of the lung arise either from the alveolar lining cells of the pulmonary parenchyma or from the mucosa of the tracheobronchial tree. The trachea, which lies in the middle mediastinum, divides into the right and left main bronchi, which extend into the right and left lungs, respectively. The bronchi then subdivide into the lobar bronchi for the upper, middle, and lower lobes on the right and the upper and lower lobes on the left. The lungs are encased in membranes called the visceral pleura. The inside of the chest cavity is lined by a similar membrane called the parietal pleura. The potential space between these two membranes is the pleural space. The mediastinum contains the heart, thymus, great vessels, and other structures between the lungs.

The great vessels include:

Aorta
Superior vena cava
Inferior vena cava
Main pulmonary artery

Intrapericardial segments of the trunk of the right and left pulmonary
    artery
Intrapericardial segments of the superior and inferior right and left pul-
    monary veins

Regional Lymph Nodes.   All regional nodes are above the diaphragm.
They include the intrathoracic, scalene, and supraclavicular nodes (Fig.
19.1). For purposes of staging, the intrathoracic nodes include the
following:

Mediastinal
Paratracheal (including those that may be designated tracheobronchial—
    that is, lower paratracheal, including azygous)
Pre- and retrotracheal (includes precarinal)
Aortic (includes aortopulmonary window, periaortic, ascending aortic, and
    phrenic)
Subcarinal
Periesophageal
Inferior pulmonary ligament

Intrapulmonary
Hilar (proximal lobar)
Peribronchial
Intrapulmonary (includes interlobar, lobar, and segmental)

Distant Metastatic Sites.   The most common metastatic sites are the
brain, bones, adrenal glands, contralateral lung, liver, pericardium, and
kidneys. However, virtually any organ can be a site of metastases.

RULES FOR CLASSIFICATION

Lung cancers are broadly classified as either non–small cell (80% of tumors) or small cell carcinomas (20% of tumors). This general histologic
distinction reflects the clinical and biologic behavior of these two tumor
types. Approximately half of all non–small cell lung cancers are either
localized or locally advanced at the time of diagnosis and are treated by
resection alone or by combined modality therapy with or without resection. By contrast, small cell lung cancers are metastatic in 80% of cases at
diagnosis. Even small cell lung cancers that are initially localized to the
hemithorax tend to metastasize early in their course and are managed
principally with systemic therapy. Less than 10% of small cell lung cancers
are detected at a very early stage when they can be treated by resection
and adjuvant chemotherapy.
    The TNM staging system described here is used primarily for non–
small cell lung cancer. Although it is supposed to be applied also to small
cell lung cancers, it is rarely used for the classification of those tumors in
routine clinical practice and in most prospective clinical trials. A more
common approach is to classify small cell lung cancers as either "limited"
or "extensive" stage. Limited stage disease is the equivalent of Stages I

through IIIB in the TNM staging system, and extensive stage small cell lung cancer is the equivalent of Stage IV disease. However, patients with pleural effusions (previously considered to have T4, Stage IIIB disease) are usually classified as having extensive stage disease. Performance status and biochemical parameters such as LDH are also used to categorize small cell lung cancers into prognostic groups.

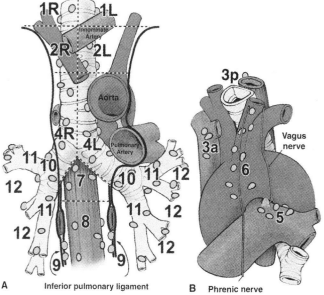

A   Inferior pulmonary ligament   **B**   Phrenic nerve

Fig. 19.1. Lymph node maps of lung

N2 nodes: All N2 nodes lie within the mediastinal pleural envelope on the ipsilateral side.

1. Highest mediastinal nodes
2. Upper paratracheal nodes
3. Prevascular and retrotracheal nodes
4. Lower paratracheal nodes
5. Subaortic nodes (aorto-pulmonary window)

6. Para-aortic nodes (ascending aorta or phrenic)
7. Subcarinal nodes
8. Paraesophageal nodes (below carina)
9. Pulmonary ligament nodes

N1 nodes: All N1 nodes lie distal to the mediastinal pleural reflection and *within the visceral pleura.*

10. Hilar nodes
11. Interlobar nodes
12. Lobar nodes bronchi

13. Segmental nodes
14. Subsegmental nodes

Illustration from ACOSOG protocol Z0030, part 1, pp. 12–13. Used by permission of the Mayo Foundation for Medical Education and Research.

Lymph node classification adapted from Mountain CF, Dresler CM: Regional lymph node classification for lung cancer staging. Chest 111:1718–1723, 1977.

Overall survival for small cell lung cancer by TNM staging based on information from the National Cancer Database is shown in Figure 19.2. For the purposes of classifying small cell lung cancers in tumor registries, the TNM system should be used.

Clinical Staging. Clinical staging is based on the non-invasive assessment of the extent of disease and typically includes a combination of medical

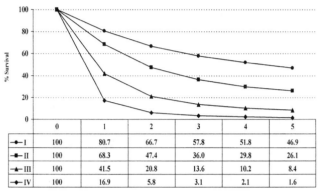

	0	1	2	3	4	5
◆ I	100	80.7	66.7	57.8	51.8	46.9
■ II	100	68.3	47.4	36.0	29.8	26.1
▲ III	100	41.5	20.8	13.6	10.2	8.4
◆ IV	100	16.9	5.8	3.1	2.1	1.6

Years Following Diagnosis

A

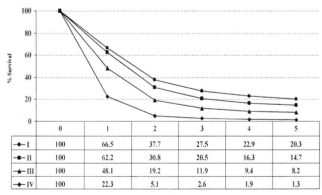

	0	1	2	3	4	5
◆ I	100	66.5	37.7	27.5	22.9	20.3
■ II	100	62.2	30.8	20.5	16.3	14.7
▲ III	100	48.1	19.2	11.9	9.4	8.2
◆ IV	100	22.3	5.1	2.6	1.9	1.3

Years Following Diagnosis

B

Fig. 19.2. Relative survival rates for non–small cell lung cancer (A) and small cell lung cancer (B) diagnosed in the United States in 1992 and 1993. Cases classified by the current staging classification, where pathologic stage group was used to classify each case when available, and clinical stage group was used otherwise. For non–small cell lung cancer, Stage I includes 30,260 patients, Stage II, 8,893 patients, Stage III 38,498 patients, and Stage IV 44,410 patients. For small cell lung cancer, Stage I includes 2,389 patients, Stage II 1,031 patients, Stage III 8,569 patients, and Stage IV 16,568 patients. Data are from the National Cancer Data Base (Commission on Cancer of the American College of Surgeons and the American Cancer Society).

history, physical examination, various imaging procedures (such as computed tomography and positron emission tomography), and laboratory tests. Information from staging procedures such as bronchoscopy, esophagoscopy, mediastinoscopy, mediastinotomy, thoracentesis, and thoracoscopy and information from exploratory thoracotomy are not included in the clinical classification, because these tests generally yield material for pathologic examination. Patients explored and found to have unresectable tumors at thoracotomy should be pathologically staged.

Lung cancer detected by sputum cytology but not seen radiographically or during bronchoscopy is known as "occult" carcinoma and is coded as TX. Occult cancers without evidence of regional lymph node involvement or distant metastasis are coded as TX, N0, M0. Any primary tumor that cannot be assessed—that is, no tumor mass present or evaluable, but lung cancer proven—is designated as TX. T2 is used when there is direct extension into the visceral pleura. T3 is used when the lesion directly invades the parietal pleura covering the mediastinum and pericardium, as well as that lining the chest wall and covering the diaphragm. Invasion of the phrenic nerve by the primary tumor is also classified as T3. Peripheral tumors directly invading the chest wall and ribs are T3 as well.

"Satellite nodules," defined as additional small tumor nodules in the same lobe as the primary tumor, are classified as T4. These nodules are in the same lobe as the primary tumor but are anatomically distinct from it. The term *satellite nodule* refers to tumor nodules identified by imaging studies such as CT scan or by gross findings at thoracotomy, but not to such nodules detected solely on pathologic examination of a resection specimen.

Pleural tumor foci that are separate from direct pleural invasion by the primary tumor should be listed as T4. A separate lesion outside the parietal pleura, in the chest wall, or in the diaphragm should be designated as M1.

Patients with a malignant pleural effusion—that is, either cytologically positive for cancer cells or clinically related to the underlying malignancy—are coded T4. However, such patients are thought to have a poor prognosis and are usually treated primarily with chemotherapy as though they had M1 disease. The T4 classification of patients who have pleural metastases requires further study and may be reconsidered in the future.

Pericardial effusion is currently classified as T4 unless clearly of benign etiology (such as viral pericarditis and congestive heart failure). A malignant pericardial effusion usually develops as a result of hematogenous or lymphatic tumor dissemination and is usually associated with a short life expectancy. Like the T4 classification for pleural metastases, the classification of pericardial metastases requires further study and may be reconsidered in the future.

Vocal cord paralysis (resulting from involvement of the recurrent branch of the vagus nerve), superior vena caval obstruction, or compression of the trachea or esophagus may be related to direct extension of the primary tumor or to lymph node involvement. The treatment options and prognosis associated with these manifestations of disease extent fall within the T4-Stage IIIB category; therefore, a classification of T4 is recommended. If the primary tumor is peripheral and clearly unrelated to vocal cord paralysis, vena caval obstruction, or compression of the trachea and esophagus, vocal cord paralysis is usually related to the presence of N2 disease in the aortopulmonary window and should be classified as such.

The designation of "Pancoast" tumors refers to the symptom complex or syndrome caused by a tumor arising in the superior sulcus of the lung that involves the inferior branches of the brachial plexus (C8 and/or T1) and the sympathetic nerve trunks, including the stellate ganglion. Some superior sulcus tumors are more anteriorly located and may cause fewer neurologic symptoms even when they are very locally advanced and encase the subclavian vessels. The extent of disease varies in these tumors, and they should be classified according to the established rules. If there is evidence of invasion of the vertebral body or spinal canal, encasement of the subclavian vessels, or unequivocal involvement of the superior branches of the brachial plexus (C8 or above), then the tumor is classified as T4. If no criteria for T4 disease pertain, the tumor is classified as T3.

Tumors directly invading the diaphragm in the absence of other signs of locally advanced disease are rare, constituting less than 1% of all cases of potentially resectable non–small cell lung cancers. These tumors are considered to be T3, but they appear to have a poor prognosis, even after complete resection and in the absence of N2 disease. The classification of such tumors may need to be re-evaluated in the future as more survival data become available.

Pathologic Staging. Pathologic staging is based on the information obtained from clinical staging, a variety of staging procedures including thoracotomy, and from examination of the resected specimen, including lymph nodes. The same classification applies to both clinical and pathologic staging. The histologic type of cancer should be recorded, because it also has a bearing on prognosis.

Multiple synchronous tumors should be considered separate primary lung cancers, and each should be staged separately. For single-patient data entry, the highest stage of disease should be recorded, with separate coding to identify multiple primary tumors. Synchronous tumors may be identified according to the criteria originally proposed by Martini and Melamed. These include multiple synchronous tumors of different histologic cell types; or two tumors of the same histologic type in separate lobes with no evidence of extrathoracic disease, of mediastinal nodal metastases, or of nodal metastases within a common nodal drainage (for example, involved interlobar nodes with right upper- and lower-lobe tumors of the same histology).

Bronchioloalveolar carcinomas may pose unique problems for staging because of their tendency to form multiple primary tumors, either synchronous or metachronous. Further investigation is required to determine the appropriate classification of multiple synchronous bronchioloalveolar carcinomas. However, at the present time, these tumors should be classified according to the rules of synchronous tumors or metastatic disease that are used for other histologic types.

DEFINITION OF TNM

Primary Tumor (T)

TX   Primary tumor cannot be assessed, or tumor proven by the presence of malignant cells in sputum or bronchial washings but not visualized by imaging or bronchoscopy

T0   No evidence of primary tumor

Tis   Carcinoma *in situ*

T1   Tumor 3 cm or less in greatest dimension, surrounded by lung or visceral pleura, without bronchoscopic evidence of invasion more proximal than the lobar bronchus,* (i.e., not in the main bronchus)

T2   Tumor with any of the following features of size or extent:
More than 3 cm in greatest dimension
Involves main bronchus, 2 cm or more distal to the carina
Invades the visceral pleura
Associated with atelectasis or obstructive pneumonitis that extends to the hilar region but does not involve the entire lung

T3   Tumor of any size that directly invades any of the following: chest wall (including superior sulcus tumors), diaphragm, mediastinal pleura, parietal pericardium; or tumor in the main bronchus less than 2 cm distal to the carina, but without involvement of the carina; or associated atelectasis or obstructive pneumonitis of the entire lung

T4   Tumor of any size that invades any of the following: mediastinum, heart, great vessels, trachea, esophagus, vertebral body, carina; or separate tumor nodules in the same lobe; or tumor with malignant pleural effusion**

Note: The uncommon superficial tumor of any size with its invasive component limited to the bronchial wall, which may extend proximal to the main bronchus, is also classified T1.

**Note*: Most pleural effusions associated with lung cancer are due to tumor. However, there are a few patients in whom multiple cytopathologic examinations of pleural fluid are negative for tumor. In these cases, fluid is non-bloody and is not an exudate. Such patients may be further evaluated by videothoracoscopy (VATS) and direct pleural biopsies. When these elements and clinical judgment dictate that the effusion is not related to the tumor, the effusion should be excluded as a staging element and the patient should be staged T1, T2, or T3.

Regional Lymph Nodes (N)

NX   Regional lymph nodes cannot be assessed

N0   No regional lymph node metastasis

N1   Metastasis to ipsilateral peribronchial and/or ipsilateral hilar lymph nodes, and intrapulmonary nodes including involvement by direct extension of the primary tumor

N2   Metastasis to ipsilateral mediastinal and/or subcarinal lymph nodes(s)

N3   Metastasis to contralateral mediastinal, contralateral hilar, ipsilateral or contralateral scalene, or supraclavicular lymph nodes(s)

Distant Metastasis (M)

MX   Distant metastasis cannot be assessed
M0   No distant metastasis
M1   Distant metastasis present

Note: M1 includes separate tumor nodule(s) in a different lobe (ipsilateral or contralateral).

STAGE GROUPING			
Occult Carcinoma	TX	N0	M0
Stage 0	Tis	N0	M0
Stage IA	T1	N0	M0
Stage IB	T2	N0	M0
Stage IIA	T1	N1	M0
Stage IIB	T2	N1	M0
	T3	N0	M0
Stage IIIA	T1	N2	M0
	T2	N2	M0
	T3	N1	M0
	T3	N2	M0
Stage IIIB	Any T	N3	M0
	T4	Any N	M0
Stage IV	Any T	Any N	M1

HISTOPATHOLOGIC TYPE

Squamous cell carcinoma
   Variants: Papillary, clear cell, small cell, basaloid
Small cell carcinoma
   Variant: Combined small cell carcinoma
Adenocarcinoma
  Acinar
  Papillary
  Bronchioloalveolar carcinoma
    Non-mucinous
    Mucinous
    Mixed mucinous and non-mucinous or indeterminate
    Solid adenocarcinoma with mucin formation
Adenocarcinoma with mixed subtypes
    Variants: Well differentiated fetal adenocarcinoma, mucinous ("colloid") adenocarcinoma, mucinous cystadenocarcinoma, signet ring adenocarcinoma, clear cell adenocarcinoma
Large cell carcinoma
    Variants: Large cell neuroendocrine carcinoma, combined large cell neuroendocrine carcinoma, basaloid carcinoma, lymphoepithelioma-like carcinoma, clear cell carcinoma, large cell carcinoma with rhabdoid phenotype

---

Note: This summarizes the classification of the four major histologic types of lung cancer from the 1999 WHO/IASLC Histologic Typing of Lung and Pleural Tumors. An important change from the previous classifications is that bronchioloalveolar carcinoma is now limited to non-invasive tumors with lepidic spread. If stromal, vascular, or pleural invasion is seen, the tumor is reclassified as adenocarcinoma, mixed subtype, with specification of the subtypes that are present.

HISTOLOGIC GRADE (G)

GX   Grade cannot be assessed
G1   Well differentiated
G2   Moderately differentiated
G3   Poorly differentiated
G4   Undifferentiated

PROGNOSTIC FACTORS

The prognostic significance of histologic cell type and anatomic extent of disease in lung cancer is generally accepted. Small cell carcinoma, characterized by rapid growth and widespread dissemination, even in clinically "early" disease is recognized as a separate entity from the non–small cell histologies—adenocarcinoma, large cell carcinoma and squamous cell carcinoma. Treatment selection and survival are significantly related to the stage and histologic classifications. It must be kept in mind that the diagnostic process will affect the accuracy of clinical staging. Series of patients in whom mediastinoscopy is required for surgical selection or those in whom a complete lymph node dissection is performed at operation will have fewer errors reported than may be reported for patients in whom these procedures are not performed.

Clinical Factors.   Performance status and severity of symptoms have prognostic significance in non–small cell carcinoma; these factors may be related either to the spread of the cancer or to associated conditions that limit treatment—for example, the cardiac and pulmonary complications associated with advancing age, as well as with tobacco use. Weight loss (more than 10% of body weight) has an adverse effect on prognosis and is predictive of recurrence in patients who have undergone resection. Differing studies have identified gender, age, and various physiologic components as indicators of a poor outcome; however, most are not reproduced in large-scale studies of well-defined lung cancer populations.

A large number of clinical, laboratory, serologic, paraneoplastic, and immune factors have been investigated for their prognostic influence on specific groups of patients with small cell carcinoma. Lactate dehydrogenase (LDH), alkaline phosphatase, albumin, hemoglobin and white blood count, and specific sites of metastasis have been identified as significant prognostic factors.

Anatomic Factors.   Each of the staging components—the primary tumor, the regional lymph nodes, and distant metastasis—has a profound effect on prognosis. The most deleterious factor is the presence of distant metastatic disease. Involvement of multiple distant sites has more serious implications than single-site metastasis, which may be responsive to available treatment in a few instances (for example, surgical treatment of solitary brain lesions and response to chemotherapy or combined regimens).

The presence or absence of regional lymph node metastasis has significant bearing on prognosis. When lymph node metastasis has progressed beyond the ipsilateral hemithorax, the outcome is very poor. Less than 3% of patients with clinical evidence of N3 disease are expected to survive 5 years or more. Survival rates for patients with metastasis limited to the ipsilateral mediastinal lymph nodes (N2) are influenced by the number and nodal levels involved (upper mediastinal, lower mediastinal, or both, and extracapsular extension).

The prognostic implications of intrapulmonary lymph node metastasis vary with the location of the nodes and the primary tumor status. Metastasis to the hilar nodes carries worse prognosis than disease limited to the lobar and segmental nodes. Involvement of N1 nodes in the presence of larger, more invasive tumors, T2 or T3, indicates a poorer outcome than expected for T1 tumors.

Biologic Factors. Research advances in the field of molecular biology have provided a new understanding of the genetic background of lung cancer. Knowledge of the role of genetic abnormalities and other biologic aberrations in tumorigenesis is the basis for many investigations of biologic markers as indicators of prognosis. In order to take marker information to clinical practice, the marker must bear a strong relationship to patient prognosis and the factor must provide additional prognostic information beyond that provided by conventional factors. No such markers are used as yet for routine staging or determination of prognosis of lung cancer, and further investigation of this area is needed.

BIBLIOGRAPHY

D'Amico TA, Aloia TA, Moore M-BH, et al: Molecular biologic substaging of Stage I lung cancer according to gender and histology. Ann Thorac Surg 69:882–886, 2000

Deschamps C, Pairolero PC, Trastek VF, Payne WS: Multiple primary lung cancers: results of surgical treatment. J Thorac Cardiovasc Surg 99:769–778, 1990

Deslauriers J, Brisson J, Cartier R, et al: Carcinoma of the lung: evaluation of satellite nodules as a factor influencing prognosis after resection. J Thorac Cardiovasc Surg 97:504–512, 1989

Ichinose Y, Yano T, Yokoyama H, Inoue T, Asoh H, Katsuda Y: The correlation between tumor size and lymphatic vessel invasion in resected peripheral stage I non-small-cell lung cancer. A potential risk of limited resection. J Thorac Cardiovasc Surg 108:684–686, 1994

Martini N, Flehinger BJ, Zaman MB, Beattie EJ, Jr.: Results of resection in non–oat cell carcinoma of the lung with mediastinal lymph node metastases. Ann Surg 198:386–397, 1983

Martini N, Melamed MR: Multiple primary lung cancers. J Thorac Cardiovasc Surg 70:606–612, 1975

Martini N, Yellin A, Ginsberg RJ, et al: Management of non–small cell lung cancer with direct mediastinal involvement. Ann Thorac Surg 58:1447–1451, 1994

Patterson GA, Piazza D, Pearson FG, et al: Significance of metastatic disease in subaortic lymph nodes. Ann Thorac Surg. 43:155–159, 1987

Pitz CCM, de la Rivière AB, Elbers HRJ, Westermann CJJ, van den Bosch JM: Results of resection of T3 non–small cell lung cancer invading the mediastinum or main bronchus. Ann Thorac Surg 62:1016–1020, 1996

Quraishi MA, Costanzi JJ, Hokanson J: The natural history of lung cancer with pericardial metastases. Cancer 51:740–742, 1983

Sagawa M, Saito Y, Takahashi S, et al: Clinical and prognostic assessment of patients with resected small peripheral lung cancer lesions. Cancer 66:2653–2657, 1990

Sagawa M, Sakurada A, Fujimura S, et al: Five-year survivors with resected pN2 non–small cell lung carcinoma. Cancer 85:864–868, 1999

Saito Y, Nagamoto N, Ota S-I, et al: Results of surgical treatment for roentgenographically occult bronchogenic squamous cell carcinoma. J Thorac Cardiovasc Surg 104:401–407, 1992

Travis WD, Colby TV, Corrin B, et al: Histologic typing of lung and pleural tumors. In World Health Organization Pathology Panel (Ed.): World Health Organization International Histological Classification of Tumors, 3rd ed. Berlin: Springer-Verlag, 5, 1999

van Velzen E, Snijder RJ, de la Rivière AB, Elbert HJJ, van den Bosch JM: Type of lymph node involvement influences survival rates of T1N1M0 non–small cell lung carcinoma: lymph node involvement by direct extension compared with lobar and hilar node metastases. Chest 110:1469–1473, 1996

Weksler B, Bains M, Burt M, et al: Resection of lung cancer invading the diaphragm. J Thorac Cardiovasc Surg 114:500–501, 1997

Werner-Wasik M, Scott C, Cox JD, et al: Recursive partitioning analysis of 1999 Radiation Therapy Oncology Group (RTOG) patients with locally-advanced non–small cell lung cancer (LA-NSCLC): identification of five groups with different survival. Int J Radiat Oncol Biol Phys 48:1475–1482, 2000

HISTOLOGIES—LUNG

8000/3	Neoplasm, malignant
8001/3	Tumor cells, malignant
8002/3	Malignant tumor, small cell type
8003/3	Malignant tumor, giant cell type
8004/3	Malignant tumor, spindle cell type
8005/3	Malignant tumor, clear cell type
8010/2	Carcinoma *in situ*, NOS
8010/3	Carcinoma, NOS
8011/3	Epithelioma, malignant
8012/3	Large cell carcinoma, NOS
8013/3	Large cell neuroendocrine carcinoma
8014/3	Large cell carcinoma with rhabdoid phenotype
8015/3	Glassy cell carcinoma
8020/3	Carcinoma, undifferentiated, NOS
8021/3	Carcinoma, anaplastic, NOS
8022/3	Pleomorphic carcinoma
8030/3	Giant cell and spindle cell carcinoma
8031/3	Giant cell carcinoma

8032/3	Spindle cell carcinoma, NOS
8033/3	Pseudosarcomatous carcinoma
8034/3	Polygonal cell carcinoma
8035/3	Carcinoma with osteoclast-like giant cells
8041/3	Small cell carcinoma, NOS
8042/3	Oat cell carcinoma
8043/3	Small cell carcinoma, fusiform cell
8044/3	Small cell carcinoma, intermediate cell
8045/3	Combined small cell carcinoma
8046/3	Non–small cell carcinoma
8050/3	Papillary carcinoma, NOS
8051/3	Verrucous carcinoma, NOS
8052/2	Papillary squamous cell carcinoma, non-invasive
8052/3	Papillary squamous cell carcinoma
8070/2	Squamous cell carcinoma *in situ,* NOS
8070/3	Squamous cell carcinoma, NOS
8071/3	Squamous cell carcinoma, keratinizing, NOS
8072/3	Squamous cell carcinoma, large cell, non-keratinizing, NOS
8073/3	Squamous cell carcinoma, small cell, non-keratinizing
8074/3	Squamous cell carcinoma, spindle cell
8075/3	Squamous cell carcinoma, adenoid
8076/2	Squamous cell carcinoma *in situ* with questionable stromal invasion
8076/3	Squamous cell carcinoma, microinvasive
8077/2	Squamous intraepithelial neoplasia, grade III
8082/3	Lymphoepithelial carcinoma
8083/3	Basaloid squamous cell carcinoma
8084/3	Squamous cell carcinoma, clear cell type
8090/3	Basal cell carcinoma, NOS
8093/3	Basal cell carcinoma, fibroepithelial
8094/3	Basosquamous carcinoma
8097/3	Basal cell carcinoma, nodular
8120/3	Transitional cell carcinoma, NOS
8122/3	Transitional cell carcinoma, spindle cell
8123/3	Basaloid carcinoma
8140/2	Adenocarcinoma *in situ,* NOS
8140/3	Adenocarcinoma, NOS
8141/3	Scirrhous adenocarcinoma
8147/3	Basal cell adenocarcinoma
8148/2	Glandular intraepithelial neoplasia, grade III
8200/3	Adenoid cystic carcinoma
8211/3	Tubular adenocarcinoma
8230/3	Solid adenocarcinoma with mucin formation
8250/3	Bronchiolo-alveolar adenocarcinoma, NOS
8251/3	Alveolar adenocarcinoma
8252/3	Bronchiolo-alveolar carcinoma, non-mucinous
8253/3	Bronchiolo-alveolar carcinoma, mucinous
8254/3	Bronchiolo-alveolar carcinoma, mixed mucinous and non-mucinous
8255/3	Adenocarcinoma with mixed subtypes
8260/3	Papillary adenocarcinoma, NOS
8310/3	Clear cell adenocarcinoma, NOS
8314/3	Lipid-rich carcinoma
8315/3	Glycogen-rich carcinoma
8320/3	Granular cell carcinoma

8323/3	Mixed cell adenocarcinoma
8333/3	Fetal adenocarcinoma
8341/3	Papillary microcarcinoma
8342/3	Papillary carcinoma, oxyphilic cell
8343/3	Papillary carcinoma, encapsulated
8430/3	Mucoepidermoid carcinoma
8440/3	Cystadenocarcinoma, NOS
8441/3	Serous cystadenocarcinoma, NOS
8450/3	Papillary cystadenocarcinoma, NOS
8452/3	Solid pseudopapillary carcinoma
8470/3	Mucinous cystadenocarcinoma, NOS
8471/3	Papillary mucinous cystadenocarcinoma
8480/3	Mucinous adenocarcinoma
8481/3	Mucin-producing adenocarcinoma
8490/3	Signet ring cell carcinoma
8525/3	Polymorphous low grade adenocarcinoma
8530/3	Inflammatory carcinoma
8550/3	Acinar cell carcinoma
8551/3	Acinar cell cystadenocarcinoma
8560/3	Adenosquamous carcinoma
8562/3	Epithelial-myoepithelial carcinoma
8570/3	Adenocarcinoma with squamous metaplasia
8571/3	Adenocarcinoma with cartilaginous and osseous metaplasia
8572/3	Adenocarcinoma with spindle cell metaplasia
8573/3	Adenocarcinoma with apocrine metaplasia
8720/3	Malignant melanoma, NOS *(primary only)*
8815/3	Solitary fibrous tumor, malignant
8940/3	Mixed tumor, malignant, NOS
8941/3	Carcinoma in pleomorphic adenoma

4

20

Pleural Mesothelioma

(Tumors metastatic to the pleura and lung tumors that have extended to the pleural surfaces are not included.)

C38.4 Pleura, NOS

SUMMARY OF CHANGES

- The AJCC has adopted the staging system proposed by the International Mesothelioma Interest Group (IMIG) in 1995. It is based on updated information about the relationships between tumor T and N status and overall survival. This staging system applies only to tumors arising in the pleura.

- T categories have been redefined.

- T1 lesions have been divided into T1a and T1b, leading to the division of Stage I into Stage IA and Stage IB.

- T3 is defined as locally advanced but potentially resectable tumor.

- T4 is defined as locally advanced, technically unresectable tumor.

- Stage II no longer involves tumors with nodal metastasis; all nodal metastasis is categorized in Stage III or Stage IV.

INTRODUCTION

Malignant mesotheliomas are relatively rare tumors that arise from the mesothelium lining the pleural, pericardial, and peritoneal cavities. They represent less than 2% of all malignant tumors. The most common risk factor for malignant mesotheliomas is previous exposure to asbestos. The latency period between asbestos exposure and the development of malignant mesothelioma is generally 20 years or more. Although peritoneal mesotheliomas are thought to occur in individuals who have had heavier exposure than those with pleural mesothelioma, there is no clearly documented relationship between the amount of asbestos exposure and the subsequent development of this neoplasm. Malignant mesotheliomas were previously thought to be virulent tumors. However, this impression was probably related to the fact that most mesotheliomas are diagnosed when they are already at an advanced stage. Recent data indicate that the clinical and biological behavior of mesotheliomas is variable and that most mesotheliomas grow relatively slowly.

All mesotheliomas are fundamentally epithelial tumors. However, their morphology ranges from a pure epithelial appearance to an entirely sarcomatoid or even desmoplastic appearance. Distinguishing the pleiomorphic histology of mesotheliomas from that of other neoplasms can be difficult, especially for the pure epithelial mesotheliomas, which may closely resemble metastatic adenocarcinoma. Therefore, confirmation of the histologic diagnosis by immunohistochemistry and/or electron microscopy is essential.

During the past 30 years, many staging systems have been proposed for malignant pleural mesothelioma. The first staging system for this disease published by the American Joint Committee on Cancer (AJCC), and simultaneously accepted by the International Union Against Cancer, appeared in the fifth edition of the *AJCC Cancer Staging Manual*. The staging system described here represents adoption of the one proposed in 1995 by the International Mesothelioma Interest Group (IMIG), which is based on updated information about the relationships between tumor T and N status and overall survival. Although this system has been validated by several surgical reports, it will probably require revision in the future as further data in larger numbers of patients become available. This staging system applies only to tumors arising in the pleura. Peritoneal and pericardial mesotheliomas are rare and do not lend themselves easily to a TNM staging system.

ANATOMY

Primary Site.   The mesothelium covers the external surface of the lungs and the inside of the chest wall. It is usually composed of flat, tightly connected cells no more than one layer thick.

Regional Lymph Nodes.   The regional lymph nodes include:

> Internal mammary
> Intrathoracic
> Scalene
> Supraclavicular

The regional lymph node map and nomenclature adopted for the mesothelioma staging system is identical to that used for lung cancer. See Chapter 19 for a detailed list of intrathoracic lymph nodes. For pN, histologic examination of a mediastinal lymphadenectomy or lymph node sampling specimen will ordinarily include regional nodes taken from the ipsilateral N1 and N2 nodal stations. Contralateral and supraclavicular nodes may be available if a mediastinoscopy or node biopsy is also performed.

Distant Metastatic Sites.   Advanced malignant pleural mesotheliomas often metastasize widely to uncommon sites, including retroperitoneal lymph nodes, the brain and spine, or even organs such as the thyroid or prostate. However, the most frequent sites of metastatic disease are the peritoneum, contralateral pleura, and lung.

RULES FOR CLASSIFICATION

This staging system serves both clinical and pathologic staging. Clinical staging depends on imaging, especially computed tomography scanning. Pathologic staging is based on surgical resection. The extent of disease before and after resection should be carefully documented. In some cases, complete N staging may not be possible, especially if technically unresectable tumor (T4) found at thoracotomy prevents access to both N1 and N2 lymph nodes.

DEFINITION OF TNM

IMIG Staging System for Diffuse Malignant Pleural Mesothelioma

Primary Tumor (T)

TX   Primary tumor cannot be assessed

T0   No evidence of primary tumor

T1   Tumor involves ipsilateral parietal pleura, with or without focal involvement of visceral pleura

T1a   Tumor involves ipsilateral parietal (mediastinal, diaphragmatic) pleura. No involvement of the visceral pleura

T1b   Tumor involves ipsilateral parietal (mediastinal, diaphragmatic) pleura, with focal involvement of the visceral pleura

T2   Tumor involves any of the ipsilateral pleural surfaces with at least one of the following:
        —confluent visceral pleural tumor (including fissure)
        —invasion of diaphragmatic muscle
        —invasion of lung parenchyma

T3*   Tumor involves any of the ipsilateral pleural surfaces, with at least one of the following:
        —invasion of the endothoracic fascia
        —invasion into mediastinal fat
        —solitary focus of tumor invading the soft tissues of the chest wall
        —non-transmural involvement of the pericardium

T4**   Tumor involves any of the ipsilateral pleural surfaces, with at least one of the following:
        —diffuse or multifocal invasion of soft tissues of the chest wall
        —any involvement of rib
        —invasion through the diaphragm to the peritoneum
        —invasion of any mediastinal organ(s)
        —direct extension to the contralateral pleura
        —invasion into the spine
        —extension to the internal surface of the pericardium
        —pericardial effusion with positive cytology
        —invasion of the myocardium
        —invasion of the brachial plexus

*T3 describes locally advanced but potentially resectable tumor

**T4 describes locally advanced, technically unresectable tumor

Regional Lymph Nodes (N)

NX   Regional lymph nodes cannot be assessed

N0   No regional lymph node metastases

N1   Metastases in the ipsilateral bronchopulmonary and/or hilar lymph node(s)

N2   Metastases in the subcarinal lymph node(s) and/or the ipsilateral internal mammary or mediastinal lymph node(s)

N3   Metastases in the contralateral mediastinal, internal mammary, or hilar lymph node(s) and/or the ipsilateral or contralateral supra-clavicular or scalene lymph node(s)

Distant Metastasis (M)

MX   Distant metastases cannot be assessed
M0   No distant metastasis
M1   Distant metastasis

STAGE GROUPING			
Stage I	T1	N0	M0
Stage IA	T1a	N0	M0
Stage IB	T1b	N0	M0
Stage II	T2	N0	M0
Stage III	T1, T2	N1	M0
	T1, T2	N2	M0
	T3	N0, N1, N2	M0
Stage IV	T4	Any N	M0
	Any T	N3	M0
	Any T	Any N	M1

HISTOPATHOLOGIC TYPE

There are four types of malignant pleural mesothelioma. They are listed here in descending order of frequency.

Epithelioid
Biphasic (at least 10% of both epithelioid and sarcomatoid components)
Sarcomatoid
Desmoplastic

In general, the pure epithelioid tumors are associated with a better prognosis than the biphasic or sarcomatoid tumors. Despite their bland histologic appearance, desmoplastic tumors appear to have the worst prognosis. The biology underlying these differences is not yet understood.

BIBLIOGRAPHY

Allen KB, Faber LP, Warren WH: Malignant pleural mesothelioma: extrapleural pneumonectomy and pleurectomy. Chest Surg Clin N Amer 4:113–126, 1994

Boutin C, Rey F, Gouvernet J, Viallat J-R, Astoul P, Ledoray V: Thoracoscopy in pleural malignant mesothelioma: a prospective study of 188 consecutive patients. Part 2: Prognosis and staging. Cancer 72:394–404, 1993

Butchart EG, Ashcroft T, Barnsley WC, Holden MP: Pleuropneumonectomy in the management of diffuse malignant mesothelioma of the pleura: experience with 29 patients. Thorax 31:15–24, 1976

Pass HI, Temeck BK, Kranda K, Steinberg SM, Feuerstein IR: Preoperative tumor volume is associated with outcome in malignant pleural mesothelioma. J Thorac Cardiovasc Surg 115:310–318, 1998

Pass HI, Temeck BK, Kranda K, et al: Phase III randomized trial of surgery with or without intraoperative photodynamic therapy and postoperative immunochemotherapy for malignant pleural mesothelioma. Ann Surg Oncol 4:628–633, 1997

Patz EF Jr., Rusch VW, Heelan R: The proposed new international TNM staging system for malignant pleural mesothelioma: application to imaging. Am J Roentgenol 166:323–327, 1996

Ruffie P, Feld R, Minkin S, et al: Diffuse malignant mesothelioma of the pleura in Ontario and Quebec: a retrospective study of 332 patients. J Clin Oncol 7:1157–1168, 1989

Rusch VW, The International Mesothelioma Interest Group: A proposed new international TNM staging system for malignant pleural mesothelioma. Chest 108:1122–1128, 1995

Rusch VW, Piantadosi S, Holmes EC: The role of extrapleural pneumonectomy in malignant pleural mesothelioma. J Thorac Cardiovasc Surg 102(1):1–9, 1991

Rusch VW, Venkatraman ES: The importance of surgical staging in the treatment of malignant pleural mesothelioma. J Thorac Cardiovasc Surg 111:815–826, 1996

Rusch VW, Venkatraman ES: Important prognostic factors in patients with malignant pleural mesothelioma, managed surgically. Ann Thorac Surg 68:1799–1804, 1999

Sugarbaker DJ, Flores RM, Jaklitsch MT, et al: Resection margins, extrapleural nodal status, and cell type determine postoperative long-term survival in trimodality therapy of malignant pleural mesothelioma: results of 183 patients. J Thorac Cardiovasc Surg 117:54–65, 1999

Sugarbaker DJ, Strauss GM, Lynch TJ, et al: Node status has prognostic significance in the multimodality therapy of diffuse, malignant mesothelioma. J Clin Oncol 11(6):1172–1178, 1993

Tammilehto L, Kivisaari L, Salminen US, Maasilta P, Mattson K: Evaluation of the clinical TNM staging system for malignant pleural mesothelioma: an assessment in 88 patients. Lung Cancer 12:25–34, 1995

HISTOLOGIES—PLEURAL MESOTHELIOMA

9050/3	Mesothelioma, malignant
9051/3	Fibrous mesothelioma, malignant
9052/3	Epithelioid mesothelioma, malignant
9053/3	Mesothelioma, biphasic, malignant

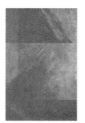

PART V
Musculoskeletal Sites

21

Bone

(Primary malignant lymphoma and multiple myeloma are not included.)

C40.0 Long bones of upper limb, scapula, and associated joints
C40.1 Short bones of upper limb and associated joints
C40.2 Long bones of lower limb and associated joints
C40.3 Short bones of lower limb and associated joints
C40.8 Overlapping lesion of bones, joints, and articular cartilage of limbs
C40.9 Bone of limb, NOS
C41.0 Bones of skull and face and associated joints
C41.1 Mandible
C41.2 Vertebral column
C41.3 Rib, sternum, clavicle, and associated joints
C41.4 Pelvic bones, sacrum, coccyx, and associated joints
C41.8 Overlapping lesion of bones, joints, and articular cartilage
C41.9 Bone, NOS

SUMMARY OF CHANGES

- T1 has changed from "Tumor confined within the cortex" to "Tumor 8 cm or less in greatest dimension."

- T2 has changed from "Tumor invades beyond the cortex" to "Tumor more than 8 cm in greatest dimension."

- T3 designation of skip metastasis is defined as "Discontinuous tumors in the primary bone site." This designation is a Stage III tumor that was not previously defined.

- M1 lesions have been divided into M1a and M1b.

- M1a is lung-only metastases.

- M1b is metastases to other distant sites, including lymph nodes.

- In the Stage Grouping, Stage IVA is M1a, and Stage IVB is M1b.

INTRODUCTION

This classification is used for all primary malignant tumors of bone except primary malignant lymphoma and multiple myeloma. Cases are categorized by histologic type (e.g., osteosarcoma, chondrosarcoma) and by histologic grade of differentiation.

ANATOMY

Primary Site.   All bones of the skeleton.

Regional Lymph Nodes.   Regional lymph metastases from bone tumors is extremely rare.

Metastatic Sites.   A metastatic site includes any site beyond the regional lymph nodes of the primary site. Spread to the lungs is frequent.

RULES FOR CLASSIFICATION

Clinical Staging.   Clinical staging includes all relevant data prior to primary definitive therapy, including physical examination, imaging, and biopsy.

The radiograph remains the mainstay in determining whether a lesion of bone requires further staging and usually is the modality that permits reliable prediction of the probable histology of a lesion of bone.

Staging of all potentially malignant tumors of bone is most accurately achieved by magnetic resonance (MR) imaging. Axial imaging, complemented by either coronal or sagittal imaging planes using T1 and T2 weighted SPIN echo sequences, most often provides accurate depiction of intra- and extraosseous tumor. To improve conspicuity in locations such as the pelvis or vertebrae, these sequences could be augmented by fat-suppressed pulse sequences. The maximum dimension of the tumor must be measured prior to any treatment.

Computerized tomography has a limited role in local staging of tumors but remains the examination of choice for evaluating the thorax for metastatic disease. In those situations, usually in flat bones such as the pelvis, scapula, or posterior elements of the vertebrae where characterization of a lesion by radiography may be incomplete or difficult because of inadequate visualization of the matrix of a lesion, CT is preferred to MR imaging. The role of CT in these circumstances is to characterize the lesion and determine whether it is potentially malignant or not, and the obtained CT images may suffice for local staging.

Technetium scintigraphy is the examination of choice for evaluating the entire skeleton to determine whether there are multiple lesions. The role of positron emission tomography (PET) in the evaluation and staging of bone sarcomas, if any, has not yet been determined.

Biopsy of the tumor completes the staging process, and the location of the biopsy must be carefully planned to allow for eventual en bloc resection of a malignant neoplasm together with the entire biopsy tract. Staging of the lesion should precede biopsy. Imaging the tumor after biopsy may compromise the accuracy of the staging process. The pathologic diagnosis is based on the microscopic examination of tissue, correlated with imaging studies.

Pathologic Staging.   Pathologic staging includes pathologic data obtained from examination of a resected specimen sufficient to evaluate the highest T category, histopathologic type and grade, regional lymph nodes as appropriate, or distant metastasis. Because regional lymph node involvement from bone tumors is rare, the pathologic stage grouping includes any of the following combinations: pT pG pN pM, or pT pG cN cM, or cT cN pM.

DEFINITION OF TNM

Primary Tumor (T)

TX   Primary tumor cannot be assessed
T0   No evidence of primary tumor
T1   Tumor 8 cm or less in greatest dimension
T2   Tumor more than 8 cm in greatest dimension
T3   Discontinuous tumors in the primary bone site

Regional Lymph Nodes (N)

NX   Regional lymph nodes cannot be assessed
N0   No regional lymph node metastasis
N1   Regional lymph node metastasis

Note: Because of the rarity of lymph node involvement in sarcomas, the designation NX may not be appropriate and could be considered N0 if no clinical involvement is evident.

Distant Metastasis (M)

MX   Distant metastasis cannot be assessed
M0   No distant metastasis
M1   Distant metastasis
M1a   Lung
M1b   Other distant sites

STAGE GROUPING

Stage IA	T1	N0	M0	G1,2 Low grade
Stage IB	T2	N0	M0	G1,2 Low grade
Stage IIA	T1	N0	M0	G3,4 High grade
Stage IIB	T2	N0	M0	G3,4 High grade
Stage III	T3	N0	M0	Any G
Stage IVA	Any T	N0	M1a	Any G
Stage IVB	Any T	N1	Any M	Any G
	Any T	Any N	M1b	Any G

HISTOLOGIC GRADE (G)

GX   Grade cannot be assessed
G1   Well differentiated—Low Grade
G2   Moderately differentiated—Low Grade
G3   Poorly differentiated—High Grade
G4   Undifferentiated—High Grade

Note: Ewing's sarcoma is classified as G4.

CLASSIFICATION OF PRIMARY MALIGNANT BONE TUMORS

I. Osteosarcoma
   A. Intramedullary high grade
      1. Osteoblastic
      2. Chondroblastic
      3. Fibroblastic
      4. Mixed
      5. Small cell
      6. Other (telangiectatic, epithelioid, chondromyxoid fibroma-like, chondroblastoma-like, osteoblastoma-like, giant cell rich)
   B. Intramedullary low grade
   C. Juxtacortical high grade (high grade surface osteosarcoma)
   D. Juxtacortical intermediate grade chondroblastic (periosteal osteosarcoma)
   E. Juxtacortical low grade (parosteal osteosarcoma)

II. Chondrosarcoma
   A. Intramedullary
      1. Conventional (hyaline/myxoid)
      2. Clear cell
      3. Dedifferentiated
      4. Mesenchymal
   B. Juxtacortical

III. Primitive neuroectodermal tumor/Ewing's sarcoma

IV. Angiosarcoma
   A. Conventional
   B. Epithelioid hemangioendothelioma

V. Fibrosarcoma/malignant fibrous histiocytoma

VI. Chordoma
   A. Conventional
   B. Dedifferentiated

VII. Adamantinoma
   A. Conventional
   B. Well differentiated–osteofibrous dysplasia-like

VIII. Other
   A. Liposarcoma
   B. Leiomyosarcoma
   C. Malignant peripheral nerve sheath tumor
   D. Rhabdomyosarcoma
   E. Malignant mesenchymoma
   F. Malignant hemangiopericytoma
   G. Sarcoma, NOS; primary malignant lymphoma; and multiple myeloma are not included.

PROGNOSTIC FACTORS

Known prognostic factors for malignant bone tumors are as follows: (1) T1 tumors have a better prognosis than T2 tumors. (2) Histopathologic low grade (G1, G2) has a better prognosis than high grade (G3,G4).

(3) Location of the primary tumor is a prognostic factor. Patients who have an anatomically resectable primary tumor have a better prognosis than those with a non-resectable tumor, and tumors of the spine and pelvis tend to have a poor prognosis. (4) The size of the primary tumor is a prognostic factor for osteosarcoma and Ewing's sarcoma. Ewing's sarcoma patients with a tumor 8 cm or less in greatest dimension have a better prognosis than those with a tumor greater than 8 cm. Osteosarcoma patients with a tumor 9 cm or less in greatest dimension have a better prognosis than those with a tumor greater than 9 cm. (5) Patients who have a localized primary tumor have a better prognosis than those with metastases. (6) Certain metastatic sites are associated with a poorer prognosis than other sites: bony and hepatic metastases convey a much worse prognosis than do lung metastases, and patients with solitary lung metastases have a better prognosis than those with multiple lung lesions. (7) Histologic response of the primary tumor to chemotherapy is a prognostic factor for osteosarcoma and Ewing's sarcoma. Those patients with a "good" response, >90% tumor necrosis, have a better prognosis than those with less necrosis. (8) Recent studies have shown that the biologic behavior of osteosarcoma and Ewing's sarcoma is related to specific molecular abnormalities identified in these neoplasms. The prognostically relevant molecular aberrations can be classified into the broad categories of gene translocations, expression of multidrug-resistance genes, expression of growth factor receptors, and mutations in cell cycle regulators. Specifically, Ewing's sarcomas having the EWS-FL1 type 1 translocation, which appears to code for a weaker transactivator, have a better prognosis than those that have other types of translocations. Studies examining the expression of the multidrug-resistance gene MDR1 and its protein product P-glycoprotein in osteosarcoma have reported conflicting results; some investigations have shown that the expression of P-glycoprotein is associated with a poor outcome, whereas a prospective analysis did not find a correlation with MDR1 RNA expression and disease progression. High levels of expression of the c-erbB-2 proto-oncogene, which encodes the human epidermal growth factor receptor 2 (HER2), in osteosarcomas, has been shown to correlate with an inferior histologic response of tumors to preoperative chemotherapy, as well as with decreased patient event-free survival. In Ewing's sarcoma, the status of the cell cycle regulators P53 and INK4A has been shown to correlate with outcome; tumors that express P53 or have a deletion of INK4A have a poorer outcome than those that do not demonstrate these abnormalities. It is anticipated that future investigations on the molecular profile of bone sarcomas will provide valuable information regarding their genesis and prognosis.

BIBLIOGRAPHY

Bacci G, Ferrari S, Bertoni F, et al: Prognostic factors in nonmetastatic Ewing's sarcoma of bone treated with adjuvant chemotherapy: analysis of 359 patients at the Istituto Ortopedico Rizzoli. J Clin Oncol 18:4–11, 2000

Baldini M, Scotlani K, Barbanti-Brodano G, et al: Expression of P-glycoprotein in high-grade osteosarcomas in relation to clinical outcome. N Engl J Med 333:1380–1385, 1995

Bieling P, Rehan N, Winkler P, et al: Tumor size and prognosis in aggressively treated osteosarcoma. J Clin Oncol 14(3):848–858, 1996

Cotterill SJ, Ahrens S, Paulussen M, et al: Prognostic factors in Ewing's tumor of bone: analysis of 975 patients from the European Intergroup Cooperative Ewing's Sarcoma Study Group. J Clin Oncol 18:3108–3114, 2000

Davis A, Bell R, Goodwin P: Prognostic factors in osteosarcoma: a critical review. J Clin Oncol 12(2):423–431, 1994

de Alva E, Antonescu CR, Panizo A, et al: Prognostic impact of P53 status in Ewing sarcoma. Cancer; 89:783–792, 2000

de Alva E, Kawai A, Healey JH, et al: EWS-FL11 fusion transcript structure is an independent determinant of prognosis in Ewing's sarcoma. J Clin Oncol 16:1248–1255, 1998

Enneking WF, Spanier S, Goodman M: A system for the surgical staging of musculoskeletal sarcoma. Clin Orth and Rel Research No. 153, 106–120, 1980

Evans R, Nesbit M, Askin F, et al: Local recurrence, rate and sites of metastases, and time to relapse as a function of treatment regimen, size of primary and surgical history in 62 patients presenting with nonmetastatic Ewing's sarcoma of the pelvic bones. Int J Radiat Oncol Biol Phys 11:129–136, 1985

Glasser DB, Lane JM, Huvos AG, et al: Survival, prognosis and therapeutic response in osteosarcoma: the Memorial Hospital experience. Cancer 67:698–708, 1992

Gorlick R, Hubos AG, Heller G, et al: Expression of HER2/erbB-2 correlates with survival in osteosarcoma. J Clin Oncol 17:2781–2788, 1999

Hornicek FJ, Gebhardt MC, Wolfe M, et al: P-glycoprotein levels predict poor outcome in patients with osteosarcoma. Clin Orthop and Rel Research 373:11–17, 2000

Mankin HJ, Mankin CJ, Simon MA: The hazards of biopsy, revisited. J Bone and Joint Surg 78A:659–663, 1996

Peabody TD, Gibbs CP, Simon MA: Evaluation and staging of musculoskeletal neoplasms. J Bone and Joint Surg 80A:1204–1218, 1998

Scully SP, Temple HT, Okeefe RJ, et al: Role of surgical resection in pelvic Ewing's sarcoma. J Clin Oncol 13(9):2336–2341, 1995

Simon MA, Bierman JS: Biopsy of bone and soft-tissue lesions. J Bone and Joint Surg 75A:616–621, 1993

Sundaram M, McDonald DJ: Magnetic resonance imaging in the evaluation of the solitary tumor of bone. Current Opinion in Radiology 2:697–702, 1990

Sundaram M, McDonald DJ: The solitary tumor or tumor-like lesion of bone. Top Magn Reson Imag 1(4):17–29, 1989

Sundaram M, McGuire MH: Computed tomography or magnetic resonance for evaluating the solitary tumor or tumor-like lesion of bone? Skeletal Radiology 17:393–401, 1988

Ward WG, Mikaelian K, Dorey F, et al: Pulmonary metastases of stage IIB extremity osteosarcoma and subsequent pulmonary metastases. J Clin Oncol 12(9):1849–1858, 1994

Wei G, Antonescu CR, de Alva E, et al: Prognostic impact of INK4A deletion in Ewing sarcoma. Cancer 89:793–799, 2000

Wuisman P, Enneking WF: Prognosis for patients who have osteosarcoma with skip metastasis. J Bone and Joint Surg 72A(1):60–68, 1990

Wunder JS, Bull SB, Aneliunas V, et al: MDR1 gene expression and outcome in osteosarcoma: a prospective, multicenter study. J Clin Oncol 18:2685–2694, 2000

HISTOLOGIES—BONE

8810/3	Fibrosarcoma, NOS
8812/3	Periosteal fibrosarcoma
8814/3	Infantile fibrosarcoma
8830/3	Malignant fibrous histiocytoma
8850/3	Liposarcoma, NOS
8890/3	Leiomyosarcoma, NOS
8900/3	Rhabdomyosarcoma, NOS
8990/3	Malignant mesenchymoma
9120/3	Angiosarcoma, NOS
9130/3	Hemangioendothelioma, malignant
9133/3	Epithelioid hemangioendothelioma, malignant
9150/3	Hemangiopericytoma, malignant
9170/3	Lymphangiosarcoma
9180/3	Osteosarcoma, NOS
9181/3	Chondroblastic osteosarcoma
9182/3	Fibroblastic osteosarcoma
9183/3	Telangiectatic osteoscarcoma
9184/3	Osteosarcoma in Paget disease of bone
9185/3	Small cell osteosarcoma
9186/3	Central osteosarcoma
9187/3	Intraosseous well differentiated osteosarcoma
9192/3	Parosteal osteosarcoma
9193/3	Periosteal osteosarcoma
9194/3	High grade surface osteosarcoma
9195/3	Intracortical osteosarcoma
9220/3	Chondrosarcoma, NOS
9221/3	Juxtacortical chondrosarcoma
9230/3	Chondroblastoma, malignant
9231/3	Myxoid chondrosarcoma
9240/3	Mesenchymal chondrosarcoma
9242/3	Clear cell chondrosarcoma
9243/3	Dedifferentiated chondrosarcoma
9250/3	Giant cell tumor of bone, malignant
9260/3	Ewing sarcoma
9261/3	Adamantinoma of long bones
9310/3	Adamantinoma, malignant
9364/3	Peripheral neuroectodermal tumor
9370/3	Chordoma, NOS
9371/3	Chondroid chordoma
9372/3	Dedifferentiated chordoma
9540/3	Malignant peripheral nerve sheath tumor
9560/3	Neurilemoma, malignant

5

22

Soft Tissue Sarcoma

(Kaposi's sarcoma, dermatofibrosarcoma protuberans, fibromatosis [desmoid tumor], and sarcoma arising from the dura mater, brain, parenchymatous organs, or hollow viscera are not included.)

C38.0 Heart
C38.1 Anterior mediastinum
C38.2 Posterior mediastinum
C38.3 Mediastinum, NOS
C38.8 Overlapping lesion of heart, mediastinum, and pleura
C47.0 Peripheral nerves and autonomic nervous system of head, face, and neck
C47.1 Peripheral nerves and autonomic nervous system of upper limb and shoulder
C47.2 Peripheral nerves and autonomic nervous system of lower limb and hip
C47.3 Peripheral nerves and autonomic nervous system of thorax
C47.4 Peripheral nerves and autonomic nervous system of abdomen

C47.5 Peripheral nerves and autonomic nervous system of pelvis
C47.6 Peripheral nerves and autonomic nervous system of trunk, NOS
C47.8 Overlapping lesion of peripheral nerves and autonomic nervous system
C47.9 Autonomic nervous system, NOS
C48.0 Retroperitoneum
C48.1 Specified parts of peritoneum
C48.2 Peritoneum, NOS
C48.8 Overlapping lesion of retroperitoneum and peritoneum
C49.0 Connective, subcutaneous, and other soft tissues of head, face, and neck
C49.1 Connective, subcutaneous, and other soft tissues of upper limb and shoulder

C49.2 Connective, subcutaneous, and other soft tissues of lower limb and hip
C49.3 Connective, subcutaneous, and other soft tissues of thorax
C49.4 Connective, subcutaneous, and other soft tissues of abdomen
C49.5 Connective, subcutaneous, and other soft tissues of pelvis
C49.6 Connective, subcutaneous, and other soft tissues of trunk, NOS
C49.8 Overlapping lesion of connective, subcutaneous, and other soft tissues
C49.9 Connective, subcutaneous, and other soft tissues, NOS

SUMMARY OF CHANGES

- Angiosarcoma and malignant mesenchymoma are no longer included in the list of histologic types for this site.

- Gastrointestinal stromal tumor and Ewing's sarcoma/primitive neuroectodermal tumor have been added to the list of histologic types for this site.

- Fibrosarcoma grade I has been replaced by fibromatosis (desmoid tumor) in the list of histologic types *not* included in this site.

- G 1–2, T2b, N0 M0 tumors have been reclassified as Stage I rather than Stage II disease.

INTRODUCTION

The staging system applies to all soft tissue sarcomas except Kaposi's sarcoma, dermatofibrosarcoma, infantile fibrosarcoma, and angiosarcoma. In addition, sarcomas arising within the confines of the dura mater, including the brain, and sarcomas arising in parenchymatous organs and from hollow viscera are not optimally staged by this system.

Data to support this staging system are based on current analyses from multiple institutions and represent the recommendations of an AJCC task force on soft tissue sarcoma. In the era of cytoreductive neoadjuvant treatments, clinical and pathologic staging may be altered in the future. Because pathologic staging drives adjuvant therapy decisions, patients should be restaged after neoadjuvant therapies have been administered.

Histologic type, grade, and tumor size and depth are essential for staging. Histologic grade of a sarcoma is one of the most important parameters of the staging system. Grade is based on analysis of various pathologic features of a tumor, such as histologic subtype, degree of differentiation, mitotic activity, and necrosis. Accurate grading requires an adequate sample of well-fixed tissue for evaluation. Accurate grading is not always possible on the basis of needle biopsies or in tumors that have been previously irradiated or treated with chemotherapy.

The current staging system does not take into account anatomic site. However, anatomic site is known to influence outcome, and therefore outcome data should be reported specifying site. Generic grouping of site is accepted. The following site groups can be used for reports that include sarcomas arising in tissues other than soft tissues (such as parenchymal organs). Extremity and superficial trunk can be combined; viscera, including all the intra-abdominal viscera, can also be combined. Where enough numbers exist, these can be reported by subdivision into the various components of the gastrointestinal tract. Lung, gastrointestinal, genitourinary, and gynecologic sarcomas should be grouped separately.

Site Groups for Soft Tissue Sarcoma
Head and neck
Extremity and superficial trunk
Gastrointestinal
Genitourinary
Visceral
Retroperitoneal
Gynecologic
Breast
Lung, pleura, mediastinum
Other

STAGING OF SOFT TISSUE SARCOMA

Inclusions. The present staging system applies to soft tissue sarcomas. Primary sarcomas can arise from a variety of soft tissues. These tissues include fibrous connective tissue, fat, smooth or striated muscle, vascular tissue, peripheral neural tissue, and visceral tissue.

Regional Lymph Nodes. Involvement of regional lymph nodes by soft tissue sarcomas is uncommon in adults. When present, regional nodal disease has prognostic significance similar to that of visceral metastatic disease.

Metastatic Sites. Metastatic sites for soft tissue sarcoma are often dependent on the original site of the primary lesion. For example, the most common site of metastatic disease for patients with extremity sarcoma is the lung, whereas retroperitoneal and gastrointestinal sarcomas often have liver as the first site of metastasis.

RULES FOR CLASSIFICATION

Clinical Staging. Clinical staging is dependent on characteristics of T, N, and M. T is divided into lesions of maximum dimension 5 cm or less and lesions of more than 5 cm in greatest dimension. Tumor size can be measured clinically or radiologically. Metastatic disease should be described according to the most likely sites of metastasis. In general, the minimal clinical staging workup of soft tissue sarcoma is accomplished by axial imaging of the involved site using MRI or CT scan and by imaging of the lungs, the most likely site for occult metastatic disease, using chest CT scans.

Pathologic Staging. Pathologic (pTNM) staging consists of the removal and pathologic evaluation of the primary tumor and clinical/radiologic evaluation for regional and distant metastases. In circumstances where it is not possible to obtain accurate measurements of the excised primary sarcoma specimen, it is acceptable to use radiologic assessment to assign a pT stage using the dimensions of the sarcoma. In examining the primary tumor, the pathologist should subclassify the lesion and assign a histopathologic grade via an accepted grading system. Occasionally, immunohistochemistry or cytogenetics may be necessary for accurate assignment of subtype.

Definition of T. Although size is currently designated as ≤5 cm or >5 cm, particular emphasis should be placed on providing size measurements (or even volume determinants) in sites other than the extremity or superficial trunk. Size should be regarded as a continuous variable, with 5 cm as merely an arbitrary division that makes it possible to dichotomize patient populations.

Depth. Depth is evaluated relative to the investing fascia of the extremity and trunk. *Superficial* is defined as lack of any involvement of the superficial investing muscular fascia in extremity or trunk lesions. For staging, all retroperitoneal and visceral lesions are considered to be deep lesions.

Depth is also an independent variable, and is defined as follows:

1. Superficial
   a. Lesion does not involve superficial fascia.
2. Deep
   a. Lesion is deep to, or involves, the superficial fascia.
   b. All intraperitoneal visceral lesions, retroperitoneal lesions intrathoracic lesions, and the majority of head and neck tumors are considered deep.
3. Depth is evaluated in relation to tumor size (T):
   a. Tumor ≤ 5 cm: T1a = superficial, T1b = deep
   b. Tumor > 5 cm: T2a = superficial, T2b = deep

Nodal Disease.   Nodal involvement is rare in adult soft tissue sarcomas and has a very poor prognosis when evident. The outcome of patients with N1 disease is similar to those with M1 disease. In the assigning of stage group, patients whose nodal status is not determined to be positive for tumor, either clinically or pathologically, should be designated as N0.

Grade.   Grade should be assigned to all sarcomas. A number of published grading systems exist; these vary in the number of tiers or grade groupings. Because many clinicians prefer a two-tiered system ("low" versus "high" grade) for recording data, the current staging system accommodates this approach. As a result, new recommendations for the translation of three- and four-tiered systems into a two-tiered system are suggested. In the most commonly employed three-tiered systems, Grade 1 will be considered "low grade" and Grades 2 and 3 "high grade." In the less common four-tiered systems, Grades 1 and 2 will be considered "low grade" and Grades 3 and 4 "high grade." However, it should be remembered that grade, like size, is a continuous variable in which arbitrary distinctions have been made to facilitate the evaluation of data.

Restaging of Recurrent Tumors.   The same staging should be used when a patient requires restaging of sarcoma recurrence. Such reports should specify whether patients have primary lesions or lesions that were previously treated and have subsequently recurred. The identification and reporting of etiologic factors such as radiation exposure and inherited or genetic syndromes are encouraged. Appropriate workup for recurrent sarcoma should include cross-sectional imaging (CT scan or MRI scan) of the tumor, a CT scan of the chest, and a tissue biopsy to confirm diagnosis prior to initiation of therapy.

DEFINITION OF TNM

Primary Tumor (T)

TX	Primary tumor cannot be assessed	
T0	No evidence of primary tumor	
T1	Tumor 5 cm or less in greatest dimension	
	T1a	superficial tumor
	T1b	deep tumor
T2	Tumor more than 5 cm in greatest dimension	
	T2a	superficial tumor
	T2b	deep tumor

Note: Superficial tumor is located exclusively above the superficial fascia without invasion of the fascia; deep tumor is located either exclusively beneath the superficial fascia, superficial to the fascia with invasion of or through the fascia, or both superficial yet beneath the fascia. Retroperitoneal, mediastinal, and pelvic sarcomas are classified as deep tumors.

Regional Lymph Nodes (N)

NX   Regional lymph nodes cannot be assessed

N0   No regional lymph node metastasis

N1*   Regional lymph node metastasis

*Note: Presence of positive nodes (N1) is considered Stage IV.

Distant Metastasis (M)

MX   Distant metastasis cannot be assessed

M0   No distant metastasis

Ml   Distant metastasis

STAGE GROUPING

Stage	T	N	M	G	G	
Stage I	T1a, 1b, 2a, 2b	N0	M0	G1–2	G1	Low
Stage II	T1a, 1b, 2a	N0	M0	G3–4	G2–3	High
Stage III	T2b	N0	M0	G3–4	G2–3	High
Stage IV	Any T	N1	M0	Any G	Any G	High or Low
	Any T	N0	M1	Any G	Any G	High or Low

HISTOLOGIC GRADE (G)

GX   Grade cannot be assessed

G1   Well differentiated

G2   Moderately differentiated

G3   Poorly differentiated

G4   Poorly differentiated or undifferentiated (four-tiered systems only)

HISTOPATHOLOGIC TYPE

Tumors included in the soft tissue category are listed below:

Alveolar soft-part sarcoma
Desmoplastic small round cell tumor
Epithelioid sarcoma
Clear cell sarcoma
Chondrosarcoma, extraskeletal
Osteosarcoma, extraskeletal
Gastrointestinal stromal tumor
Ewing's sarcoma/primitive neuroectodermal tumor
Fibrosarcoma
Leiomyosarcoma
Liposarcoma
Malignant fibrous histiocytoma
Malignant hemangiopericytoma
Malignant peripheral nerve sheath tumor
Rhabdomyosarcoma
Synovial sarcoma
Sarcoma, NOS

TABLE 22.1. Five-year survival rates in extremity soft tissue sarcoma

Stage	N	Freedom from Local Recurrence	Disease-free Survival	Overall Survival
I	137	88.04%	86.13%	90.00%
II	491	81.97%	71.68%	80.89%
III	469	83.44%	51.77%	56.29%

Local recurrence, disease-free survival, and overall survival by stage. Source: Memorial Sloan-Kettering Cancer Center (MSKCC) for the time period of 7/1/82 to 6/30/00.

The following histologic types are *not* included: angiosarcoma, dermatofibrosarcoma protuberans, inflammatory myofibroblastic tumor, fibromatosis (desmoid tumor), mesothelioma, sarcomas arising in tissues apart from soft tissue (e.g., parenchymal organs). Malignant mesenchymoma has been deleted because it is a diagnostic term that is no longer used.

PROGNOSTIC FACTORS

Neurovascular and Bone Invasion. In earlier staging systems, neurovascular and bone invasion by soft tissue sarcomas had been included as a determinant of stage. It is not included in the current staging system, and no plans are proposed to add it at the present time. Nevertheless, neurovascular and bone invasion should always be reported where possible, and further studies are needed to determine whether or not such invasion is an independent prognostic factor.

Molecular Markers. Molecular markers and genetic abnormalities are being evaluated as determinants of outcome. At the present time, however, insufficient data exist to include specific molecular markers in the staging system.

For the present time, molecular and genetic markers should be considered as important information to aid in histopathologic diagnosis, rather than as determinants of stage.

Validation. The current staging system has the capacity to discriminate the overall survival of patients with soft tissue sarcoma. Patients with Stage I lesions are at low risk for disease-related mortality, whereas Stages II and III entail progressively greater risk (Table 22.1). These figures are based on large numbers [patients in Stage I ($n = 137$); patients in Stage II ($n = 491$); patients in Stage III ($n = 469$)] of patients with primary tumors treated at a single institution. Patients with nodal or disseminated metastases have a poor prognosis. Validation of this staging system is also illustrated by the fact that the local recurrence rate is similar for all three stages (Table 22.1). For this reason, any of these patients can be incorporated into studies that examine the consequences of adjuvant therapy for local recurrence.

BIBLIOGRAPHY

Billingsley KG, Burt ME, Jara E, Ginsberg RJ, Woodruff JM, Leung DHY, et al: Pulmonary metastases from soft tissue sarcoma: analysis of patterns of disease and postmetastasis survival. Ann Surg 229(5):602–610, 1999

Brennan MF: Staging of soft tissue sarcomas. Ann Surg Oncol 6:8–9, 1999

Coindre JM. Pathology and grading of soft tissue sarcomas. Cancer Treat Res 67:1–22, 1993

Coindre JM, Terrier P, Bui NB, Bonichon F, Collin CF, Le Doussal V, et al: Prognostic factors in adult patients with locally controlled soft tissue sarcoma: a study of 546 patients from the French Federation of Cancer Centers Sarcoma Group. J Clin Oncol 14(3):869–877, 1996

Fleming JB, Berman R, Cheng S, Chen NP, Hunt K, Feig BW, et al: Long-term outcome of patients with American Joint Committee on Cancer Stage IIB extremity soft tissue sarcoma. J Clin Oncol 17(9):2772–2780, 1999

Fong V, Coit DG, Woodruff JM, et al: Lymph node metastasis from soft tissue sarcoma: analysis of data from a prospective database of 1772 sarcoma patients. Ann Surg 217:72, 1993

Gaynor JJ, Tan CC, Casper ES, Collin CF, Friedrich C, Shiu MH, et al: Refinement of clinicopathologic staging for localized soft tissue sarcoma of the extremity: a study of 423 adults. J Clin Oncol 10:1317–1329, 1993

Geer RJI, Woodruff JM, Casper ES, et al: Management of small soft tissue sarcoma of the extremity in adults. Arch Surg 127:1285–1289, 1992

Guillou L, Coindre JM, Bonichon F, Bui NB, Terrier P, Collin CF, et al: Comparative study of the National Cancer Institute and French Federation of Cancer Centers Sarcoma Group grading systems in a population of 410 adult patients with soft tissue sarcoma. J Clin Oncol 15:350–362, 1997

Heslin MJ, Lewis JJ, Nadler E, Newman E, Woodruff JM, Casper ES, et al: Prognostic factors associated with long-term survival for retroperitoneal sarcoma: implications for management. J Clin Oncol 15(8):2832–2839, 1997

Pisters PWT, Leung DHY, Woodruff JM, Shi W, Brennan MF. Analysis of prognostic factors in 1041 patients with localized soft tissue sarcomas of the extremities. J Clin Oncol 14:1679–1689, 1996

Pisters PWT, Pollock RE: Prognostic factors in soft tissue sarcoma. In Gospodarowicz M, O'Sullivan B (Eds.) UICC: prognostic factors in cancer. New York: Wiley, in press

Van Glabbeke M, van Oosterom AT, Oosterhuis JW, Mouridsen H, Crowther D, Somers R, Verwij J, Santoro A, Buesa J, Tursz T: Prognostic factors for the outcome of chemotherapy in advanced soft tissue sarcoma: an analysis of 2185 patients treated with anthracycline-containing first-line regimens—European Organization for Research and Treatment of Cancer Soft Tissue and Bone Sarcoma group study. J Clin Oncol 17(1):150–157, 1999

Weiss, SW, Goldblum, JR: Enzinger and Weiss's soft tissue tumor, 4th ed. Philadelphia: Mosby-Harcourt Brace, 2001

HISTOLOGIES—SOFT TISSUE SARCOMA

8800/3	Sarcoma, NOS
8804/3	Epithelioid sarcoma
8806/3	Desmoplastic small round cell tumor
8810/3	Fibrosarcoma
8830/3	Malignant fibrous histiocytoma
8850/3	Liposarcoma

HISTOLOGIES—SOFT TISSUE SARCOMA (CONT.)

8890/3	Leiomyosarcoma
8900/3	Rhabdomyosarcoma
8936/3	Gastrointestinal stromal tumor
9040/3	Synovial sarcoma
9044/3	Clear cell sarcoma
9150/3	Malignant hemangiopericytoma
9180/3	Osteosarcoma
9220/3	Chondrosarcoma
9260/3	Ewing's sarcoma
9540/3	Malignant peripheral nerve sheath tumor
9581/3	Alveolar soft-part sarcoma
9743/3	Primitive neuroectodermal tumor

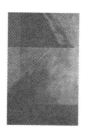

PART VI
Skin

6

23

Carcinoma of the Skin

(Excluding Eyelid, Vulva, and Penis)

C44.0 Skin of lip, NOS
C44.2 External ear
C44.3 Skin of other and unspecified parts of face
C44.4 Skin of scalp and neck

C44.5 Skin of trunk
C44.6 Skin of upper limb and shoulder
C44.7 Skin of lower limb and hip

C44.8 Overlapping lesion of skin
C44.9 Skin, NOS
C63.2 Scrotum, NOS

SUMMARY OF CHANGES

• The definition of TNM and the Stage Grouping for this chapter have not changed from the Fifth Edition.

INTRODUCTION

This chapter applies to non-melanomatous cancers of the skin, which are predominantly basal cell carcinomas and squamous cell carcinomas. Skin cancers are largely related to solar exposure and are relatively common, although their frequency varies with geographic latitude and population at risk. For example, they occur in 729 individuals per 100,000 population in Hawaii but in only 195 per 100,000 in the northern United States. Higher rates are found in Australia and New Zealand, and the incidence generally is rising rapidly. Basal cell carcinomas are the most common cancer in humans, and are four to five times more common than squamous cell carcinomas of the skin. For the most part, non-melanomatous skin cancers have a good prognosis and nearly always can be treated with curative intent. Refer to Chapter 40 for staging of carcinoma of the eyelid and to Chapter 24 for malignant melanoma of the skin.

ANATOMY

Primary Site. The skin is made up of three layers: an outermost epidermis, a middle dermis, and an inner subcutis. The epidermis consists predominantly of stratified squamous epithelium, the outermost layer of which is keratinized. The innermost layer consists primarily of germinative cells and melanocytes. The dermis is made up of connective tissue and elastic fibers immersed in an amorphous matrix of mucoproteins and mucopolysaccharides. The subcutis is predominantly adipose tissue. The sebaceous and other glands of the skin, as well as hair follicles—collectively called adnexal structures—are found in the dermis and subjacent subcutis. All of the components of the skin (epidermis, dermis, and adnexal structures within the subcutis) can give rise to malignant neoplasms.

Cancers of the skin most commonly arise on those surfaces exposed to sunlight (including the face, ears, hands, and scalp, especially in balding men), and the role of sunlight in the induction of cutaneous cancer has been well described. Approximately four-fifths of all cutaneous squamous cell cancers and approximately two-thirds of all basal cell cancers occur in unprotected sun-exposed skin of lightly pigmented persons. Squamous cell carcinoma can also arise in skin that was previously scarred or ulcerated— that is, at sites of burns and chronic ulcers. Radiation in other than ultra-violet forms, chemicals, and genetic syndromes are also proven causes of cutaneous carcinomas.

Skin cancers rarely cause symptoms. Signs vary depending on the local site of origin and whether the precursor lesion is an actinic keratosis or a cutaneous ulcer. Squamous cell tumors developing at the site of actinic keratoses usually begin as hyperkeratotic papules or plaques or as ulcers. Induration, which is usually absent in actinic keratoses, may develop early in squamous cell cancer. Further progression is associated with thickening of the plaque, ulceration, and bleeding. Tumors that arise in cutaneous ulcers or burn scars present as an expanding mass at the site. High-risk tumors (higher local recurrence rate or high risk for metastasis) are found on the lip, scalp, ears, eyelids, and nose.

Basal cell carcinomas initially appear clinically as firm, translucent papules coursed by telangiectatic blood vessels. Central areas of crusting and depression, associated with ulceration, usually occur late. Bleeding, however, may be described in early as well as late lesions. Pigmentation occurs uncommonly and may lead clinically to confusion with cutaneous melanoma. Morpheaform basal cell carcinoma (basal cell carcinoma with a fibrotic component) may look and feel like localized patches of sclero-derma, or a scar, and is generally without telangiectasia or measurable elevation.

Primary Growth.   Local extension is the predominant mode of growth of non-melanomatous skin cancers. Basal cell carcinomas that remain un-treated for long periods will eventually erode adjacent structures, such as bone, and into local vasculature. Perineural invasion in morpheaform basal cell cancers is often observed, and it is associated with a high rate of in-complete excision and recurrence. Squamous cell carcinoma may also in-vade the perineural space, and this feature is associated with increased local recurrence. Squamous cell carcinoma may also penetrate into other local structures, including muscle, bone, and vasculature.

Regional Lymph Nodes.   Skin cancers characteristically spread by local extension. Involvement of regional lymph nodes infrequently occurs and is usually associated with large size and invasiveness into the dermis and subcutaneous fat. Which specific lymph node chains are involved depends on the location of the primary lesion, because tumor cells are passively borne along with the "draining" lymphatic fluid, usually to the geograph-ically closest node(s). In this context, for tumors of the lower torso or lower extremities, the inguinal nodes are considered the regional basin and should be designated N1. For pN (pathologic staging), histologic exami-nation of a regional lymphadenectomy specimen should include careful examination of all resected nodes.

Hematogenously Borne Metastases. Basal cell and squamous cell cancers that arise in actinically damaged skin are relatively slow growing and rarely metastasize. Metastases are more likely to arise from squamous cell tumors that originate in scars or ulcers. Tumors that metastasize have often been present for a long time before metastases are observed. The most common visceral metastatic site is the lung, especially for squamous cell carcinomas. Other sites of distant spread are unusual. Non-melanoma skin cancers arising in transplant patients may be more aggressive and may metastasize more readily and more widely.

RULES FOR CLASSIFICATION

The clinical and pathologic classifications are identical. However, pathologic staging uses the symbol p as a prefix.

Clinical Staging. The assessment of skin cancer is based on inspection and palpation of the involved area and the regional lymph nodes. Imaging studies of the underlying bony structures are important for any lesion that appears fixed to underlying fascia, muscle, or bone.

Pathologic Staging. Complete resection of the entire site is required. Confirmation of lymph node involvement is also necessary when involvement is suspected. The degree of malignancy of squamous cell cancer of the skin generally is related to the degree of anaplasia within the tumor. Low-grade tumors show considerable cell differentiation, uniform cell size, infrequent cellular mitoses and nuclear irregularity, and intact intercellular bridges. High-grade tumors show little differentiation, are often of spindle cell in character, show necrosis, exhibit high mitotic activity, and are often deeply invasive. Depth of invasion can often be correlated with degree of tumor aggressiveness.

DEFINITION OF TNM

Definitions for clinical (cTNM) and pathologic (pTNM) classifications are the same.

Primary Tumor (T)

TX   Primary tumor cannot be assessed
T0   No evidence of primary tumor
Tis Carcinoma *in situ*
T1   Tumor 2 cm or less in greatest dimension
T2   Tumor more than 2 cm, but not more than 5 cm, in greatest dimension
T3   Tumor more than 5 cm in greatest dimension
T4   Tumor invades deep extradermal structures (i.e., cartilage, skeletal muscle, or bone)

Note: In case of multiple simultaneous tumors, the tumor with the highest T category will be classified and the number of separate tumors will be indicated in parentheses, e.g., T2 (5).

Regional Lymph Nodes (N)

NX   Regional lymph nodes cannot be assessed
N0   No regional lymph node metastasis
N1   Regional lymph node metastasis

Distant Metastasis (M)

MX   Distant metastasis cannot be assessed
M0   No distant metastasis
M1   Distant metastasis

STAGE GROUPING

Stage	T	N	M
Stage 0	Tis	N0	M0
Stage I	T1	N0	M0
Stage II	T2	N0	M0
	T3	N0	M0
Stage III	T4	N0	M0
	Any T	N1	M0
Stage IV	Any T	Any N	M1

HISTOPATHOLOGIC TYPE

The classification applies only to carcinomas of the skin, primarily squamous cell and basal cell varieties. It also applies to the adenocarcinomas that develop from sweat or sebaceous glands and to a spindle cell variant of squamous cell carcinoma. There should be microscopic verification of the disease to permit grouping of cases by histologic type. A form of *in situ* squamous cell carcinoma or intraepidermal squamous cell carcinoma is often referred to as Bowen disease. This lesion should be coded as Tis. Squamous cell tumors may also be described as verrucous.

HISTOLOGIC GRADE (G)

GX   Grade cannot be assessed
G1   Well differentiated
G2   Moderately differentiated
G3   Poorly differentiated
G4   Undifferentiated

PROGNOSTIC FACTORS

In squamous cell carcinoma, tumor aggressiveness correlates well with tumor size, duration, location, origin, and degree of anaplasia. Large tumors are usually present for longer periods or are rapidly growing. Long-standing tumors tend to grow extensively and to invade other structures, such as local vasculature, nervous tissue, or soft tissue. Tumors of the scalp, ears, lips, nose, eyelids, or soft tissues readily invade subcutaneous tissue and have a greater risk of subclinical tumor extension.

Anaplastic squamous cell carcinomas readily tend to invade locally and to metastasize earlier than well-differentiated tumors, regardless of location.

Although they have been noted in cases of large ulcerated and recurrent lesions, metastases from basal cell carcinomas are rare. However, basal cell cancers are often locally destructive.

BIBLIOGRAPHY

Alam M, Ratner D: Primary care: cutaneous squamous-cell carcinoma. N Engl J Med 344(13):975–983, 2001

Callen JP, Headington J: Bowen's and non-Bowen's squamous intraepithelial neoplasia of the skin. Arch Dermatol 116:422–426, 1980

Chuang T-Y, Reizner GT, Elpern DJ, et al: Squamous cell carcinoma in Kauai, Hawaii. Int J. Dermatol 34:393–397, 1995

Czarnecki D, Collins M, Meehan C, et al: Basal cell carcinoma in temperate and tropical Australia. Int J Cancer 50:874–875, 1992

Czarnecki D, Obrien T, Meehan CJ: Nonmelanoma skin cancer: number of cancers and their distribution in outpatients. Int J Dermatol 33:416–417, 1994

Czarnecki D, Staples M, Mar A, et al: Metastases from squamous cell carcinomas of the skin in southern Australia. Dermatology 189:52–54, 1994

Karagas MR, Greenberg RE, Spencer SK, et al: Increase in incidence rates of basal cell and squamous cell skin cancer in New Hampshire, USA. Int J Cancer 81:555–559, 1999

Kwa RE, Campana K, Moy RL: Biology of cutaneous squamous cell carcinoma. J Am Acad Dermatol 26:1–26, 1992

Lawrence N, Cottel WI: Squamous cell carcinoma of the skin with perineural invasion. J Am Acad Dermatol 31:30–33, 1994

Lund HZ: How often does squamous cell carcinoma of the skin metastasize? Arch Dermatol 92:635–637, 1965

McDonald CJ: Malignant neoplasms of the skin. In Calabresi P, Schein PS (Eds.): Medical oncology. New York: McGraw-Hill, 517–543, 1993

Moan J, Dahlback A: The relationship between skin cancers, solar radiation and ozone depletion. Br J Cancer 65:916–921, 1992

Rowe DE, Carrol RJ, Day CL: Prognostic factors for local recurrence, metastasis, and survival rate in squamous cell carcinoma of the skin, ear and lip. J Am Acad Dermatol 26:976–990, 1992

Scotto J, Fears TR, Fraumeni JF: Incidence of nonmelanoma skin cancer in the United States. NIH Publication No. 83–2433. Washington, DC: U.S. Department of Health and Human Services, 1983.

HISTOLOGIES—CARCINOMA OF THE SKIN

8010/2	Carcinoma *in situ*, NOS
8010/3	Carcinoma, NOS
8011/3	Epithelioma, malignant
8012/3	Large cell carcinoma, NOS
8013/3	Large cell neuroendocrine carcinoma
8014/3	Large cell carcinoma with rhabdoid phenotype
8015/3	Glassy cell carcinoma
8020/3	Carcinoma, undifferentiated, NOS
8021/3	Carcinoma, anaplastic, NOS
8022/3	Pleomorphic carcinoma

8030/3	Giant cell and spindle cell carcinoma
8031/3	Giant cell carcinoma
8032/3	Spindle cell carcinoma, NOS
8033/3	Pseudosarcomatous carcinoma
8034/3	Polygonal cell carcinoma
8035/3	Carcinoma with osteoclast-like giant cells
8041/3	Small cell carcinoma, NOS
8042/3	Oat cell carcinoma
8043/3	Small cell carcinoma, fusiform cell
8044/3	Small cell carcinoma, intermediate cell
8045/3	Combined small cell carcinoma
8046/3	Non–small cell carcinoma
8050/2	Papillary carcinoma *in situ*
8050/3	Papillary carcinoma, NOS
8051/3	Verrucous carcinoma, NOS
8052/2	Papillary squamous cell carcinoma non-invasive
8052/3	Papillary squamous cell carcinoma
8070/2	Squamous cell carcinoma *in situ*, NOS
8070/3	Squamous cell carcinoma, NOS
8071/3	Squamous cell carcinoma, keratinizing, NOS
8072/3	Squamous cell carcinoma, large cell
8073/3	Squamous cell carcinoma, small cell, non-keratinizing
8074/3	Squamous cell carcinoma, spindle cell
8075/3	Squamous cell carcinoma, adenoid
8076/2	Squamous cell carcinoma *in situ* with questionable stromal invasion
8076/3	Squamous cell carcinoma, microinvasive
8077/2	Squamous intraepithelial neoplasia, grade III
8078/3	Squamous cell carcinoma with horn formulation
8080/2	Queyrat erythroplasia
8081/2	Bowen disease
8082/3	Lymphoepithelial carcinoma
8083/3	Basaloid squamous cell carcinoma
8084/3	Squamous cell carcinoma, clear cell type
8090/3	Basal cell carcinoma
8091/3	Multifocal superficial basal cell carcinoma
8092/3	Infiltrating basal cell carcinoma, NOS
8093/3	Basal cell carcinoma, fibroepithelial
8094/3	Basosquamous carcinoma
8095/3	Metatypical carcinoma
8097/3	Basal cell carcinoma, nodular
8098/3	Adenoid basal carcinoma
8102/3	Trichilemmocarcinoma
8110/3	Pilomatrix carcinoma
8140/2	Adenocarcinoma *in situ*, NOS
8140/3	Adenocarcinoma, NOS
8141/3	Scirrhous adenocarcinoma
8190/3	Trabecular adenocarcinoma
8200/3	Adenoid cystic carcinoma
8201/3	Cribriform carcinoma, NOS
8247/3	Merkel cell carcinoma
8390/3	Skin appendage carcinoma
8400/3	Sweat gland adenocarcinoma
8401/3	Apocrine adenocarcinoma
8402/3	Nodular hidradenoma, malignant

8403/3	Malignant eccrine spiradenoma
8407/3	Sclerosing sweat duct carcinoma
8408/3	Eccrine papillary adenocarcinoma
8409/3	Eccrine poroma, malignant
8410/3	Sebaceous adenocarcinoma
8413/3	Eccrine adenocarcinoma
8420/3	Ceruminous adenocarcinoma
8430/3	Mucoepidermoid carcinoma
8440/3	Cystadenocarcinoma, NOS
8490/3	Signet ring cell carcinoma
8560/3	Adenosquamous carcinoma
8562/3	Epithelial-myoepithelial carcinoma
8570/3	Adenocarcinoma with squamous metaplasia
8571/3	Adenocarcinoma with cartilaginous and osseous metaplasia
8572/3	Adenocarcinoma with spindle cell metaplasia
8573/3	Adenocarcinoma with apocrine metaplasia
8940/3	Mixed tumor, malignant, NOS
8941/3	Carcinoma in pleomorphic adenoma

6

24

Melanoma of the Skin

C44.0 Skin of lip, NOS
C44.1 Eyelid
C44.2 External ear
C44.3 Skin of other and unspecified parts of face
C44.4 Skin of scalp and neck
C44.5 Skin of trunk
C44.6 Skin of upper limb and shoulder

C44.7 Skin of lower limb and hip
C44.8 Overlapping lesion of skin
C44.9 Skin, NOS
C51 Vulva
C51.0 Labium majus
C51.1 Labium minus
C51.2 Clitoris
C51.8 Overlapping lesion of vulva

C51.9 Vulva, NOS
C60 Penis
C60.0 Prepuce
C60.1 Glans penis
C60.2 Body of penis
C60.8 Overlapping lesion of penis
C60.9 Penis, NOS
C63.2 Scrotum, NOS

SUMMARY OF CHANGES

- Melanoma thickness and ulceration, but not level of invasion, are used in the T category (except for T1 melanomas).

- The number of metastatic lymph nodes, rather than their gross dimensions and the delineation of clinical occult (i.e., "microscopic") vs. clinically apparent (i.e., "macroscopic") nodal metastases, are used in the N category.

- The site of distant metastases and the presence of elevated serum lactic dehydrogenase (LDH) are used in the M category.

- All patients with Stage I, II, or III disease are upstaged when a primary melanoma is ulcerated.

- Satellite metastases around a primary melanoma and in-transit metastases have been merged into a single staging entity that is grouped into Stage IIIc disease.

- A new convention for defining clinical and pathologic staging has been developed that takes into account the new staging information gained from intraoperative lymphatic mapping and sentinel node excision.

6

INTRODUCTION

Melanoma of the skin continues to increase in frequency, with 47,700 new cases and 9,200 deaths in the year 2000.[1] Melanoma can arise from skin anywhere on the body. It occurs most commonly in fair-skinned persons, especially those with a history of significant sun exposure.

A completely revised melanoma staging system is described herein, along with operational definitions. In addition, a major database analysis of prognostic factors involving 17,600 patients from 13 cancer centers and organizations was performed to validate the staging categories and groupings.[2] Within each stage grouping and its subgroups, there is a uniform risk for distant metastases and a uniform survival probability. This revised version of melanoma staging more accurately reflects the prognosis and natural history of melanoma and will therefore be more applicable to treatment planning and clinical trials involving melanoma.

The major differences between the new version of the melanoma staging system and the version that appeared in the Fifth Edition are summarized in Table 24.1. The chapter summary above outlines the major revisions, while more details about the staging rationale and interpretation have been published elsewhere.[3–5]

ANATOMY

Primary Sites. Cutaneous melanoma can occur anywhere on the skin. It occurs most commonly on the extremities in females and on the trunk in males. Melanomas located on the palms, soles, and nailbeds (acral lentiginous melanoma), although they occur infrequently, are distinctive because they can occur in individuals of any ethnic origin and in persons with no history of significant sun exposure.

Regional Lymph Nodes. The regional lymph nodes are the most common site of metastases. The widespread use of cutaneous lymphoscintigraphy, lymphatic mapping, and sentinel lymph node biopsies has greatly enhanced the ability to identify the presence or absence of, and to stage, nodal metastases. Intralymphatic regional metastases may also become clinically manifest either as satellite metastases (defined arbitrarily as intralymphatic metastases occurring within 2 cm of the primary melanoma) or as in-transit metastases (defined arbitrarily as intralymphatic metastases occurring more than 2 cm from the primary melanoma but before the first echelon of regional lymph nodes). By convention, the term *regional nodal metastases* refers to disease confined to one nodal basin or two contiguous nodal basins, as in patients with nodal disease in combinations of femoral/iliac, axillary/supraclavicular, cervical/supraclavicular, axillary/femoral, or bilateral axillary or femoral metastases.

Metastatic Sites. Melanoma can metastasize to virtually any organ site. Metastases most commonly occur in the skin or soft tissues, the lung, and the liver.

RULES FOR CLASSIFICATION

The primary difference between the definitions of clinical and pathologic stage grouping is whether the regional lymph nodes are staged by clinical/radiologic exam or by pathological exam (after partial or complete lymphadenectomy).

Clinical Staging. By convention, clinical staging should be performed after complete excision of the primary melanoma (including microstaging) and after information about metastases to either regional or distant anatomic sites has been obtained after clinical, radiologic, and laboratory assessment. The microstaging of a primary melanoma is performed after an

TABLE 24.1. Differences between the previous (1997) version and the present (2002) version of the melanoma staging system (adapted from Balch et al.[3])

Factor	Old System	New System	Comments
Thickness	Secondary prognostic factor; thresholds of 0.75, 1.50, 4.0 mm	Primary determinant of T staging; thresholds of 1.0, 2.0, 4.0 mm	Correlation of metastatic risk is a continuous variable
Level of invasion	Primary determinant of T staging	Used only for defining T1 melanomas	Correlation only significant for thin lesions; variability in interpretation
Ulceration	Not included	Included as a second determinant of T and N staging	Signifies a locally advanced lesion; dominant prognostic factor for grouping Stages I, II, and III
Satellite metastases	In T category	In N category	Merged with in-transit lesions
Thick melanomas (> 4.0 mm)	Stage III	Stage IIC	Stage III defined as regional metastases
Dimensions of nodal metastases	Dominant determinant of N staging	Not used	No evidence of significant prognostic correlation
Number of nodal metastases	Not included	Primary determinant of N staging	Thresholds of 1 vs. 2–3 vs. ≥ 4 nodes
Metastatic tumor burden	Not included	Included as a second determinant of N staging	Clinically occult ("microscopic") vs. clinically apparent ("macroscopic") nodal volume
Lung metastases	Merged with all other visceral metastases	Separate category as M1b	Has a somewhat better prognosis than other visceral metastases
Elevated serum LDH	Not included	Included as a second determinant of M staging	
Clinical vs. pathologic staging	Did not account for sentinel node technology	Sentinel node results incorporated into definition of pathologic staging	Large variability in outcome between clinical and pathologic staging; pathologic staging encouraged prior to entry into clinical trials

6

excisional biopsy of a primary melanoma, with pathologic assessment of tumor thickness (Breslow method), level of invasion (Clark method), and any ulceration of the overlying epidermis. All of these parameters are used in melanoma staging.

Clinical Stages I and II are confined to those patients who have no evidence of metastases, at either regional or distant sites, based on clinical, radiologic, and/or laboratory evaluation. Stage III melanoma patients are those with clinical or radiologic evidence of regional metastases, either metastases in the regional lymph nodes or intralymphatic metastases manifesting as either satellite or in-transit metastases. Clinical Stage III groupings rely on clinical and/or radiologic assessment of the regional lymph nodes, which is inherently difficult, especially with respect to assessing both the presence and the number of metastatic nodes. Therefore, no subgroup definitions of clinically staged patients with nodal or intralymphatic regional metastases have been made. They are all categorized as clinical Stage III disease. Clinical Stage IV melanoma patients have metastases at any distant site and are not substaged further.

Pathologic Staging. Pathologic staging uses all of the same staging information described above under Clinical Staging *plus* information gained from pathologic evaluation of the regional lymph nodes after partial (i.e., sentinel) or complete lymphadenectomy (i.e., after elective or therapeutic lymph node dissection), along with pathologic confirmation of metastases identified by clinical or radiological examinations.

Pathologic Stage I melanoma and Stage II melanoma comprise those patients who have no evidence of regional or distant metastases, based on absence of nodal metastases after careful pathologic examination of the regional lymph nodes, and absence of distant metastases, based on routine clinical and radiologic examination. Pathologic Stage III melanoma patients have pathologic evidence of regional metastases, either in the regional lymph nodes or the intralymphatic sites. The quantitative classification for pathologic nodal status requires that pathologists perform a careful examination of the surgically resected nodal basin and report on the actual number of lymph nodes examined and the number of nodal metastases identified. Pathologic Stage IV melanoma patients have histologic documentation of metastases at one or more distant sites.

With the widespread use of sentinel node lymphadenectomy, it is clear that there is considerable stage migration of patients who have previously been staged as "node negative" but who in fact had undetected nodal metastases. These previously understaged Stage III patients have revealed an extraordinary heterogeneity of metastatic risk for Stage III melanoma. Thus the survival rates among various subgroups of pathologic Stage III patients vary widely, ranging from 9% to 63% 10-year survival.[2]

DEFINITION OF TNM

Patients with melanoma *in situ* are categorized as Tis. Those patients with melanoma presentations that are indeterminate or cannot be microstaged should be categorized as Tx. The T category of melanoma is classified primarily by measuring the thickness of the melanoma as defined by Dr. Alexander Breslow.[6,7] The T category thresholds of melanoma thickness are defined in whole integers (i.e., at 1.0, 2.0, and 4.0 mm). Melanoma ulceration is the absence of an intact epidermis overlying the primary melanoma, assessed by histopathologic examination.[8–10] The level of invasion, as defined by Dr. Wallace Clark,[11] is used to define subcategories of T1 melanomas but not for thicker melanomas (i.e., T2, T3, or T4).

Regional metastases most commonly present in the regional lymph nodes. The actual number of nodal metastases identified by the pathologist must be reported for staging purposes. A second staging definition is related to tumor burden: microscopic vs. macroscopic. Thus those patients without clinical or radiologic evidence of lymph node metastases, but who have pathologically documented nodal metastases, are defined by convention as exhibiting "microscopic" or "clinically occult" nodal metastases. In contrast, melanoma patients with both clinical evidence of nodal metastases *and* pathologic examination documenting the number of nodal metastases (after therapeutic lymphadenectomy) are defined by convention as having "macroscopic" or "clinically apparent" nodal metastases. Regional metastases also include intralymphatic metastases, defined as the presence of clinical or microscopic satellites around a primary melanoma, and/or in-transit metastases between the primary melanoma and the regional lymph nodes.

Distant metastases are staged primarily by the organ or site(s) in which they are located. A second factor in staging is the presence or absence of an elevated serum LDH. An elevated serum LDH should be used only when there are two or more determinations obtained more than 24 hours apart, because an elevated serum LDH on a single determination can be falsely positive as a result of hemolysis or other factors unrelated to melanoma metastases.

Primary Tumor (T)

TX — Primary tumor cannot be assessed (e.g., shave biopsy or regressed melanoma)

T0 — No evidence of primary tumor

Tis — Melanoma *in situ*

T1 — Melanoma ≤ 1.0 mm in thickness with or without ulceration

T1a — Melanoma ≤ 1.0 mm in thickness and level II or III, no ulceration

T1b — Melanoma ≤ 1.0 mm in thickness and level IV or V or with ulceration

T2 — Melanoma 1.01–2 mm in thickness with or without ulceration

T2a — Melanoma 1.01–2.0 mm in thickness, no ulceration

T2b — Melanoma 1.01–2.0 mm in thickness, with ulceration

T3 — Melanoma 2.01–4 mm in thickness with or without ulceration

T3a — Melanoma 2.01–4.0 mm in thickness, no ulceration

T3b — Melanoma 2.01–4.0 mm in thickness, with ulceration

T4 — Melanoma greater than 4.0 mm in thickness with or without ulceration

T4a — Melanoma > 4.0 mm in thickness, no ulceration

T4b — Melanoma > 4.0 mm in thickness, with ulceration

Regional Lymph Nodes (N)

NX   Regional lymph nodes cannot be assessed

N0   No regional lymph node metastasis

N1   Metastasis in one lymph node

N1a   Clinically occult (microscopic) metastasis

N1b   Clinically apparent (macroscopic) metastasis

N2   Metastasis in two to three regional nodes or intralymphatic regional metastasis without nodal metastases

N2a   Clinically occult (microscopic) metastasis

N2b   Clinically apparent (macroscopic) metastasis

N2c   Satellite or in-transit metastasis *without* nodal metastasis

N3   Metastasis in four or more regional nodes, or matted metastatic nodes, or in-transit metastasis or satellite(s) *with* metastasis in regional node(s)

Distant Metastasis (M)

MX   Distant metastasis cannot be assessed

M0   No distant metastasis

M1   Distant metastasis

M1a   Metastasis to skin, subcutaneous tissues or distant lymph nodes

M1b   Metastasis to lung

M1c   Metastasis to all other visceral sites or distant metastasis at any site associated with an elevated serum lactic dehydrogenase (LDH)

STAGE GROUPING

Patients with primary melanomas with no evidence of regional or distant metastases (either clinically or pathologically) are divided into two stages: Stage I for early-stage patients with "low risk" for metastases and melanoma-specific mortality and Stage II for those with "intermediate risk" for metastases and melanoma-specific mortality. There are no substages for clinical Stage III melanoma, because criteria for subgrouping can be inaccurate. Pathologic Stage III patients with regional metastases make up a very heterogeneous group that has been divided into three subgroups according to prognostic risk. Stage IIIA patients have up to three microscopic nodal metastases arising from a non-ulcerating primary melanoma and have an "intermediate risk" for distant metastases and melanoma-specific survival. Stage IIIB patients have up to three macroscopic nodal metastases arising from a non-ulcerating melanoma, or have up to three microscopic nodal metastases arising from an ulcerating melanoma, or have intralymphatic metastases without nodal metastases. They constitute a "high-risk" group prognostically. The remaining patients are Stage IIIC and are at "very high risk" for distant metastases and melanoma-specific mortality. The presence of melanoma ulceration "upstages" the prognosis of Stage I, II, and III patients compared to patients with melanomas of equivalent thickness without ulceration or those with nodal metastases arising from a non-ulcerating melanoma. There are no subgroups of Stage IV melanoma.

CLINICAL STAGE GROUPING

Stage 0	Tis	N0	M0
Stage IA	T1a	N0	M0
Stage IB	T1b	N0	M0
	T2a	N0	M0
Stage IIA	T2b	N0	M0
	T3a	N0	M0
Stage IIB	T3b	N0	M0
	T4a	N0	M0
Stage IIC	T4b	N0	M0
Stage III	Any T	N1	M0
	Any T	N2	M0
	Any T	N3	M0
Stage IV	Any T	Any N	M1

Note: Clinical staging includes microstaging of the primary melanoma and clinical/radiological evaluation for metastases. By convention, it should be used after complete excision of the primary melanoma with clinical assessment for regional and distant metastases.

6

PATHOLOGIC STAGE GROUPING

Stage 0	Tis	N0	M0
Stage IA	T1a	N0	M0
Stage IB	T1b	N0	M0
	T2a	N0	M0
Stage IIA	T2b	N0	M0
	T3a	N0	M0
Stage IIB	T3b	N0	M0
	T4a	N0	M0
Stage IIC	T4b	N0	M0
Stage IIIA	T1–4a	N1a	M0
	T1–4a	N2a	M0
Stage IIIB	T1–4b	N1a	M0
	T1–4b	N2a	M0
	T1–4a	N1b	M0
	T1–4a	N2b	M0
	T1–4a/b	N2c	M0
Stage IIIC	T1–4b	N1b	M0
	T1–4b	N2b	M0
	Any T	N3	M0
Stage IV	Any T	Any N	M1

Note: Pathologic staging includes microstaging of the primary melanoma and pathologic information about the regional lymph nodes after partial or complete lymphadenectomy. Pathologic Stage 0 or Stage IA patients are the exception; they do not require pathologic evaluation of their lymph nodes.

HISTOPATHOLOGIC TYPE

Melanoma *in situ*
Malignant melanoma, NOS
Superficial spreading melanoma
Nodular melanoma
Lentigo maligna melanoma
Acral lentiginous melanoma,
Desmoplastic melanoma,
Epithelioid cell melanoma
Spindle cell melanoma
Balloon cell melanoma
Blue nevus, malignant
Malignant melanoma in giant pigmented nevus

The following histologies are no longer appropriate for or relevant to the staging of melanoma:

Malignant melanoma, regressing
Meningeal melanomatosis
Amelanotic melanoma
Malignant melanoma in junctional nevus
Precancerous melanosis
Mucosal lentiginous melanoma
Mixed epithelioid and spindle cell melanoma
Spindle cell melanoma, type A
Spindle cell melanoma, type B
Lentigo maligna

PROGNOSTIC FACTORS AND SURVIVAL RESULTS

A summary of survival rates and the demographics of the melanoma patient database used to validate the staging criteria have been published.[2,3] Fifteen-year survival rates for patients with Stages I to IV melanoma are shown in Fig. 24.1.

The AJCC Melanoma Database, which consists of prospectively accumulated melanoma outcome data merged into a single database for the purpose of validating the proposed revisions to the melanoma staging system,[2] includes 17,600 patients with complete clinical and pathologic information for analyzing all of the factors required for the proposed TNM classification and stage grouping.

Ten-year survival rates for each of the T categories are shown in Fig. 24.2. Survival rates for patients with an ulcerated melanoma are proportionately lower than those for patients with a non-ulcerated melanoma of equivalent T category but are remarkably similar to those for patients with a non-ulcerated melanoma of the next highest T category (Fig. 24.2 and Table 24.2). The level of invasion does not reflect prognosis as accurately as tumor thickness, for reasons that have been discussed in

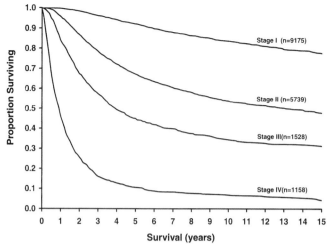

Fig. 24.1. Fifteen-year survival curves for the melanoma staging system, comparing localized melanoma (Stages I and II), regional metastases (Stage III), and distant metastases (Stage IV).[3] The numbers in parentheses are the numbers of patients from the AJCC melanoma staging database used to calculate the survival rates. The differences between the curves are highly significant ($p < 0.0001$).

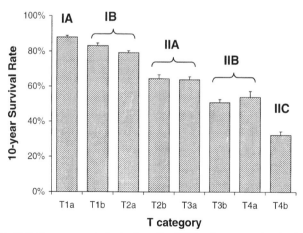

Fig. 24.2. Ten-year survival rates from the AJCC melanoma staging database comparing the different T categories and the stage groupings for Stages I and II melanoma.[3] Note that the stage groupings involve upstaging to account for melanoma ulceration, where thinner melanomas with ulceration are grouped with the next greatest T substage for non-ulcerated melanomas.

TABLE 24.2. Five-year survival rates of pathologically staged patients (adapted from Balch et al.[2])

	IA	IB	IIA	IIB	IIC	IIIA	IIIB	IIIC
Ta: Non-ulcerated Melanoma	T1a	T2a	T3a	T4a		N1a	N1b	N3
	95%	89%	79%	67%		N2a	N2b	
						67%	54%	28%
Tb: Ulcerated Melanoma		T1b	T2b	T3b	T4b		N1a	N1b
		91%	77%	63%	45%		N2a	N2b
								N3
							52%	24%

previous publications.[4,5,8,12–15] Nevertheless, level of invasion did provide additional prognostic discrimination in the specific subgroup of thin (i.e., T1) melanomas.[2]

In a multivariate analysis of 13,581 patients with localized melanoma (either clinically or pathologically), the two most significant independent characteristics of the primary melanoma were tumor thickness and ulceration (Table 24.3). Indeed, no other feature of the melanoma or of the patient with localized melanoma had the predictive capability of these two factors. Other statistically significant prognostic factors were patient age, site of the primary melanoma, level of invasion, and gender (Table 24.3).

Complete clinical and histopathologic data were available for 1151 patients with lymph node metastases. A Cox multivariate analysis demonstrated that three factors were most significant (with $p < 0.0001$): (1) the number of metastatic nodes, (2) the tumor burden at the time of staging (i.e., microscopic vs. macroscopic), and (3) the presence or absence of ulceration of the primary melanoma (Table 24.4). There was a significantly lower survival (calculated from the time the primary melanoma was diagnosed) for those patients who presented with macroscopic (i.e., palpable) nodal metastases (pN1b, N2b) than for those with microscopic (i.e., non-palpable) nodal metastases, (pN1a, N2a), even after accounting for lead-time bias ($p < 0.0001$). (Fig. 24.3, Table 24.5). Diminishing 5-year survival with increasing tumor burden based on increasing number of

TABLE 24.3. Cox regression analysis for 13,581 melanoma patients without evidence of nodal or distant metastases (adapted from Balch et al.[2])

Variable	Chi-Square Value (Wald)	P-Value	Risk Ratio	95% C.I.*
Thickness	244.3	< 0.00001	1.558	1.473–1.647
Ulceration	189.5	< 0.00001	1.901	1.735–2.083
Age	45.6	< 0.00001	1.101	1.071–1.132
Site	41.0	< 0.00001	1.338	1.224–1.463
Level	32.7	< 0.00001	1.214	1.136–1.297
Gender	15.1	0.001	0.836	0.764–0.915

*CI, confidence interval

TABLE 24.4. Cox regression analysis for 1,151 Stage III (nodal metastases) patients (adapted from Balch et al.[2])

Variable	Chi-Square Value (Wald)	P-Value	Risk Ratio	95% C.I.
Number of metastatic nodes	57.616	< 0.00001	1.257	1.185–1.334
Tumor burden	40.301	< 0.00001	1.792	1.497–2.146
Ulceration	23.282	< 0.00001	1.582	1.313–1.906
Site	17.843	0.0001	1.461	1.225–1.746
Age	13.369	0.0003	1.118	1.053–1.187
Thickness	1.964	0.1611	1.091	0.966–1.233
Level	0.219	0.6396	1.033	0.901–1.186
Gender	0.006	0.9407	1.007	0.836–1.213

metastatic nodes present was observed for all subgroups ($p < 0.0001$) (Table 24.5).

Ulceration of a primary melanoma was the only primary-tumor feature that still predicted an adverse outcome in Stage III disease (Table 24.5, Fig. 24.3). When all three of the most important prognostic factors were

6

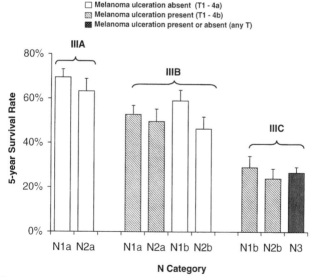

Fig. 24.3. Five-year survival rates from the AJCC melanoma staging database, comparing the different N categories and the stage groupings for Stage III melanoma[3]. The survival results are significantly different when the primary melanoma is ulcerated compared to the equivalent N category of patients without ulceration. See Tables 24.1 and 24.2 for definitions.

TABLE 24.5. Five-year survival rates for Stage III (nodal metastases) patients stratified by number of metastatic nodes, ulceration, and tumor burden (adapted from Balch et al.[2])

Melanoma Ulceration	Microscopic % ± S.E.			Macroscopic % ± S.E.		
	1+ Nodes	2–3 Nodes	> 3+ Nodes	1+ Nodes	2–3 Nodes	> 3+ Nodes
Absent	69 ± 3.7 (n = 252)	63 ± 5.6 (n = 130)	27 ± 9.3 (n = 57)	59 ± 4.7 (n = 122)	46 ± 5.5 (n = 93)	27 ± 4.6 (n = 109)
Present	52 ± 4.1 (n = 217)	50 ± 5.7 (n = 111)	37 ± 8.8 (n = 46)	29 ± 5.0 (n = 98)	25 ± 4.4 (n = 109)	13 ± 3.5 (n = 104)

n indicates the number of patients

taken into account, 5-year survival rates were remarkably heterogeneous ranging from 69% in Stage IIIA patients who had three or fewer microscopic nodal metastases arising from a non-ulcerating primary to 13% for Stage IIIC patients who had four or more metastatic nodal metastases arising from an ulcerated primary melanoma (Table 24.5).

Intralymphatic metastases portend a very poor prognosis.[5,16,17] The available data show no substantial difference in survival outcome for these two anatomically defined entities (satellite metastases and in-transit metastases).[5] Therefore, they are both assigned to a separate N2c classification in the absence of synchronous nodal metastases, because both have a prognosis equivalent to that of multiple nodal metastases. Furthermore, the available data demonstrate that patients with a combination of satellites/in-transit metastases and nodal metastases have a worse outcome than patients who experience either event alone, so these patients are assigned to the N3 classification regardless of the number of synchronous metastatic nodes.

The prognostic influence of different distant metastatic sites was analyzed in 1,158 Stage IV patients, using various combinations of sites of metastases. The most significant differences in 1-year survival rates were noted when lung metastases were compared to all other visceral sites and non-visceral sites (i.e., skin, subcutaneous, distant lymph nodes) (Fig. 24.4). Although it is uncommon in staging classifications to include serum factors prognostically, serum LDH was among the most predictive factors of poor outcome in all published studies where it was analyzed in a multivariate analysis, even after accounting for site and number of metastases.[18–23]

Significant differences were identified when survival rates for melanoma patients who were clinically staged were compared to those whose nodal disease was staged pathologically.[3] These survival differences

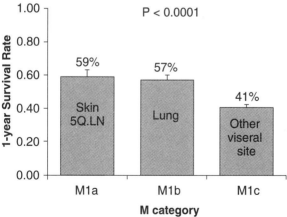

Fig. 24.4. One-year survival rates from the AJCC melanoma staging database comparing the different M categories.[3] See Table 24.1 for definitions. There is a significant difference when skin, subcutaneous and lung metastases are compared to all other sites (p < 0.0001).

between clinically and pathologically staged patients were statistically significant among all T substages except T4b (Table 24.6). These results highlight the compelling prognostic value of knowing the nodal status, as identified by lymphatic mapping and sentinel lymphadenectomy, in those situations where accurate staging is important.

The prognostic factors used to validate the melanoma staging system should be the primary stratification criteria and the end-results reporting criteria of melanoma clinical trials. It is recommended that all melanoma patients who have clinically negative regional lymph nodes and may be considered for later entry into surgical and adjuvant therapy clinical trials should have pathologic staging with sentinel lymphadenectomy to ensure prognostic homogeneity within assigned treatment groups. In this way, investigators will be better able to discern between the natural-history impact and the treatment impact being studied in melanoma clinical trials. Moreover, the use of a consistent set of criteria will facilitate the comparability of melanoma clinical trials and thereby accelerate the progress of multidisciplinary melanoma treatment approaches.

MELANOMA GROWTH PATTERNS

The data used to derive the TNM categories were largely based on melanomas with superficial spreading and nodular growth patterns. There is

TABLE 24.6. Five-year survival rates for 5,346 patients with clinically negative nodal metastases who were pathologically staged after either RND or SLN (adapted from Balch et al.[3])

T stage	Path Nodes (N)	5-Year Survival, % ± S.E.	P-value*
T1a	N− ($n = 379$)	94 ± 2.0	0.0035
	N+ ($n = 15$)	64 ± 17.7	
T1b	N− ($n = 319$)	90 ± 2.5	0.0039
	N+ ($n = 18$)	76 ± 14.9	
T2a	N− ($n = 1480$)	94 ± 0.8	< 0.0001
	N+ ($n = 150$)	73 ± 5.6	
T2b	N− ($n = 408$)	83 ± 2.3	< 0.0001
	N+ ($n = 62$)	56 ± 8.8	
T3a	N− ($n = 808$)	86 ± 1.6	< 0.0001
	N+ ($n = 177$)	59 ± 6.0	
T3b	N− ($n = 639$)	72 ± 2.1	< 0.0001
	N+ ($n = 176$)	49 ± 4.5	
T4a	N− ($n = 203$)	75 ± 3.9	0.0116
	N+ ($n = 66$)	61 ± 7.4	
T4b	N− ($n = 330$)	53 ± 3.1	0.2403
	N+ ($n = 116$)	44 ± 5.5	

*The p-value based on the comparison of survival curves using the log rank test.
RND: regional lymph node dissection
SLN: sentinel lymphadenectomy

some evidence that other growth patterns, namely lentigo maligna melanoma, acral lentiginous melanoma, and desmoplastic melanoma, may have a different etiology and natural history.[24–29] At present, the same staging criteria should be used for melanomas with these growth patterns, even though their prognosis may differ somewhat from the more commonly occurring superficial spreading and nodular growth patterns.

REFERENCES

1. NCI Fact Book. Bethesda, MD, National Cancer Institute, 2000
2. Balch C, Soong SJ, Gershenwald JE, Thompson JF, Reintgen DS, Cascinelli N, Urist MM, McMasters KM, Ross MI, Kirkwood JM, Atkins MB, Thompson JA, Coit DG, Byrd D, Desmond R, Zhang Y, Liu PY, Lyman GH, Morabito A: Prognostic factors analysis of 17,600 melanoma patients. Validation of the AJCC melanoma staging system. J Clin Oncol, 19:3622–3634, 2001
3. Balch C, Buzaid AC, Soong SJ, Atkins MB, Cascinelli N, Coit DG, Fleming ID, Gershenwald JE, Houghton A, Kirkwood JM, McMasters KM, Mihm MF, Morton DL, Reintgen DS, Ross MI, Sober AJ, Thompson JA, Thompson JF: Final version of the AJCC staging system for cutaneous melanoma. J Clin Oncol, 19:3635–3648, 2001
4. Balch CM, Buzaid AC, Atkins MB, et al: A new American Joint Committee on Cancer staging system for cutaneous melanoma. Cancer 88:1484–1491, 2000
5. Buzaid AC, Ross MI, Balch CM, et al: Critical analysis of the current American Joint Committee on Cancer staging system for cutaneous melanoma and proposal of a new staging system. J Clin Oncol 15:1039–1051, 1997
6. Breslow A: Thickness, cross-sectional areas and depth of invasion in the prognosis of cutaneous melanoma. Ann Surg 172:902–908, 1970
7. Breslow A: Tumor thickness, level of invasion and node dissection in stage I cutaneous melanoma. Ann Surg 182:572–575, 1975
8. Balch CM, Murad TM, Soong SJ, et al: A multifactorial analysis of melanoma: prognostic histopathological features comparing Clark's and Breslow's staging methods. Ann Surg 188:732–742, 1978
9. Balch CM, Wilkerson JA, Murad TM, et al: The prognostic significance of ulceration of cutaneous melanoma. Cancer 45:3012–3017, 1980
10. McGovern VJ, Shaw HM, Milton GW, et al: Ulceration and prognosis in cutaneous malignant melanoma. Histopathology 6:399–407, 1982
11. Clark WH Jr, From L, Bernardino EA, Mihm MC: The histogenesis and biological behavior of primary human malignant melanoma of the skin. Cancer Research 29:705–727, 1969
12. Breslow A: Problems in the measurement of tumor thickness and level of invasion in cutaneous melanoma. Hum Pathol 8:1–2, 1977
13. Breslow A: Tumor thickness in evaluating prognosis of cutaneous melanoma [letter]. Ann Surg 187:440, 1978
14. Prade M, Sancho-Garnier H, Cesarini JP, et al: Difficulties encountered in the application of Clark classification and the Breslow thickness measurement in cutaneous malignant melanoma. Int J Cancer 26:159–163, 1980
15. Lock-Andersen J, Hou-Jensen K, Hansen JP, et al: Observer variation in histological classification of cutaneous malignant melanoma. Scand J Plast Reconstr Surg Hand Surg 29:141–148, 1995
16. Cascinelli N, Bufalino R, Marolda R, et al: Regional non-nodal metastases of cutaneous melanoma. Eur J Surg Oncol 12:175–80, 1986

6

17. Day CJ, Harrist T, Gorstein F, et al: Malignant melanoma: Prognostic significance of "microscopic satellites" in the reticular dermis and subcutaneous fat. Ann Surg 194:108–112, 1981

18. Eton O, Legha SS, Moon TE, et al: Prognostic factors for survival of patients treated systemically for disseminated melanoma. J Clin Oncol 16:1103–1111, 1998

19. Keilholz U, Conradt C, Legha SS, et al: Results of interleukin-2-based treatment in advanced melanoma: A case record-based analysis of 631 patients. J Clin Oncol 16:2921–2929, 1998

20. Deichmann M, Benner A, Bock M, et al: S100-Beta, melanoma-inhibiting activity, and lactate dehydrogenase discriminate progressive from nonprogressive American Joint Committee on Cancer stage IV melanoma. J Clin Oncol 17:1891–1896, 1999

21. Agrawal S, Yao T-J, Coit DG: Surgery for melanoma metastatic to the gastrointestinal tract. Ann Surg Oncol 6:336–344, 1999

22. Sirott M, Bajorin D, Wong G, et al: Prognostic factors in patients with metastatic malignant melanoma. A multivariate analysis. Cancer 72:3091–3098, 1993

23. Franzke A, Probst-Kepper M, Buer J, et al: Elevated pretreatment serum levels of soluble vascular cell adhesion molecule 1 and lactate dehydrogenase as predictors of survival in cutaneous metastatic malignant melanoma. Brit J Cancer 78:40–45, 1998

24. Cascinelli N, Zurrida S, Galimberti V, et al: Acral lentiginous melanoma. A histological type without prognostic significance. J Dermatol Surg Oncol 20:817–822, 1994

25. McGovern VJ, Shaw HM, Milton GW, et al: Is malignant melanoma arising in a Hutchinson's melanotic freckle a separate disease entity? Histopathology 4:235–242, 1980

26. Kuchelmeister C, Schaumburg-Lever G, Garbe C: Acral cutaneous melanoma in Caucasians: clinical features, histopathology and prognosis in 112 patients. Br J Dermatol 143:275–280, 2000

27. Urist MM, Balch CM, Soong SJ, et al: Head and neck melanoma in 534 clinical Stage I patients. A prognostic factors analysis and results of surgical treatment. Ann Surg 200:769–775, 1984

28. Slingluff CL Jr, Vollmer R, Seigler HF: Acral melanoma: a review of 185 patients with identification of prognostic variables. J Surg Oncol 45:91–98, 1990

29. Balch CM: Cutaneous melanoma: prognosis and treatment results worldwide. Semin Surg Oncol 8:400–414, 1992

HISTOLOGIES—MALIGNANT MELANOMA OF THE SKIN

8720/2	Melanoma *in situ*
8720/3	Malignant melanoma, NOS
8721/3	Nodular melanoma
8722/3	Balloon cell melanoma
8742/3	Lentigo maligna melanoma
8743/3	Superficial spreading melanoma
8744/3	Acral lentiginous melanoma, malignant
8745/3	Desmoplastic melanoma, malignant
8761/3	Malignant melanoma in giant pigmented nevus
8771/3	Epithelioid cell melanoma
8772/3	Spindle cell melanoma
8780/3	Blue nevus, malignant

PART VII
Breast

7

25

Breast

C50.0 Nipple
C50.1 Central portion of breast
C50.2 Upper inner quadrant of breast

C50.3 Lower inner quadrant of breast
C50.4 Upper outer quadrant of breast
C50.5 Lower outer quadrant of breast

C50.6 Axillary tail of breast
C50.8 Overlapping lesion of breast
C50.9 Breast, NOS

SUMMARY OF CHANGES

- Micrometastases are distinguished from isolated tumor cells on the basis of size and histologic evidence of malignant activity.

- Identifiers have been added to indicate the use of sentinel lymph node dissection and immunohistochemical or molecular techniques.

- Major classifications of lymph node status are designated according to the number of involved axillary lymph nodes as determined by routine hematoxylin and eosin staining (preferred method) or by immunohistochemical staining.

- The classification of metastasis to the infraclavicular lymph nodes has been added as N3.

- Metastasis to the internal mammary nodes, based on the method of detection and the presence or absence of axillary nodal involvement, has been reclassified. Microscopic involvement of the internal mammary nodes detected by sentinel lymph node dissection using lymphoscintigraphy but not by imaging studies or clinical examination is classified as N1. Macroscopic involvement of the internal mammary nodes as detected by imaging studies (excluding lymphoscintigraphy) or by clinical examination is classified as N2 if it occurs in the absence of metastases to the axillary lymph nodes or as N3 if it occurs in the presence of metastases to the axillary lymph nodes.

- Metastasis to the supraclavicular lymph nodes has been reclassified as N3 rather than M1.

INTRODUCTION

This staging system for carcinoma of the breast applies to infiltrating (including microinvasive) and *in situ* carcinomas. Microscopic confirmation of the diagnosis is mandatory, and the histologic type and grade of carcinoma should be recorded.

ANATOMY

Primary Site. The mammary gland, situated on the anterior chest wall, is composed of glandular tissue with a dense fibrous stroma. The glandular tissue consists of lobules that group together into 15–25 lobes arranged approximately in a spoke-like pattern. Multiple major and minor ducts connect the milk-secreting lobular units to the nipple. Small milk ducts course throughout the breast, converging into larger collecting ducts that open into the lactiferous sinus at the base of the nipple. Most cancers form initially in the terminal duct lobular units of the breast. Glandular tissue is more abundant in the upper outer portion of the breast; as a result, half of all breast cancers occur in this area.

Chest Wall. The chest wall includes ribs, intercostal muscles, and serratus anterior muscle, but not the pectoral muscles.

Regional Lymph Nodes. The breast lymphatics drain by way of three major routes: axillary, transpectoral, and internal mammary. Intramammary lymph nodes are coded as axillary lymph nodes for staging purposes. Supraclavicular lymph nodes are classified as regional lymph nodes for staging purposes. Metastasis to any other lymph node, including cervical or contralateral internal mammary lymph nodes, is classified as distant (M1) (refer to Fig. 25.1.)

The regional lymph nodes are as follows:

1. Axillary (ipsilateral): interpectoral (Rotter's) nodes and lymph nodes along the axillary vein and its tributaries that may be (but are not required to be) divided into the following levels:
   a. Level I (low-axilla): lymph nodes lateral to the lateral border of pectoralis minor muscle.

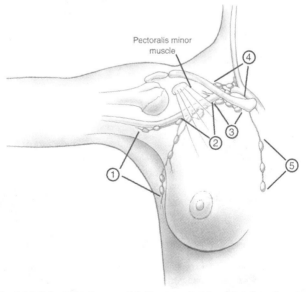

Fig. 25.1. Schematic diagram of the breast and regional lymph nodes. ① Low axillary, Level I; ② Mid-axillary, Level II; ③ High axillary, apical, Level III; ④ Supraclavicular; ⑤ Internal mammary nodes.

b. Level II (mid-axilla): lymph nodes between the medial and lateral borders of the pectoralis minor muscle and the interpectoral (Rotter's) lymph nodes.

c. Level III (apical axilla): lymph nodes medial to the medial margin of the pectoralis minor muscle, including those designated as apical.

2. Internal mammary (ipsilateral): lymph nodes in the intercostal spaces along the edge of the sternum in the endothoracic fascia.

3. Supraclavicular: lymph nodes in the supraclavicular fossa, a triangle defined by the omohyoid muscle and tendon (lateral and superior border), the internal jugular vein (medial border), and the clavicle and subclavian vein (lower border). Adjacent lymph nodes outside of this triangle are considered to be lower cervical nodes (M1).

Metastatic Sites. Tumor cells may be disseminated by either the lymphatic or the blood vascular system. The four major sites of involvement are bone, lung, brain, and liver, but tumor cells are also capable of metastasizing to many other sites.

RULES FOR CLASSIFICATION

Clinical Staging. Clinical staging includes physical examination, with careful inspection and palpation of the skin, mammary gland, and lymph nodes (axillary, supraclavicular, and cervical), imaging, and pathologic examination of the breast or other tissues as appropriate to establish the diagnosis of breast carcinoma. The extent of tissue examined pathologically for clinical staging is not so great as that required for pathologic staging (see Pathologic Staging below). Imaging findings are considered elements of staging if they are collected within 4 months of diagnosis in the absence of disease progression or through completion of surgery(ies), whichever is longer. Such imaging findings would include the size of the primary tumor and of chest wall invasion, and the presence or absence of regional or distant metastasis. Imaging findings and surgical findings obtained after a patient has been treated with neoadjuvant chemotherapy, hormonal therapy, immunotherapy, or radiation therapy are not considered elements of initial staging.

Pathologic Staging. Pathologic staging includes all data used for clinical staging, plus data from surgical exploration and resection as well as pathologic examination of the primary carcinoma, regional lymph nodes, and metastatic sites (if applicable), including not less than excision of the primary carcinoma with no macroscopic tumor in any margin of resection by pathologic examination. A cancer can be classified pT for pathologic stage grouping if there is only microscopic, but not macroscopic, involvement at the margin. If there is tumor in the margin of resection by macroscopic examination, the cancer is coded pTX because the total extent of the primary tumor cannot be assessed. If the primary tumor is invasive and not only microinvasive, resection of at least the low axillary lymph nodes (Level I)—that is, those lymph nodes located lateral to the lateral border of the pectoralis minor muscle—should be performed for pathologic (pN) classification. Such a resection will ordinarily include six or more lymph nodes. Alternatively, one or more sentinel lymph nodes may be resected and examined for pathologic classification. Certain histologic tumor types (pure tubular carcinoma < 1 cm, pure mucinous carcinoma < 1 cm, and microinvasive carcinoma) have a very low incidence of axillary lymph node metastasis and do not usually require an axillary lymph node dissection. Cancerous nodules in the axillary fat adjacent to the breast, without histologic evidence of residual lymph node tissue, are classified as regional lymph node metastases (N). Pathologic stage grouping includes any of the following combinations of pathologic and clinical classifications: pT pN pM, or pT pN cM, or cT cN pM. If surgery occurs after the patient has received neoadjuvant chemotherapy, hormonal therapy, immunotherapy, or radiation therapy, the prefix "y" should be used with the TNM classification, e.g., ypTNM.

TNM CLASSIFICATION

Primary Tumor (T)

Determining Tumor Size
The clinical measurement used for classifying the primary tumor (T) is the one judged to be most accurate for that particular case (that is, physical examination or imaging such as mammography or ultrasound). The pathologic tumor size for the T classification is a measurement of *only the invasive component.* For example, if there is a 4.0-cm intraductal component and a 0.3-cm invasive component, the tumor is classified T1a. The size of the primary tumor is measured for T classification before any tissue is removed for special studies, such as for estrogen receptors. In patients who have received multiple core biopsies, measuring only the residual lesion may result in significantly underclassifying the T component and thus understaging the tumor. In such cases, original tumor size should be reconstructed on the basis of a combination of imaging and all histologic findings.

Tis Classification
Carcinoma *in situ*, with no evidence of an invasive component, is classified as Tis, with a subclassification indicating type. Cases of ductal carcinoma *in situ* and cases with both ductal carcinoma *in situ* and lobular carcinoma *in situ* are classified Tis (DCIS). Lobular carcinoma *in situ* is increasingly defined as a risk factor for subsequent breast cancer, although there is some evidence that it may occasionally be a precursor of invasive lobular carcinoma. For example, this may be the case with LCIS with more atypical cytology (pleomorphic) as well as more extensive and locally distorting examples of well-developed LCIS.[1] Regardless of this controversy, LCIS is reported as a malignancy by national database registrars and should be designated as such in this classification system—e.g., Tis (LCIS). Paget's disease of the nipple without an associated tumor mass (clinical) and invasive carcinoma (pathologic) is classified Tis (Paget's). Paget's disease with a demonstrable mass (clinical) anywhere within that breast or an

invasive component (pathologic) is classified according to the size of the tumor mass or invasive component.

Microinvasion of Breast Carcinoma
Microinvasion is the extension of cancer cells beyond the basement membrane into the adjacent tissues with no focus more than 0.1 cm in greatest dimension. When there are multiple foci of microinvasion, the size of only the largest focus is used to classify the microinvasion. (Do not use the sum of all the individual foci.) The presence of multiple foci of microinvasion should be noted and/or quantified, as it is with multiple larger invasive carcinomas.

Multiple Simultaneous Ipsilateral Primary Carcinomas
The following guidelines are used in classifying multiple simultaneous ipsilateral primary (infiltrating, macroscopically measurable) carcinomas. These criteria do not apply to one macroscopic carcinoma associated with multiple separate microscopic foci. Most conservatively, tumors are defined as arising independently only if they occur in different quadrants of the breast.

1. Use the largest primary carcinoma to designate T classification. Do not assign a separate T classification for the smaller tumor(s).
2. Enter into the record that this is a case of multiple simultaneous ipsilateral primary carcinomas. The outcome of such cases should be analyzed separately.

Simultaneous Bilateral Breast Carcinomas
Each carcinoma is staged as a separate primary carcinoma in a separate organ.

7

Inflammatory Carcinoma
Inflammatory carcinoma is a clinicopathologic entity characterized by diffuse erythema and edema (peau d'orange) of the breast, often without an underlying palpable mass. These clinical findings should involve the majority of the skin of the breast. Classically, the skin changes arise quickly in the affected breast. Thus the term *inflammatory carcinoma* should not be applied to a patient with neglected locally advanced cancer of the breast presenting late in the course of her disease. On imaging, there may be a detectable mass and characteristic thickening of the skin over the breast. This clinical presentation is due to tumor emboli within dermal lymphatics, which may or may not be apparent on skin biopsy. The tumor of inflammatory carcinoma is classified T4d. It is important to remember that inflammatory carcinoma is primarily a clinical diagnosis. Involvement of the dermal lymphatics alone does not indicate inflammatory carcinoma in the absence of clinical findings. In addition to the clinical picture, however, a biopsy is still necessary to demonstrate cancer either within the dermal lymphatics or in the breast parenchyma itself.

Skin of Breast
Dimpling of the skin, nipple retraction, or any other skin change except those described under T4b and T4d may occur in T1, T2, or T3 without changing the classification.

Regional Lymph Nodes (N)

Macrometastasis

Cases in which regional lymph nodes cannot be assessed (previously removed or not removed for pathologic examination) are designated NX or pNX. Cases in which no regional lymph node metastasis is detected are designated N0 or pN0.

In patients who are clinically node-positive, N1 designates metastasis to one or more movable ipsilateral axillary lymph nodes, N2a designates metastasis to axillary lymph nodes that are fixed to each other (matted) or to other structures, and N3a indicates metastasis to ipsilateral infraclavicular lymph nodes. Metastasis to the ipsilateral internal mammary nodes are designated as N2b when they are detected by imaging studies (including CT scan and ultrasound, but excluding lymphoscintigraphy) or by clinical examination and when they do not occur in conjunction with metastasis to the axillary lymph nodes. Metastases to the ipsilateral internal mammary nodes are designated as N3b when they are detected by imaging studies or by clinical examination and when they occur in conjunction with metastasis to the axillary lymph nodes. Metastasis to the ipsilateral supraclavicular lymph nodes are designated as N3c regardless of the presence or absence of axillary or internal mammary nodal involvement.

In patients who are pathologically node-positive with one or more tumor deposits greater than 2 mm, cases with 1 to 3 positive axillary lymph nodes are classified pN1a, cases with 4 to 9 positive axillary lymph nodes are classified pN2a, and cases with 10 or more positive axillary lymph nodes are classified pN3a. Cases with histologically confirmed metastasis to the internal mammary nodes, detected by sentinel lymph node dissection but not by imaging studies (excluding lymphoscintigraphy) or clinical examination, are classified as pN1b if occurring in the *absence* of metastasis to the axillary lymph nodes and as pN1c if occurring in the *presence* of metastases to 1 to 3 axillary lymph nodes. (If 4 or more axillary lymph nodes are involved, the classification pN3b is used.) Clinical involvement with histologic confirmation of the internal mammary nodes by imaging studies (excluding lymphoscintigraphy) in the absence or presence of axillary nodal metastases are classified as pN2b and pN3b, respectively. Histologic evidence of metastasis in ipsilateral supraclavicular lymph node(s) is classified as pN3c. A classification of pN3, regardless of primary tumor size or grade, is classified as Stage IIIC. A case in which the classification is based only on sentinel lymph node dissection is given the additional designation (sn) for "sentinel node"—for example, pN1 (sn). For a case in which an initial classification is based on a sentinel lymph node dissection but a standard axillary lymph node dissection is subsequently performed, the classification is based on the total results of the axillary lymph node dissection (that is, including the sentinel node).

Isolated Tumor Cells and Micrometastases

Isolated tumor cells (ITCs) are defined as single cells or small clusters of cells not greater than 0.2 mm in largest dimension, usually with no histologic evidence of malignant activity (such as proliferation or stromal reaction). If an additional immunohistochemical examination was made for ITCs in a patient with histologically negative lymph nodes, the regional lymph nodes should be designated as pN0(i−) or pN0(i+), as appropriate.

Micrometastases are defined as tumor deposits greater than 0.2 mm but not greater than 2.0 mm in largest dimension that may have histologic evidence of malignant activity (such as proliferation or stromal reaction). Cases in which only micrometastases are detected (none greater than 2 mm) are classified pN1mi. The classification is designated as (i+) for "immunohistochemical" if micrometastasis was detected only by IHC [e.g., pN1mi (i+)].

If histologically and immunohistochemically negative lymph nodes are examined for evidence of metastasis using molecular methods [reverse transcriptase–polymerase chain reaction (RT-PCR)], the regional lymph nodes are classified as pN0(mol−) or pN0(mol+), as appropriate.

Distant Metastasis (M)

Cases where distant metastasis cannot be assessed are designated MX, cases in which there is no distant metastasis are designated M0, and cases in which one or more distant metastases are identified are designated M1. A negative clinical history and examination are sufficient to designate a case as M0; extensive imaging or other testing is not required. Note that positive supraclavicular lymph nodes are now classified as N3 rather than M1.

DEFINITION OF TNM

Primary Tumor (T)

Definitions for classifying the primary tumor (T) are the same for clinical and for pathologic classification. If the measurement is made by physical examination, the examiner will use the major headings (T1, T2, or T3). If other measurements, such as mammographic or pathologic measurements, are used, the subsets of T1 can be used. Tumors should be measured to the nearest 0.1 cm increment.

TX	Primary tumor cannot be assessed
T0	No evidence of primary tumor
Tis	Carcinoma *in situ*
Tis (DCIS)	Ductal carcinoma *in situ*
Tis (LCIS)	Lobular carcinoma *in situ*
Tis (Paget's)	Paget's disease of the nipple with no tumor

Note: Paget's disease associated with a tumor is classified according to the size of the tumor.

T1	Tumor 2 cm or less in greatest dimension
T1mic	Microinvasion 0.1 cm or less in greatest dimension
T1a	Tumor more than 0.1 cm but not more than 0.5 cm in greatest dimension
T1b	Tumor more than 0.5 cm but not more than 1 cm in greatest dimension
T1c	Tumor more than 1 cm but not more than 2 cm in greatest dimension
T2	Tumor more than 2 cm but not more than 5 cm in greatest dimension

T3	Tumor more than 5 cm in greatest dimension
T4	Tumor of any size with direct extension to (a) chest wall or (b) skin, only as described below
T4a	Extension to chest wall, not including pectoralis muscle
T4b	Edema (including peau d'orange) or ulceration of the skin of the breast, or satellite skin nodules confined to the same breast
T4c	Both T4a and T4b
T4d	Inflammatory carcinoma

Regional Lymph Nodes (N)

Clinical

NX	Regional lymph nodes cannot be assessed (e.g., previously removed)
N0	No regional lymph node metastasis
N1	Metastasis to movable ipsilateral axillary lymph node(s)
N2	Metastases in ipsilateral axillary lymph nodes fixed or matted, or in clinically apparent* ipsilateral internal mammary nodes in the *absence* of clinically evident axillary lymph node metastasis
N2a	Metastasis in ipsilateral axillary lymph nodes fixed to one another (matted) or to other structures
N2b	Metastasis only in clinically apparent* ipsilateral internal mammary nodes and in the *absence* of clinically evident axillary lymph node metastasis
N3	Metastasis in ipsilateral infraclavicular lymph node(s) with or without axillary lymph node involvement, or in clinically apparent* ipsilateral internal mammary lymph node(s) and in the *presence* of clinically evident axillary lymph node metastasis; or metastasis in ipsilateral supraclavicular lymph node(s) with or without axillary or internal mammary lymph node involvement
N3a	Metastasis in ipsilateral infraclavicular lymph node(s)
N3b	Metastasis in ipsilateral internal mammary lymph node(s) and axillary lymph node(s)
N3c	Metastasis in ipsilateral supraclavicular lymph node(s)

Clinically apparent is defined as detected by imaging studies (excluding lymphoscintigraphy) or by clinical examination or grossly visible pathologically.

Pathologic (pN)[a]

pNX	Regional lymph nodes cannot be assessed (e.g., previously removed, or not removed for pathologic study)
pN0	No regional lymph node metastasis histologically, no additional examination for isolated tumor cells (ITC)

Note: Isolated tumor cells (ITC) are defined as single tumor cells or small cell clusters not greater than 0.2 mm, usually detected only by immunohistochemical (IHC) or molecular methods but which may be verified on H&E stains. ITCs do not usually show evidence of malignant activity e.g., proliferation or stromal reaction.

pN0(i−)	No regional lymph node metastasis histologically, negative IHC
pN0(i+)	No regional lymph node metastasis histologically, positive IHC, no IHC cluster greater than 0.2 mm
pN0(mol−)	No regional lymph node metastasis histologically, negative molecular findings (RT-PCR)[b]
pN0(mol+)	No regional lymph node metastasis histologically, positive molecular findings (RT-PCR)[b]

[a]Classification is based on axillary lymph node dissection with or without sentinel lymph node dissection. Classification based solely on sentinel lymph node dissection without subsequent axillary lymph node dissection is designated (sn) for "sentinel node," e.g., pN0(i+) (sn).

[b]RT-PCR: reverse transcriptase/polymerase chain reaction.

pN1	Metastasis in 1 to 3 axillary lymph nodes, and/or in internal mammary nodes with microscopic disease detected by sentinel lymph node dissection but not clinically apparent**
pN1mi	Micrometastasis (greater than 0.2 mm, none greater than 2.0 mm)
pN1a	Metastasis in 1 to 3 axillary lymph nodes
pN1b	Metastasis in internal mammary nodes with microscopic disease detected by sentinel lymph node dissection but not clinically apparent**
pN1c	Metastasis in 1 to 3 axillary lymph nodes and in internal mammary lymph nodes with microscopic disease detected by sentinel lymph node dissection but not clinically apparent.** (If associated with greater than 3 positive axillary lymph nodes, the internal mammary nodes are classified as pN3b to reflect increased tumor burden)
pN2	Metastasis in 4 to 9 axillary lymph nodes, or in clinically apparent* internal mammary lymph nodes in the *absence* of axillary lymph node metastasis
pN2a	Metastasis in 4 to 9 axillary lymph nodes (at least one tumor deposit greater than 2.0 mm)
pN2b	Metastasis in clinically apparent* internal mammary lymph nodes in the *absence* of axillary lymph node metastasis
pN3	Metastasis in 10 or more axillary lymph nodes, or in infraclavicular lymph nodes, or in clinically apparent* ipsilateral internal mammary lymph nodes in the *presence* of 1 or more positive axillary lymph nodes; or in more than 3 axillary lymph nodes with clinically negative microscopic metastasis in internal mammary lymph nodes; or in ipsilateral supraclavicular lymph nodes

7

pN3a	Metastasis in 10 or more axillary lymph nodes (at least one tumor deposit greater than 2.0 mm), or metastasis to the infraclavicular lymph nodes
pN3b	Metastasis in clinically apparent* ipsilateral internal mammary lymph nodes in the *presence* of 1 or more positive axillary lymph nodes; or in more than 3 axillary lymph nodes and in internal mammary lymph nodes with microscopic disease detected by sentinel lymph node dissection but not clinically apparent**
pN3c	Metastasis in ipsilateral supraclavicular lymph nodes

Clinically apparent is defined as detected by imaging studies (excluding lymphoscintigraphy) or by clinical examination.

**Not clinically apparent* is defined as not detected by imaging studies (excluding lymphoscintigraphy) or by clinical examination.

Distant Metastasis (M)

MX	Distant metastasis cannot be assessed
M0	No distant metastasis
M1	Distant metastasis

STAGE GROUPING

Stage 0	Tis	N0	M0
Stage I	T1*	N0	M0
Stage IIA	T0	N1	M0
	T1*	N1	M0
	T2	N0	M0
Stage IIB	T2	N1	M0
	T3	N0	M0
Stage IIIA	T0	N2	M0
	T1*	N2	M0
	T2	N2	M0
	T3	N1	M0
	T3	N2	M0
Stage IIIB	T4	N0	M0
	T4	N1	M0
	T4	N2	M0
Stage IIIC	Any T	N3	M0
Stage IV	Any T	Any N	M1

---

*T1 includes T1mic

Note: Stage designation may be changed if post-surgical imaging studies reveal the presence of distant metastases, provided that the studies are carried out within 4 months of diagnosis in the absence of disease progression and provided that the patient has not received neoadjuvant therapy.

HISTOPATHOLOGIC TYPE

The histopathologic types are the following:

In situ Carcinomas
NOS (not otherwise specified)
Intraductal
Paget's Disease and intraductal

Invasive Carcinomas
NOS
Ductal
Inflammatory
Medullary, NOS
Medullary with lymphoid stroma
Mucinous
Papillary (predominantly micropapillary pattern)
Tubular
Lobular
Paget's Disease and infiltrating
Undifferentiated
Squamous cell
Adenoid cystic
Secretory
Cribriform

HISTOLOGIC GRADE (G)

All invasive breast carcinomas with the exception of medullary carcinoma should be graded. The Nottingham combined histologic grade (Elston-Ellis modification of Scarff-Bloom-Richardson grading system) is recommended.[2,3] The grade for a tumor is determined by assessing morphologic features (tubule formation, nuclear pleomorphism, and mitotic count), assigning a value of 1 (favorable) to 3 (unfavorable) for each feature, and adding together the scores for all three categories. A combined score of 3–5 points is designated as grade 1; a combined score of 6–7 points is grade 2; a combined score of 8–9 points is grade 3.

HISTOLOGIC GRADE (NOTTINGHAM COMBINED HISTOLOGIC GRADE IS RECOMMENDED)

GX   Grade cannot be assessed
G1   Low combined histologic grade (favorable)
G2   Intermediate combined histologic grade (moderately favorable)
G3   High combined histologic grade (unfavorable)

CONSIDERATIONS FOR EVIDENCE-BASED CHANGES TO THE *AJCC CANCER STAGING MANUAL*, 6TH EDITION

Should histologic grade (Nottingham combined histologic grade recommended) be incorporated into the TNM classification system?
It was first recognized by Hansemann in 1890 that the morphological appearance of tumors was associated with the degree of malignancy,[4] and the

first formal grading of morphologic features in breast cancer occurred 35 years later.[5] Since then, the histologic grading of invasive breast carcinoma has been clearly shown to provide significant prognostic information.[2,6–9] Different approaches to histologic grading have been described and used. Though all of these approaches offer some degree of prognostic information, there are varying levels of agreement among them, and this makes clinical studies difficult to compare. In addition, grading is by nature subjective, and there can be substantial differences in assessment even when the same grading system is used.[10–13]

Several observers have pointed out that observer variation in estimating histologic grade may have only a small adverse effect in estimating prognosis, especially if the variation in outcome is greater than the variation among observers.[8,14] This may be true in a general way, but it should be remembered that the inclusion of histologic grade in the AJCC staging system will affect data collection and coding for national cancer registrars. Institute-to-institute reproducibility will be an important requirement for data inclusion in these large databases.

The modification of the Bloom and Richardson grading system by Elston and Ellis (the Nottingham combined histologic grade)[2] was designed to make grading criteria more quantitative. Three morphologic features (percentage of tubule formation, degree of nuclear pleomorphism, and accurate mitotic count in a defined field area) are evaluated semiquantitatively, and a numerical score for each is used in calculating the overall grade. Elston and Ellis compiled long-term survival information from 1,831 patients for whom a Nottingham combined histologic grade was assessed, and they found a very strong correlation with prognosis ($p < 0.0001$). In subsequent studies, better interobserver agreement was obtained with the Nottingham combined histologic grade than with previous systems,[15–17] and it is recommended in the College of American Pathologists Consensus Statement.[3] Thus the Nottingham combined histologic grade is strongly recommended in this revision for the histologic grading of tumors.

Even with this more quantitative approach, significant variation in results can stem from technical variations in processing the tumor tissue. The time lag between surgical excision and fixation can vary greatly from one case to another (from 10 min to 4 hr in one published study[18]). A time lag of as little as 2 hours can result in mitotic rate decreases of 10% to 30%,[19,20] and a delay of 24 hours can result in a striking decline of more than 75%.[21] Even with fixation times standardized, the type of fixative used can also be an important element; some commonly used fixatives contribute to suboptimal cell morphology.[17,18] Precise guidelines about these technical details will be important in ensuring data comparability across institutes.

Thus histologic grading has prognostic value, and improved reproducibility is possible with the Nottingham combined histologic grade. The question of how to add grading to the existing TNM classification system remains. Because large tumors (T3, T4) nearly always carry a recommendation for adjuvant therapy, and because many such tumors tend to be high grade, the addition of grading information would not be expected to have a significant effect on treatment planning for this group. Most conservatively, grading should be considered in those cases where it would influence treatment decisions most heavily—that is, for small (T1,T2) node-negative tumors. It is unfortunate, therefore, that available evidence about the interaction between tumor size and histologic grade as they relate to patient outcome is disappointingly meager for these small tumors.

Table 25.1 shows the results of eight retrospective studies that analyzed outcome data on the basis of histologic grade in small tumors.[8,14,18,22–26] Because of the variety of follow-up times, grading systems, patient samples, and measured outcomes, it is difficult to extract a consistent picture from these studies. All studies showed a difference between Grade 1 and Grade 3, but the positioning of the Grade 2 intermediate tumors varied, sometimes clustering with Grade 1 and at other times clustering with Grade 3. In those studies that specifically used the Nottingham combined histologic grade,[18,24,26] Grade 2 either clustered with Grade 3 or else was intermediate between Grades 1 and 3 for a variety of outcomes. Three studies specifically looked at T1a/b tumors.[23–25] These studies used three different histologic grading systems and three different outcomes, but they nonetheless showed somewhat smaller outcome differences between Grade 1 and Grade 3 than other studies that included larger tumors.

These tentative observations, coupled with the overall sparseness and variability of the information, strongly suggest that the available data are not yet mature enough to offer guidance in incorporating histologic grade into the staging system for breast cancer. Because the evidence indicating that histologic grade is an important prognostic factor in breast cancer is so robust, it seems certain that emerging data will support the incorporation of grade into the AJCC staging system in the near future.

Should the classification of pathologic lymph node status in node-negative patients be amplified to include information about isolated tumor cells detected by immunohistochemical techniques?

Isolated tumor cells (ITCs) are defined as single tumor cells or small clusters of cells that are not greater than 0.2 mm in size and that usually show no histologic evidence of malignant activity (such as proliferation or stromal reaction). Although there is a growing feeling that ITCs detected by immunohistochemical staining may be prognostically relevant, their clinical significance has not yet been demonstrated. Even with larger clusters of single cells, it is not clear whether a finding of ITC would justify an axillary lymph node dissection. This is especially true for ITCs found in sentinel lymph nodes in cases where the primary tumor is very small and the probability of metastasis in a nonsentinel lymph node seems to be virtually zero.[27]

Clearly, organized large-scale data collection is essential for determining the clinical significance of ITCs. For this reason, a uniform shorthand is now suggested for describing pN0 patients where there has been immunohistochemical examination for ITCs. The added designation of "i+" or "i−" indicates that immunohistochemical staining was performed with positive or negative results.

TABLE 25.1. Histologic grade and outcome in patients with early-stage breast cancer.

Authors	Patient Description	Number of patients	Follow-up (years)	Grading System[a]	Outcome Measured[b]	Outcome		
						Grade 1	Grade 2	Grade 3
Rosen et al., 1989[21]	T1, N0	644	20	NS	Relapse	10%	23%	30%
Henson et al., 1991[7]	T1, N0 or T0,N1	22,616	10	NS	Relative survival	95%	91%	84%[c]
	T1/2, N1 or T2, N0		10	NS	Relative survival	82%	71%	63%[c]
Rosner & Lane, 1991[22]	T1a/b	113	7	BR	DFR	100%[d]		91%
	T1c	125	7	BR	DFR	91%[d]		79%
	T2	132	7	BR	DFR	65%[d]		70%
Genestie et al., 1998[17]	T1/2, N0/1	877	5	N	OS	96%	88%	80%
					MFS	91%	81%	78%
Kollias et al., 1999[23]	T1a/b, N0	318	10	N	OS	95%	91%	91%
Leitner et al., 1999[24]	T1a/b	218	7	WHO	RFS	100%	97%	88%
Reed et al., 2000[25]	T1/2, N0	228	10	N	RFS	90%	70%	69%
					OS	94%	86%	78%
Lundin et al., 2001[13]	T1, N0	665	5	WHO	DDFS	98%	86%	87%
	T2, N0	244	5	WHO	DDFS	96%	78%	69%

[a]NS: grading system not specified; BR: Bloom-Richardson; N: Nottingham combined histologic grade; WHO: World Health Organization

[b]DFR: disease-free rate; OS: overall survival; MFS: metastasis-free survival; RFS: relapse-free survival; DDFS: distant-disease-free survival

[c]Original Grades 3 and 4 showed no significant difference and were collapsed into Grade 3 for this review.

[d]Original Grades 1 and 2 were collapsed into one category in the original study.

Should micrometastases (pN1mi) detected by immunohistochemical staining and not verified by H&E staining be classified as pN1?

Micrometastases are defined as tumor deposits greater than 0.2 mm and no greater than 2.0 mm in size. Unlike isolated tumor cells, micrometastases may show histologic evidence of metastatic activity, such as proliferation or stromal reaction. The use of immunohistochemical techniques (IHC) to detect occult micrometastases has increased dramatically with the growing acceptance of sentinel lymph node dissection. The reported incidence of nodal micrometastases detected by IHC in patients who are histologically node-negative has ranged from 12% to 29%.[28-32]

The unresolved issue is whether micrometastases detected by IHC and not verified by standard histologic staining have a significant impact on patient outcome. Retrospective studies have reported decreases in disease-free survival ranging from 10% to 22% in some subgroups of patients where micrometastatic axillary disease was detected by immunohistochemical techniques. A significant percentage of histologically node-negative patients ultimately experience distant recurrence and die of their disease, and it has been suggested that some of this subgroup of patients may be those with occult micrometastases in the axillary nodes, but bone marrow and other metastases may occur with no axillary involvement.[30,31,33]

The premise that H&E verification is required to validate the metastatic potential of lesions detected by IHC is under increasing scrutiny. Cell deposits identified only by IHC are increasingly being used to make clinical recommendations without H&E verification. The size of the micrometastatic focus may prove to be critical; a 1-mm IHC-positive lesion may contain as many as 500,000 cells, and this would clearly meet the proliferation requirement for metastatic potential, regardless of H&E verification. Nonetheless, verification by H&E staining is recommended by the College of American Pathologists, because it provides more definitive cytologic and histologic evidence of malignancy than is usually available from immunostained preparations and avoids overinterpretation of staining artifacts.

Should size criteria be used to distinguish between isolated tumor cells and micrometastases?

Isolated tumor cells should theoretically be distinguishable from micrometastases on the basis of metastatic characteristics, such as proliferation or stromal reaction.[34] This distinction can be highly subjective, however, and replication among pathologists and among institutions may be difficult. This revision incorporates size criteria to assist in making this distinction, with isolated tumor cell groups defined as not greater than 0.2 mm in diameter and micrometastases defined as greater than 0.2 mm and not greater than 2.0 mm in diameter. The use of 2.0 mm as an upper size limit for micrometastases, originally proposed by Huvos and colleagues in 1971,[35] is consistent with standards already used in the AJCC staging system. The use of 0.2 mm as a lower limit was selected because it significantly reduces the likelihood that ITCs will be recorded as micrometastases, without making it necessary to estimate actual cell number counts in ITCs. The resulting classification of patients with metastatic tumor deposits no greater than 0.2 mm as pN0 is consistent with the low recurrence rates typically seen in this patient group.

How should RT-PCR be used in the detection of small tumor deposits?
An even finer level of resolution in the detection of isolated tumor cells and micrometastases is potentially available with the use of reverse transcriptase–polymerase chain reaction (RT-PCR). Verbanac and colleagues[36] recently reported that this technique was able to identify a neoplastic marker in a significant percentage of sentinel nodes that were negative for disease by both histologic and immunohistochemical staining. This is not altogether surprising, given that RT-PCR is theoretically capable of identifying single cells. However, it seems unlikely that such cells would become clinically important. There is evidence that such highly sensitive tests produce false positive results. Furthermore, because an entire block of lymph node tissue is digested in preparation for RT-PCR, it would be technically challenging to determine the exact size of the original lesion.

Pending further developments in this area, this edition of the *AJCC Cancer Staging Manual* will classify any lesion identified by RT-PCR alone as pN0 (the classification it would have had using standard histologic staining) for the purposes of staging. All cases that were histologically negative for regional lymph node metastasis and in which an additional examination for tumor cells was made with RT-PCR will have the appended designation (mol +) or (mol −), as appropriate.

Should the classification of pathological lymph node status in node-positive (all nodes with deposits greater than 0.2 mm) patients be changed to reflect more clearly the prognostic significance of number of affected nodes?
In past editions of the *AJCC Cancer Staging Manual,* the TNM system has used similar definitions for clinical lymph node status and pathological lymph node status. This has had the unfortunate result of assigning number of affected lymph nodes to subcategories of the pN1 classification, effectively ignoring this important prognostic indicator.

In this revision, patients with 1 to 3 positive axillary lymph nodes (with at least one tumor deposit greater than 2 mm and all tumor deposits greater than 0.2 mm) are classified as pN1a, patients with 4 to 9 positive axillary lymph nodes are classified as pN2a, and patients with 10 or more positive axillary lymph nodes are classified as pN3a. This recognition of the prognostic importance of the absolute number of involved lymph nodes is in keeping with current clinical practice and is supported by a large body of clinical data. The decision to separate patients with 1 to 3 positive nodes from patients with 4 or more positive nodes is consistent with survival data reported by Carter and colleagues (see Fig. 25.2).[37] These researchers examined 5-year survival rates by tumor size and lymph node status in 24,740 breast cancer cases recorded in the Surveillance, Epidemiology, and End Results (SEER) Program of the National Cancer Institute. In each size group of tumors (< 2 cm, 2–5 cm, > 5 cm) they found an inverse relationship between overall survival and number of positive nodes. In patients with tumors < 2 cm in size, for example, the relative 5-year survival was 96.3% for patients with negative nodes, 87.4% for

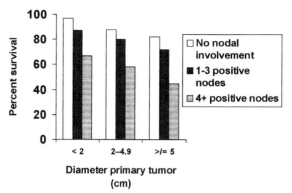

Fig. 25.2. Five-year relative survival of breast cancer as a function of both tumor diameter and number of positive axillary lymph nodes. (From Carter, et al: Relation of tumor size, lymph node status, and survival in 24,740 breast cancer cases. Cancer 63:181–187, 1989. Reprinted by permission of Wiley-Liss, Inc., a subsidiary of John Wiley & Sons, Inc.)

patients with 1 to 3 positive nodes, and 66.0% for patients with 4 or more positive nodes.

The decision to separate patients with 10 or more positive nodes into the N3a category, though somewhat more arbitrary, is based on the recognition that survival rates continue to decrease with increasing numbers of positive axillary lymph nodes. In a survey of 20,547 cases of breast carcinoma collected by the American College of Surgeons, Nemoto and colleagues[38] demonstrated that expected survival declined linearly with increasing number of axillary lymph nodes that were positive by histologic examination, up to a total of 21 positive nodes (Fig. 25.3). The specific breakpoint used here ($\geq$ 10) is in common usage. (See, for example, the report on the NSABP B-11 protocol in Paik et al.[39] and various other clinical studies.[40–42])

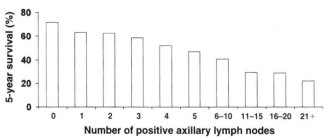

Fig. 25.3. Survival of 20,547 women with breast cancer according to the number of histologically involved axillary nodes. (Data from Nemoto et al: Management and survival of female breast cancer: results of a national survey by the American College of Surgeons. Cancer 45:2917–2924, 1980.)

The change in classification of axillary lymph node-positive patients reorganizes the pathologic staging system to reflect more closely the current practice standards used by clinicians in stratifying patients for prognosis and treatment decisions.

Should a finding of positive internal mammary lymph nodes retain a current classification of N3?

Data from the National Cancer Data Base (1985–1991) were analyzed to compare 5-year relative survival rates in all Stage IIIB breast cancer patients versus only Stage IIIB cancer patients with positive internal mammary nodes (N3)(L.L. Douglas, personal communication). For all Stage IIIB cancers ($n = 9775$), the relative 5-year survival rate was 47.6% with a 99% confidence interval of 45.7–49.5. For Stage IIIB cases with N3 only ($n = 717$), the relative survival rate was 45.2% with a 99% confidence interval of 38.6–51.9. This suggests no survival difference between N3 patients and the Stage IIIB group as a whole. In a separate report, Veronesi and colleagues[43] reported the results of a randomized trial carried out from 1964 to 1968 in which T1–3, N0–1 breast cancer patients were treated with a Halsted mastectomy or with an extended mastectomy that included removal of the internal mammary nodes. In the 342 patients treated with extended mastectomy, the 5-year overall survival rate was 44% in patients with positive internal mammary nodes, compared with 78% in patients with negative internal mammary nodes. These survival rates are consistent with those taken from the National Cancer Data Base.

A problem with these reports is that neither one considers the independent survival effects of positive internal mammary lymph nodes (IM) in the absence of positive axillary lymph nodes (AX). Table 25.2 shows the results of five studies that compared survival rates in patients who were IM−/AX+, IM+/AX−, and IM+/AX+.[44–48] Although the survival rates in the first two categories were similar, there was a significant decrease in survival in patients who were IM+ and AX+.

On the basis of these findings, this revision classifies clinically positive internal mammary lymph nodes that are detected by imaging studies (including CT scan or ultrasound, but excluding lymphoscintigraphy) or by clinical examination as N2b when they occur in the *absence* of positive axillary lymph nodes and as N3b when they occur in the *presence* of posi-

TABLE 25.2. Survival rates in breast cancer patients as a function of nodal status in the axillary and internal mammary lymph nodes

		% Survival		
Author	N	IM−/AX+	IM+/AX−	Both positive
Bucalossi et al., 1971[43]	610	56	79	28
Caceres, 1967[44]	425	52	56	24
Li & Shen, 1983[45]	1242	60	73	38
Urban & Marjani, 1971[46]	500	68	64	54
Veronesi et al., 1983[47]	995	72	88	56

IM: Internal mammary lymph nodes; AX: axillary lymph nodes

tive axillary lymph nodes. In cases where proven microscopic disease is detected in the internal mammary lymph nodes, the classification is based on whether the disease was clinically occult. For positive internal mammary nodes with microscopic disease detected by sentinel lymph node dissection but not by imaging studies (excluding lymphoscintigraphy), the pathologic classification is pN1b in the *absence* of positive axillary lymph nodes and is pN1c in the *presence* of 1 to 3 positive axillary lymph nodes. Positive internal mammary nodes discovered by sentinel lymph node dissection but in the presence of 4 or more positive axillary lymph nodes are considered pN3b to reflect the increased tumor burden. For positive internal mammary nodes with histologic macroscopic disease detected by imaging studies (excluding lymphoscintigraphy) or by clinical examination, the classification is pN2b in the *absence* of positive axillary lymph nodes and is pN3b in the *presence* of positive axillary lymph nodes.

Should a finding of positive supraclavicular lymph nodes be classified as N3 rather than M1?

As early as 1907, it was recognized that clinically evident supraclavicular lymph nodes (SCLN) conferred a poor prognosis for breast cancer patients.[49] Clinical studies carried out from 1966 to 1995 reported 5-year survival rates ranging from 5% to 34% (median 18%).[50] The bad prognosis led to the conclusion that SCLN metastasis qualified as distant metastasis (M1) rather than as an advanced regional lymph node metastasis (N3), and this change was incorporated into the 1997 revision of the *AJCC Cancer Staging Manual*.[51]

An examination of these earlier studies reveals a bias against treating patients aggressively when a positive SCLN was treated as a distant metastasis. Because patients with distant metastases are considered incurable, most studies used only locoregional therapy (surgery and/or irradiation) in the treatment of SCLN-positive patients, and such therapy was considered palliative.

A recent study by Brito and colleagues[52] provides evidence that aggressive treatment of SCLN-positive patients results in outcomes comparable to those in patients with locally advanced breast cancer (LABC, Stage IIIB) without distant metastasis. In this study, 70 patients with SCLN-positive LABC received intensive treatment that included induction chemotherapy, surgery, post-surgical chemotherapy, and irradiation. At a median follow-up time of 8.5 years, there was no difference in disease-free survival or overall survival in LABC patients with positive SCLN and no other sign of distant metastasis compared with Stage IIIB patients without distant metastasis. Both Stage IIIB and SCLN-positive patients differed significantly in overall survival when compared with Stage IV patients (Fig. 25.4). These findings indicate that classifying SCLN as a distant metastasis may be a disservice to patients, because it implies incurability and may lead to suboptimal therapy. Patients with ipsilateral SCLN metastases and no other distant metastases should be classified as N3 rather than M1, because their clinical course and outcomes are similar to patients with stage IIIB LABC. To clarify the significance of N3 disease, the new category Stage IIIC has been instituted for any T, N3 that includes pN3a, pN3b, or pN3c.

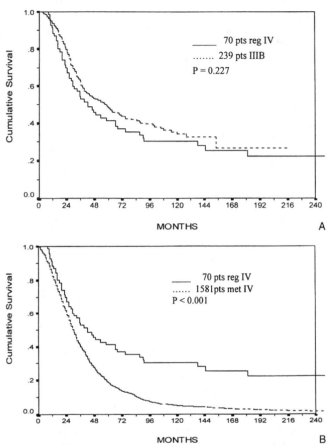

Fig. 25.4. (A) Estimated overall survival for patients with Stage IIIB breast cancer compared with regional Stage IV breast cancer (ipsilateral supraclavicular adenopathy without evidence of distant disease). **(B)** Estimated overall survival for patients with regional Stage IV breast cancer (ipsilateral supraclavicular adenopathy without evidence of distant disease) compared with patients with Stage IV breast cancer (distant metastases). (Reprinted from Brito et al: Long-term results of combined-modality therapy for locally advanced breast cancer with ipsilateral supraclavicular metastases: The University of Texas M. D. Anderson Cancer Center experience. J Clin Oncol 19(3):628–633, 2001 with permission.)

Are there other prognostic factors that are powerful enough to consider for inclusion in the TNM grading system?

Prognostic factors provide information about potential patient outcome in the absence of systemic therapy. These factors tend to reflect biologic characteristics of the tumor, such as proliferation, invasiveness, and metastatic capacity. Prognostic factors must be carefully distinguished from predictive factors, which reflect response to a particular therapeutic agent or combination of agents.

A clinically useful prognostic factor is one that is statistically significant (its prognostic value only rarely occurs by chance), independent (it retains its prognostic value when combined with other factors), and clinically relevant (it has a major impact on prognostic accuracy). Axillary lymph node status has been shown definitively to be the single most important prognostic factor for disease-free and overall survival in breast cancer patients.[3]

In the Fifth Edition of the *AJCC Cancer Staging Manual,*[51] it was reported that approximately 80 potential prognostic variables had been identified for human breast cancer. Since that time, additional factors have been suggested (various growth factors with their receptors and binding proteins; proteases, including cathepsin-D, urokinase-type plasminogen activator, and matrix metalloproteinases). Simultaneously, some factors that were once considered promising have yielded ambiguous or disappointing results in outcome studies (p53, HER2/neu), often because technical approaches have not been standardized and data are difficult to compare between studies.

In addition to axillary lymph node status, the College of American Pathologists Consensus Report[3] and the clinical practice guidelines from the American Society of Clinical Oncology[53,54] have identified tumor size, histopathologic grade, and mitotic index as clinically useful prognostic factors. (This revision recommends the routine use of the Nottingham combined histologic grading system, which incorporates mitotic index into the measurement of tumor grade.) DNA ploidy was reported to be an unreliable prognostic marker in both studies. Estrogen receptor status, although a good predictive factor for response to hormonal therapy, is a relatively weak prognostic factor. Promising results have been reported in some cases for p53, but lack of standardization and data comparability are ongoing problems. Similar problems affect the use of HER2/neu as a prognostic factor, although it should be routinely measured in patients to predict the likelihood of their response to Herceptin® should they relapse after standard adjuvant therapy. Factors such as Ki-67 continue to have technical problems that limit interuser reproducibility.

It is expected that ongoing studies will provide more definitive evidence about the clinical usefulness of many of these factors. These studies should also contribute to the standardization of assay systems and analytic approaches that will be required to achieve reproducibility among different researchers and different institutions. Such studies of promising new prognostic factors should simultaneously measure and report proven factors—particularly size, nodal status, and histologic grade—to indicate how much the new factors reflect the classic ones.

REFERENCES

1. Page DL, Kidd TE, Dupont WD, Simpson JF, Rogers LW: Lobular neoplasia of the breast: higher risk for subsequent invasive cancer predicted by more extensive disease. Hum Pathol ; 22:1232–1239, 1991
2. Elston CW, Ellis IO: Pathological prognostic factors in breast cancer. I. The value of histologic grade in breast cancer: experience from a large study with long-term follow-up. Histopathology 19:403–410, 1991

3. Fitzgibbons PL, Page DL, Weaver D, et al: Prognostic factors in breast cancer. College of American pathologists consensus statement 1999. Arch Pathol Lab Med 124:966–978, 2000

4. Hansemann von D: Über assymetrische zelltheilung in epithelkrebsen und deren biologische bedeutung. Virchows Arch Pathol Anat 119:299–326, 1890

5. Greenough RB: Varying degrees of malignancy in cancer of the breast. J Cancer Res 9:452–463, 1925

6. Bloom HJG, Richardson WW. Histologic grading and prognosis in breast cancer. Br J Cancer 9:359–377, 1957

7. Le Doussal V, Tubiana-Hulin M, Friedman S, et al: Prognostic value of histologic grade nuclear components of Scarff-Bloom-Richardson (SBR): an improved score modification based on multivariate analysis of 1262 invasive ductal breast carcinomas. Cancer 64:1914–1921, 1989

8. Henson DE, Ries L, Freedman LS, Carriaga M: Relationship among outcome, stage of disease, and histologic grade for 22,616 cases of breast cancer. Cancer 68:2142–2149, 1991

9. Neville AM, Bettelheim R, Gelber RD, et al: Factors predicting treatment responsiveness and prognosis in node-negative breast cancer. J Clin Oncol 10:696–705, 1992

10. Delides GS, Garas G, Georgouli G, et al: Intralaboratory variations in the grading of breast carcinoma. Arch Pathol Lab Med 106:126–128, 1982

11. Stenkvist B, Bengtsson E, Eriksson O, et al: Histopathological systems of breast cancer classification: reproducibility and clinical significance. J Clin Pathol 36:392–398, 1983

12. Gilchrist KW, Kalish L, Gould VE, et al: Interobserver reproducibility of histopathological features in Stage II breast cancer: an ECOG study. Breast Cancer Res Treat 5:3–10, 1985

13. Harvey JM, de Klerk NH, Sterrett GH: Histologic grading in breast cancer: interobserver agreement, and relation to other prognostic factors including ploidy. Pathology 24:63–68, 1992

14. Lundin J, Lundin M, Holli K, et al: Omission of histologic grading from clinical decision making may result in overuse of adjuvant therapies in breast cancer: results from a nationwide study. J Clin Oncol 19:28–36, 2001

15. Dalton LW, Page DL, Dupont WD: Histologic grading of breast carcinoma. A reproducibility study. Cancer 73:2765–2770, 1994

16. Frierson HF, Wolber RA, Berean KW, et al: Interobserver reproducibility of the Nottingham modification of the Bloom and Richardson histologic grading scheme for infiltrating ductal carcinoma. Am J Clin Pathol 103:195–198, 1995

17. Robbins P, Pinder S, de Klerk N, et al: Histologic grading of breast carcinomas: a study of interobserver agreement. Hum Pathol 26:873–879, 1995

18. Genestie C, Zafrani B, Asselain B, et al: Comparison of the prognostic value of Scarff-Bloom-Richardson and Nottingham histologic grades in a series of 825 cases of breast cancer: major importance of the mitotic count as a component of both grading systems. Anticancer Res 18:571–576, 1998

19. Donhuijsen K, Schmidt U, Hirche H, et al: Changes in mitotic rate and cell cycle fractions caused by delayed fixation. Hum Pathol 21:709–714, 1990

20. Cross SS, Start RD, Smith JHF: Does delay in fixation affect the number of mitotic figures in processed tissue? J Clin Pathol 43:597–599, 1990

21. Start RD, Flynn MS, Cross SS, et al: Is the grading of breast carcinomas affected by a delay in fixation? Virch Arch A Pathol Anat 419:475–477, 1991

22. Rosen PP, Groshen S, Saigo PE, et al: Pathological prognostic factors in Stage I (T1N0M0) and Stage II (T1N1M0) breast carcinoma: a study of 644 patients with median follow-up of 18 years. J Clin Oncol 7:1239–1251, 1989

23. Rosner D, Lane WW: Should all patients with node-negative breast cancer receive adjuvant therapy? Cancer 68:1482–1494, 1991

24. Kollias J, Murphy CA, Elston CW, et al: The prognosis of small primary breast cancers. Eur J Cancer 35:908–912, 1999

25. Leitner SP, Swern AS, Weinberger D, et al: Predictors of recurrence for patients with small (one centimeter or less) localized breast cancer (T1a,bN0M0). Cancer 76:2266–2274, 1995

26. Reed W, Hannisdal E, Boehler PJ, et al: The prognostic value of p53 and c-erb B-2 immunostaining is overrated for patients with lymph node negative breast cancer. Cancer 88:804–813, 2000

27. Czerniecki BH, Scheff AM, Callans LS, et al: Immunohistochemistry with pancytokeratins improves the sensitivity of sentinel lymph node biopsy in patients with breast carcinoma. Cancer 1089–1103, 1999

28. Trojani M, de Mascarel I, Bonichon F, et al: Micrometastases to axillary lymph nodes from carcinoma of breast: detection by immunohistochemistry and prognostic significance. Br J Cancer 55:303–306, 1987

29. Senmak DD, Meineke TA, Knechtges DS, Anderson J. Prognostic significance of cytokeratin-positive breast cancer metastases. Mod Pathol 2:516–520, 1989

30. Chen ZL, Wen DR, Coulson WF, et al: Occult metastases in the axillary lymph nodes of patients with breast cancer node negative by clinical and histologic examination and conventional histology. Dis Markers 9:238–248, 1991

31. de Mascarel I, Bonichon F, Coindre JM, et al: Prognostic significance of breast cancer axillary lymph node micrometastases assessed by two special techniques: re-evaluation with longer follow-up. Br J Cancer 66:523–527, 1992

32. Hainsworth PI, Tjandra JJ, Stillwell RG, et al: Detection and significance of occult metastases in node-negative breast cancer. Br J Surg 80:459–463, 1993

33. Clare SE, Sener SF, Wilkens W, et al: Prognostic significance of occult lymph node metastases in node-negative breast cancer. Ann Surg Oncol 4:447–451, 1997

34. Hermanek P, Hutter RVP, Sobin LH, Wittekind C: Classification of isolated tumor cells and micrometastasis. Cancer 86:2668–2673, 1999

35. Huvos AG, Hutter RVP, Berg JW: Significance of axillary macrometastases and micrometastases in mammary cancer. Ann Surg 173:44–46, 1971.

36. Verbanac KM, Fleming TP, Min CH, et al: RT-PCR increases detection of breast cancer sentinel lymph node micrometastases. [Abstract 125]. 22nd Annual San Antonio Breast Cancer Symposium, 1999

37. Carter CL, Allen C, Henson DE: Relation of tumor size, lymph node status, and survival in 24,740 breast cancer cases. Cancer 63:181–187, 1989

38. Nemoto T, Vana J, Bedwani RN, et al: Management and survival of female breast cancer: results of a national survey by the American College of Surgeons. Cancer 45:2917–2924, 1980

39. Paik S, Bryant J, Park C, et al: erbB-2 and response to doxorubicin in patients with axillary lymph node–positive, hormone receptor–negative breast cancer. J Natl Cancer Inst 90:1361–1370, 1998

40. Crump M, Goss PE, Prince M, Girouard C: Outcome of extensive evaluation before adjuvant therapy in women with breast cancer and 10 or more positive axillary lymph nodes. J Clin Oncol 14:66–69, 1996

7

41. Diab SG, Hilsenbeck SG, de Moor C, et al: Radiation therapy and survival in breast cancer patients with 10 or more positive axillary lymph nodes treated with mastectomy. J Clin Oncol 16:1655–1660, 1998

42. Fountzilas G, Nicolaides C, Aravantinos G, et al: Dose-dense adjuvant chemotherapy with epirubicin monotherapy in patients with operable breast cancer and > 10 positive axillary lymph nodes: a feasibility study. Oncology 55:508–12, 1998

43. Veronesi U, Marubini E, Mariani L, et al: The dissection of internal mammary nodes does not improve the survival of breast cancer patients: 30-year results of a randomized trial. Eur J Cancer 35:1320–1325, 1999

44. Bucalossi P, Veronesi U, Zingo L, Cantu C: Enlarged mastectomy for breast cancer: review of 1,213 cases. Am J Roentgenol Radium Ther Nucl Med 111:119–122, 1971

45. Caceres E: An evaluation of radical mastectomy and extended radical mastectomy for cancer of the breast. Surg Gynecol Obstetrics 123:337–241, 1967

46. Li KYY, Shen Z-Z: An analysis of 1,242 cases of extended radical mastectomy. Breast, Diseases of the Breast 10:10–19, 1984

47. Urban JA, Marjani MA: Significance of internal mammary lymph node metastases in breast cancer. Am J Roentgenol Radium Ther Nucl Med 111:130–136, 1971

48. Veronesi U, Cascinelli N, Bufalino R, et al: Risk of internal mammary lymph node metastases and its relevance on prognosis of breast cancer patients. Ann Surg 198:681–684, 1983

49. Halsted WS: The results of radical operations for the cure of cancer of the breast. Ann Surg 46:1–5, 1907

50. Debois JM: The significance of a supraclavicular node metastasis in patients with breast cancer: a literature review. Strahlenther Onkol 173:1–12, 1997

51. AJCC cancer staging manual, 5th ed. Philadelphia: Lippincott-Raven, 1997

52. Brito RA, Valero VV, Buzdar AU, et al: Long-term results of combined-modality therapy for locally advanced breast cancer with ipsilateral supraclavicular metastases: The University of Texas M. D. Anderson Cancer Center experience. J Clin Oncol 19:628–633, 2001

53. American Society of Clinical Oncology: Clinical practice guidelines for the use of tumor markers in breast and colorectal cancer. J Clin Oncol 14:2843–2877, 1996

54. American Society of Clinical Oncology: 1997 update of recommendations for the use of tumor markers in breast and colorectal cancer. J Clin Oncol 16:793–795, 1998

HISTOLOGIES—BREAST

8010/2	Carcinoma *in situ,* NOS
8010/3	Carcinoma, NOS
8020/3	Carcinoma undifferentiated, NOS
8070/3	Squamous cell carcinoma, NOS
8200/3	Adenoid cystic carcinoma
8201/2	Cribriform carcinoma *in situ*
8201/3	Cribriform carcinoma, NOS
8211/3	Tubular adenocarcinoma
8480/3	Mucinous adenocarcinoma
8500/2	Intraductal carcinoma, noninfiltrating, NOS
8500/3	Infiltrating duct carcinoma, NOS
8501/2	Comedocarcinoma, noninfiltrating

8502/3	Secretory carcinoma of breast
8503/2	Noninfiltrating intraductal papillary adenocarcinoma
8510/3	Medullary carcinoma, NOS
8520/2	Lobular carcinoma *in situ,* NOS
8520/3	Lobular carcinoma, NOS
8522/2	Intraductal carcinoma and lobular carcinoma *in situ*
8530/3	Inflammatory carcinoma
8540/3	Paget's disease, mammary
8541/3	Paget's disease and infiltrating duct carcinoma of breast
8543/2	Paget's disease and intraductal carcinoma of breast
8980/3	Carcinosarcoma, NOS
9020/3	Phyllodes tumor, malignant

7

PART VIII
Gynecologic Sites

Cervix uteri, corpus uteri, ovary, vagina, vulva, fallopian tube, and gestational trophoblastic tumors are the sites included in this section. Cervix uteri and corpus uteri were among the first sites to be classified by the TNM system. The League of Nations stages for carcinoma of the cervix were first introduced more than 70 years ago, and since 1937 the Fédération Internationale de Gynécologie et d'Obstétrique (FIGO) has continued to modify these staging systems and collect outcomes data from throughout the world. The TNM categories have therefore been defined to correspond to the FIGO stages. Some amendments have been made in collaboration with FIGO, and the classifications now published have the approval of FIGO, the American Joint Committee on Cancer (AJCC), and all other national TNM committees of the International Union Against Cancer (UICC).

8

26

Vulva

(Mucosal malignant melanoma is not included.)

C51.0 Labium majus	C51.2 Clitoris	C51.9 Vulva, NOS
C51.1 Labium minus	C51.8 Overlapping lesion of vulva	

SUMMARY OF CHANGES

- The definition of TNM and the Stage Grouping for this chapter have not changed from the Fifth Edition.

ANATOMY

Primary Site.   The vulva is the anatomic area immediately external to the vagina. It includes the labia and the perineum. The tumor may extend to involve the vagina, urethra or anus. It may be fixed to the pubic bone.

Regional Lymph Nodes.   The femoral and inguinal nodes are the sites of regional spread. For pN, histologic examination of an inguinal lymphadenectomy specimen will ordinarily include six or more lymph nodes. Negative pathologic examination of a lesser number of nodes still mandates a pN0 designation. The concept of sentinel lymph node mapping where only one or two key nodes are removed is currently being investigated.

Metastatic Sites.   The metastatic sites include any site beyond the area of the regional lymph nodes. Tumor involvement of pelvic lymph nodes, including internal iliac, external iliac, and common iliac lymph nodes, is considered distant metastasis.

RULES FOR CLASSIFICATION

Clinical Staging.   Cases should be classified as carcinoma of the vulva when the primary site of the growth is in the vulva. Tumors present on the vulva as secondary growths from either a genital or an extragenital site should be excluded. This classification does not apply to mucosal malignant melanoma. There should be histologic confirmation of the tumor.

Pathologic Staging.   FIGO uses surgical/pathologic staging for vulvar cancer. Stage should be assigned at the time of definitive surgical treatment or prior to radiation or chemotherapy if either of these is the initial mode of therapy. The stage cannot be changed on the basis of disease progression or recurrence or on the basis of response to initial radiation or chemotherapy that precedes primary tumor resection.

DEFINITION OF TNM

The definitions of the T categories correspond to the stages accepted by the Fédération Internationale de Gynécologie et d'Obstétrique (FIGO). Both systems are included for comparison.

Primary Tumor (T)

TNM Categories	FIGO Stages	
TX		Primary tumor cannot be assessed
T0		No evidence of primary tumor
Tis	0	Carcinoma *in situ* (preinvasive carcinoma)
T1	I	Tumor confined to the vulva or vulva and perineum, 2 cm or less in greatest dimension
T1a	IA	Tumor confined to the vulva or vulva and perineum, 2 cm or less in greatest dimension, and with stromal invasion no greater than 1 mm*
T1b	IB	Tumor confined to the vulva or vulva and perineum, 2 cm or less in greatest dimension, and with stromal invasion greater than 1 mm*
T2	II	Tumor confined to the vulva or vulva and perineum, more than 2 cm in greatest dimension
T3	III	Tumor of any size with contiguous spread to the lower urethra and/or vagina or anus
T4	IVA	Tumor invades any of the following: upper urethra, bladder mucosa, rectal mucosa, or is fixed to the pubic bone

Note: The depth of invasion is defined as the measurement of the tumor from the epithelial-stromal junction of the adjacent most superficial dermal papilla to the deepest point of invasion.

Regional Lymph Nodes (N)

NX		Regional lymph nodes cannot be assessed
N0		No regional lymph node metastasis
N1	III	Unilateral regional lymph node metastasis
N2	IVA	Bilateral regional lymph node metastasis

Every effort should be made to determine the site and laterality of lymph node metastases. However, if "regional lymph node metastases, NOS" is the final diagnosis, then the patient should be staged as N1.

Distant Metastasis (M)

MX		Distant metastasis cannot be assessed
M0		No distant metastasis
M1	IVB	Distant metastasis (including pelvic lymph node metastasis)

STAGE GROUPING

Stage 0	Tis	N0	M0
Stage I	T1	N0	M0
Stage IA	T1a	N0	M0
Stage IB	T1b	N0	M0
Stage II	T2	N0	M0
Stage III	T1	N1	M0
	T2	N1	M0
	T3	N0	M0
	T3	N1	M0
Stage IVA	T1	N2	M0
	T2	N2	M0
	T3	N2	M0
	T4	Any N	M0
Stage IVB	Any T	Any N	M1

HISTOPATHOLOGIC TYPE

Squamous cell carcinoma is the most frequent form of cancer of the vulva. This classification does not apply to malignant melanoma.

The common histopathologic types are:

Vulvar intraepithelial neoplasia, grade III
Squamous cell carcinoma *in situ*
Squamous cell carcinoma
Verrucous carcinoma
Paget's disease of vulva
Adenocarcinoma, NOS
Basal cell carcinoma, NOS
Bartholin's gland carcinoma

HISTOLOGIC GRADE (G)

GX   Grade cannot be assessed
G1   Well differentiated
G2   Moderately differentiated
G3   Poorly differentiated
G4   Undifferentiated

PROGNOSTIC FACTORS

Vulvar cancer is a surgically staged malignancy. Surgical-pathologic staging provides specific information about primary tumor size and lymph node status, which are the most important prognostic factors in vulvar cancer. Other commonly evaluated items, such as histologic type, differentiation, DNA ploidy, and S-phase fraction analysis, as well as age, are not uniformly identified as important prognostic factors in vulvar cancer.

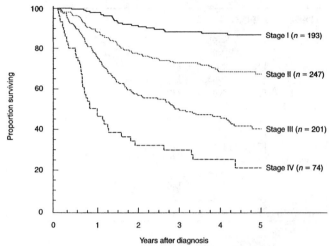

FIG. 26.1. Carcinoma of the vulva, patients treated in 1993–1995. Survival by FIGO stage (epidermoid invasive cancer only), $n = 715$. (Reprinted with permission from Beller U, Sideri M, Maisonneuve P et al: Carcinoma of the vulva. FIGO Annual Report. J Epid Biostat 2001; 6(1):153–174, 2001.)

OUTCOMES RESULTS

Overall survival data from the FIGO Annual Report for patients treated mostly with radical surgery are shown in Fig. 26.1.

BIBLIOGRAPHY

Beller U, Sideri M, Maisonneuve P, et al: Carcinoma of the vulva. FIGO Annual Report. J Epid Biostat 6:153–174, 2001

Grendys EC Jr., Fiorica JV: Innovations in the management of vulvar carcinoma. Current Opin Obstet Gynecol 12:15–20, 2000

Magrina JF, Gonzalez-Bosquet J, Weaver AL, et al: Squamous cell carcinoma of the vulva stage IA: long-term results. Gynecol Oncol 76:24–27, 2000

Moore DH, Thomas GM, Montana GS, et al: Preoperative chemoradiation for advanced vulvar cancer: a phase II study of the Gynecologic Oncology Group. Int J Rad Oncol Biol Phys 42:79–85, 1998

Nash JD, Curry S. Vulvar cancer. Surg Oncol Clinics North Am 7:335–346, 1998

HISTOLOGIES—VULVA

8010/3	Bartholin's gland carcinoma
8051/3	Verrucous carcinoma, NOS
8070/2	Squamous cell carcinoma *in situ*, NOS
8070/3	Squamous cell carcinoma, NOS
8077/2	Squamous intraepithelial neoplasia, grade III
8090/3	Basal cell carcinoma, NOS
8140/3	Adenocarcinoma, NOS
8542/3	Paget's disease of vulva
8560/3	Adenosquamous carcinoma

27

Vagina

C52.9 Vagina, NOS

SUMMARY OF CHANGES

- The definition of TNM and the Stage Grouping for this chapter have not changed from the Fifth Edition.

ANATOMY

Primary Site. The vagina extends from the vulva upward to the uterine cervix. It is lined by squamous epithelium with only rare glandular structures. The vagina is drained by lymphatics toward the pelvic nodes in its upper two-thirds and toward the inguinal nodes in its lower third.

Regional Lymph Nodes. The upper two-thirds of the vagina is drained by lymphatics to the pelvic nodes, including

> Obturator
> Internal iliac (hypogastric)
> External iliac
> Pelvic, NOS

The lower third of the vagina is drained to the groin nodes, including:

> Inguinal
> Femoral

Metastatic Sites. The most common sites of distant spread include the aortic lymph nodes, lungs, and skeleton.

RULES FOR CLASSIFICATION

There should be histologic verification of the disease. The classification applies to primary carcinoma only. Cases should be classified as carcinoma of the vagina when the primary site of the growth is in the vagina. Tumors present in the vagina as secondary growths from either genital or extragenital sites should not be included. A growth that involves the cervix, including the external os, should always be assigned to carcinoma of the cervix. A growth limited to the urethra should be classified as carcinoma of the urethra. Tumor involving the vulva and extending to the vagina should be classified as carcinoma of the vulva.

Clinical Staging. FIGO uses clinical staging for cancer of the vagina. All data available prior to first definitive treatment should be used. The results of biopsy or fine-needle aspiration of inguinal/femoral or other nodes may be included in the clinical staging. The rules of staging are similar to those for carcinoma of the cervix.

Pathologic Staging. In addition to data used for clinical staging, information available from examination of the resected specimen, including pelvic and retroperitoneal lymph nodes, is to be used. The pT, pN, and pM categories correspond to the T, N, and M categories.

DEFINITION OF TNM

The definitions of the T categories correspond to the stages accepted by the Fédération Internationale de Gynécologie et d'Obstétrique (FIGO). Both systems are included for comparison.

Primary Tumor (T)

TNM Categories	FIGO Stages	
TX		Primary tumor cannot be assessed
T0		No evidence of primary tumor
Tis	0	Carcinoma in situ
T1	I	Tumor confined to vagina
T2	II	Tumor invades paravaginal tissues but not to pelvic wall
T3	III	Tumor extends to pelvic wall*
T4	IVA	Tumor invades mucosa of the bladder or rectum and/or extends beyond the true pelvis (bullous edema is not sufficient evidence to classify a tumor as T4)

*Pelvic wall is defined as muscle, fascia, neurovascular structures, or skeletal portions of the bony pelvis.

Regional Lymph Nodes (N)

NX		Regional lymph nodes cannot be assessed
N0		No regional lymph node metastasis
N1	IVB	Pelvic or inguinal lymph node metastasis

Distant Metastasis (M)

MX		Distant metastasis cannot be assessed
M0		No distant metastasis
M1	IVB	Distant metastasis

STAGE GROUPING

Stage 0	Tis	N0	M0
Stage I	T1	N0	M0
Stage II	T2	N0	M0
Stage III	T1–T3	N1	M0
	T3	N0	M0
Stage IVA	T4	Any N	M0
Stage IVB	Any T	Any N	M1

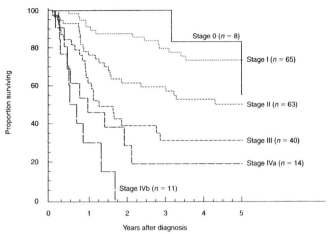

FIG. 27.1. Carcinoma of the vagina, patients treated in 1993–1995. Survival by FIGO stage, $n = 201$. (Reprinted with permission from Beller U, Sideri M, Maisonneuve P et al: Carcinoma of the vagina. FIGO Annual Report. J Epid Biostat 6(1):141–152 2001.)

HISTOPATHOLOGIC TYPE

Squamous cell carcinoma is the most common type of cancer occurring in the vagina. Approximately 10% of vaginal cancers are adenocarcinoma; melanoma and sarcoma occur rarely.

HISTOLOGIC GRADE (G)

GX   Grade cannot be assessed
G1   Well differentiated
G2   Moderately differentiated
G3   Poorly differentiated
G4   Undifferentiated

PROGNOSTIC FACTORS

The most significant prognostic factor is anatomic staging, which reflects the extent of invasion into the surrounding tissue or of metastatic spread.

OUTCOMES RESULTS

Overall survival data from large series are not available because of the rarity of this malignancy. However, FIGO 5-year survival data by clinical stage in patients managed with a variety of modalities are shown in Fig. 27.1.

BIBLIOGRAPHY

Beller U, Sideri M, Maisonneuve P, et al: Carcinoma of the vagina. FIGO Annual Report. J Epid Biostat 6:141–152, 2001

Foroudi F, Bull CA, Gebski V: Primary invasive cancer of the vagina: outcome and complications of therapy. Austral Radiol 43:472–475, 1999

Goodman A. Primary vaginal cancer. Surg Oncol Clinics North Am 7:347–361, 1998

Pingley S, Shrivastava SK, Sarin R, et al: Primary carcinoma of the vagina: Tata Memorial Hospital Experience. Intl J Radiat Oncol Biol Physics 46:101–108, 2000

Stock RG, Chen AS, Seski J. A 30-year experience in the management of primary carcinoma of the vagina: analysis of prognostic factors and treatment modalities. Gynecol Oncol 56:45–52, 1995

Sulak P, Barnhill D, Heller P, et al: Nonsquamous cancer of the vagina. Gynecol Oncol 29:346–353, 1988

HISTOLOGIES—VAGINA

8010/2	Carcinoma *in situ*, NOS
8010/3	Carcinoma, NOS
8052/2	Papillary squamous cell carcinoma, non-invasive
8052/3	Papillary squamous cell carcinoma
8070/2	Squamous cell carcinoma *in situ*, NOS
8070/3	Squamous cell carcinoma, NOS
8071/3	Squamous cell carcinoma, keratinizing, NOS
8072/3	Squamous cell carcinoma, large cell, non-keratinizing, NOS
8076/2	Squamous cell carcinoma *in situ* with questionable stromal invasion
8076/3	Squamous cell carcinoma, microinvasive
8077/2	Squamous intraepithelial neoplasia, grade III
8082/3	Lymphoepithelial carcinoma
8084/3	Squamous cell carcinoma, clear cell type
8140/2	Adenocarcinoma *in situ*, NOS
8140/3	Adenocarcinoma, NOS
8570/3	Adenocarcinoma with squamous metaplasia
8572/3	Adenocarcinoma with spindle cell metaplasia
8800/3	Sarcoma, NOS
8801/3	Spindle cell sarcoma

28

Cervix Uteri

C53.0 Endocervix
C53.1 Exocervix

C53.8 Overlapping lesion of cervix uteri

C53.9 Cervix uteri

SUMMARY OF CHANGES

• The definition of TNM and the Stage Grouping for this chapter have not changed from the Fifth Edition.

ANATOMY

Primary Site. The cervix is the lower third of the uterus. It is roughly cylindrical in shape and projects into the upper vagina. The endocervical canal is lined by glandular or columnar epithelium. Through the cervix runs the endocervical canal, which is the passageway connecting the vagina with the uterine cavity. The vaginal portion of the cervix, known as the exocervix, is covered by squamous epithelium. The squamocolumnar junction is usually located at the external cervical os, where the endocervical canal begins. Cancer of the cervix may originate from the squamous epithelium of the exocervix or the glandular epithelium of the canal.

Regional Lymph Nodes. The cervix is drained by parametrial, cardinal and uterosacral ligament routes into the following regional lymph nodes:

> Parametrial
> Paracervical
> Obturator
> Internal iliac (hypogastric)
> External iliac
> Common iliac
> Sacral
> Presacral

Metastatic Sites. The most common sites of distant spread include the aortic and mediastinal nodes, lungs, and skeleton. Para-aortic node involvement is considered distant metastasis and is coded M1.

RULES FOR CLASSIFICATION

The classification applies only to carcinoma. There should be histologic confirmation of the disease.

Clinical Staging. Because many patients with cervical cancer are treated by radiation and never undergo surgical-pathologic staging, clinical staging of all patients provides uniformity and is therefore preferred. FIGO staging of cervical cancer is clinical.

The clinical stage should be determined prior to the start of definitive therapy. The clinical stage must not be changed because of subsequent findings once treatment has started. When there is doubt about to which stage a particular cancer should be allocated, the lesser stage should be utilized. Careful clinical examination should be performed in all cases, preferably by an experienced examiner and with the patient under anesthesia. The following examinations are recommended for staging purposes: palpation, inspection, colposcopy, endocervical curettage, hysteroscopy, cystoscopy, proctoscopy, intravenous urography, and X-ray examination of the lungs and skeleton. Suspected involvement of the bladder mucosa or rectal mucosa must be confirmed by biopsy and histology. Fine-needle aspiration cytology of palpable nodes or masses may be used, but laparoscopic or radiologically guided biopsy or aspiration is not to be used for clinical staging. The results of additional examinations such as computerized tomography (CT), magnetic resonance imaging (MRI), positron emission tomography (PET), lymphangiography, arteriography, and venography may *not* be used to determine clinical staging because these techniques are not universally available. They may, however, be used to develop a treatment plan.

Pathologic Staging. In cases treated by surgical procedures, the pathologist's findings in the removed tissues can be the basis for extremely accurate statements on the extent of disease. These findings should not be allowed to change the clinical staging but should be recorded in the manner described for the pathologic staging of disease. The pTNM nomenclature is appropriate for this purpose and corresponds to the T, N, and M categories. Infrequently, hysterectomy is carried out in the presence of unsuspected invasive cervical carcinoma. Such cases cannot be clinically staged or included in therapeutic statistics; they should be reported separately.

DEFINITION OF TNM

The definitions of the T categories correspond to the stages accepted by the Fédération Internationale de Gynécologie et d'Obstétrique (FIGO). Both systems are included for comparison.

Primary Tumor (T)

TNM Categories	FIGO Stages	
TX		Primary tumor cannot be assessed
T0		No evidence of primary tumor
Tis	0	Carcinoma *in situ*

T1	I	Cervical carcinoma confined to uterus (extension to corpus should be disregarded)
*T1a	IA	Invasive carcinoma diagnosed only by microscopy. Stromal invasion with a maximum depth of 5.0 mm measured from the base of the epithelium and a horizontal spread of 7.0 mm or less. Vascular space involvement, venous or lymphatic, does not affect classification
T1a1	IA1	Measured stromal invasion 3.0 mm or less in depth and 7.0 mm or less in horizontal spread
T1a2	IA2	Measured stromal invasion more than 3.0 mm and not more than 5.0 mm with a horizontal spread 7.0 mm or less
T1b	IB	Clinically visible lesion confined to the cervix or microscopic lesion greater than T1a/IA2
T1b1	IB1	Clinically visible lesion 4.0 cm or less in greatest dimension
T1b2	IB2	Clinically visible lesion more than 4.0 cm in greatest dimension
T2	II	Cervical carcinoma invades beyond uterus but not to pelvic wall or to lower third of vagina
T2a	IIA	Tumor without parametrial invasion
T2b	IIB	Tumor with parametrial invasion
T3	III	Tumor extends to pelvic wall and/or involves lower third of vagina, and/or causes hydronephrosis or non-functioning kidney
T3a	IIIA	Tumor involves lower third of vagina, no extension to pelvic wall
T3b	IIIB	Tumor extends to pelvic wall and/or causes hydronephrosis or non-functioning kidney
T4	IVA	Tumor invades mucosa of bladder or rectum, and/or extends beyond true pelvis (bullous edema is not sufficient to classify a tumor as T4)

*All macroscopically visible lesions—even with superficial invasion—are T1b/IB.

Regional Lymph Nodes (N)

NX		Regional lymph nodes cannot be assessed
N0		No regional lymph node metastasis
N1		Regional lymph node metastasis

Distant Metastasis (M)

MX		Distant metastasis cannot be assessed
M0		No distant metastasis
M1	IVB	Distant metastasis

STAGE GROUPING

Stage 0	Tis	N0	M0
Stage I	T1	N0	M0
Stage IA	T1a	N0	M0
Stage IA1	T1a1	N0	M0
Stage IA2	T1a2	N0	M0
Stage IB	T1b	N0	M0
Stage IB1	T1b1	N0	M0
Stage IB2	T1b2	N0	M0
Stage II	T2	N0	M0
Stage IIA	T2a	N0	M0
Stage IIB	T2b	N0	M0
Stage III	T3	N0	M0
Stage IIIA	T3a	N0	M0
Stage IIIB	T1	N1	M0
	T2	N1	M0
	T3a	N1	M0
	T3b	Any N	M0
Stage IVA	T4	Any N	M0
Stage IVB	Any T	Any N	M1

HISTOPATHOLOGIC TYPE

Cases should be classified as carcinoma of the cervix if the primary growth is in the cervix. All carcinomas should be included. Grading is encouraged but is not a basis for modifying the stage groupings. When surgery is the primary treatment, the histologic findings permit the case to have pathologic staging, and the pTNM nomenclature is to be used. The histopathologic types are

Cervical intraepithelial neoplasia, grade III
Squamous cell carcinoma *in situ*
Squamous cell carcinoma
    Invasive
    Keratinizing
    Non-keratinizing
    Verrucous
Adenocarcinoma *in situ*
Adenocarcinoma, invasive
Endometrioid adenocarcinoma
Clear cell adenocarcinoma
Adenosquamous carcinoma
Adenoid cystic carcinoma
Adenoid basal cell carcinoma
Small cell carcinoma
Neuroendocrine
Undifferentiated carcinoma

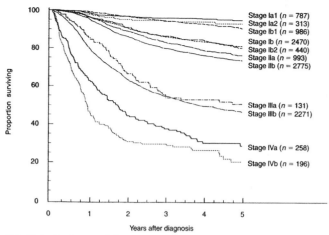

FIG. 28.1. Carcinoma of the cervix uteri: patients treated in 1993–1995. Survival by FIGO stage, $n = 11,620$. (Reprinted with permission from Benedet JL, Odicino F, Maisonneuve P et al: Carcinoma of the cervix. FIGO Annual Report. J Epid Biostat 6:5–44, 2001.)

HISTOLOGIC GRADE (G)

GX Grade cannot be assessed
G1 Well differentiated
G2 Moderately differentiated
G3 Poorly differentiated
G4 Undifferentiated

PROGNOSTIC FACTORS

Current data suggest that more than 90% of squamous cervical cancer contains human papilloma virus (HPV) DNA, most frequently types 16 and 18. In addition to extent or stage of disease, prognostic factors include histology and tumor differentiation. Small cell, neuroendocrine, and clear cell lesions have a worse prognosis, as do poorly differentiated cancers. Women with cervical cancer who are infected with human immunodeficiency virus (HIV) are defined as having autoimmune deficiency syndrome (AIDS), and they have a very poor prognosis, often with rapidly progressive cancer.

OUTCOMES RESULTS

The overall survival by stage of more than 11,000 patients treated from 1993 to 1995 is shown in Figure 28.1.

BIBLIOGRAPHY

Benedet JL, Odicino F, Maisonneuve P, et al: Carcinoma of the cervix. FIGO Annual Report. J Epid Biostat 6:5–44, 2001

Bodurka-Bevers D, Morris M, Eifel PJ, et al: Posttherapy surveillance of women with cervical cancer: an outcomes analysis. Gynecol Oncol 78:187–193, 2000

Coucke PA, Maingon P, Ciernik IF, et al: A survey on staging and treatment in uterine cervical carcinoma in the Radiotherapy Cooperative Group of the European Organization for Research and Treatment of Cancer. Rad Oncol 54:221–228, 2000

Koh WJ, Panwala K, Greer B: Adjuvant therapy for high-risk, early stage cervical cancer. Semin Rad Oncol 10:51–60, 2000

Perez CA, Grigsby PW, Chao KS, et al: Tumor size, irradiation dose, and long-term outcome of carcinoma of uterine cervix. Intl J Rad Oncol, Biol, Physics 41:307–317, 1998

Zaino RJ. Glandular lesions of the uterine cervix. Mod Pathol 13:261–274, 2000

HISTOLOGIES—CERVIX UTERI

8020/3	Carcinoma, undifferentiated, NOS
8041/3	Small cell carcinoma, NOS
8051/3	Verrucous carcinoma, NOS
8070/2	Squamous cell carcinoma *in situ*, NOS
8070/3	Squamous cell carcinoma, NOS
8071/3	Squamous cell carcinoma, keratinizing, NOS
8072/3	Squamous cell carcinoma, large cell, non-keratinizing, NOS
8073/3	Squamous cell carcinoma, small cell, non-keratinizing
8077/2	Squamous intraepithelial neoplasia, grade III
8098/3	Adenoid basal carcinoma
8140/2	Adenocarcinoma *in situ*, NOS
8140/3	Adenocarcinoma, NOS
8200/3	Adenoid cystic carcinoma
8246/3	Neuroendocrine carcinoma, NOS
8310/3	Clear cell adenocarcinoma, NOS
8380/3	Endometrioid adenocarcinoma, NOS
8560/3	Adenosquamous carcinoma

29

Corpus Uteri

C54.0 Isthmus uteri
C54.1 Endometrium
C54.2 Myometrium

C54.3 Fundus uteri
C54.8 Overlapping lesion of
corpus uteri

C54.9 Corpus uteri
C55.9 Uterus, NOS

SUMMARY OF CHANGES

- The definition of TNM and the Stage Grouping for this chapter have not changed from the Fifth Edition.

ANATOMY

Primary Site. The upper two-thirds of the uterus above the level of the internal cervical os is referred to as the uterine corpus. The oviducts (fallopian tubes) and the round ligaments enter the uterus at the upper and outer corners (cornu) of the pear-shaped organ. The portion of the uterus that is above a line connecting the tubo-uterine orifices is referred to as the uterine fundus. The lower third of the uterus is called the cervix and lower uterine segment. Tumor involvement of the endocervical mucosa and/or the stroma of the endocervix is prognostically important and affects staging (T2). The location of the tumor must be carefully evaluated and recorded by the pathologist. The depth of tumor invasion into the myometrium is also of prognostic significance and should be included in the pathology report. Extension of the tumor through the myometrial wall of the uterus into the parametrium occurs on occasion and constitutes regional extension (T3a). Involvement of the ovaries (T3a) by direct extension or metastases or extension to the vagina (T3b) occurs relatively infrequently.

Regional Lymph Nodes. The regional lymph nodes are paired and each of the paired sites should be examined. The regional nodes are:

Obturator
Internal iliac (hypogastric)
External iliac
Common iliac
Para-aortic
Presacral
Parametrial
Pelvic lymph nodes, NOS

For adequate evaluation of the regional lymph nodes, sampling of para-aortic and bilateral obturator nodes and at least one other regional node group should be documented in either or both of the operative and surgical pathology reports.

Parametrial nodes are not commonly detected unless a radical hysterectomy is performed for cases with gross cervical stromal invasion.

Metastatic Sites.   The vagina and lung are the common metastatic sites. Intra-abdominal metastases occur frequently in advanced disease.

RULES FOR CLASSIFICATION

The classification applies only to carcinoma and malignant mixed mesodermal tumors. There should be histologic verification and grading of the tumor.

Clinical Staging.   If the surgeon feels that systematic regional lymph node sampling imposes an unfavorable risk-to-benefit ratio, clinical assessment of the pertinent node groups (obturator, para-aortic groups, internal iliac, common iliac, and external iliac) should be performed and specifically annotated in the operative report and recorded as cN.

A small number of patients may be treated with primary radiation therapy. In such cases, patients should be staged with the clinical staging system adopted by FIGO (Fédération Internationale de Gynécologie et d'Obstétrique) in 1971. The designation of that staging system must be recorded (cT).

Pathologic Staging.   FIGO uses surgical/pathologic staging for corpus uteri cancer. Stage should be assigned at the time of definitive surgical treatment or prior to radiation or chemotherapy if those are the initial modes of therapy. The stage should not be changed on the basis of disease progression or recurrence or on the basis of response to initial radiation or chemotherapy that precedes primary tumor resections. Ideally, the depth of myometrial invasion (in millimeters) should be recorded, along with the thickness of the myometrium at that level (recorded as a percentage of myometrial invasion).

The presence of carcinoma in the regional lymph nodes is a clinically critical prognostic variable. Multiple studies have confirmed the inaccuracy of clinical assessment of regional nodal metastasis in many anatomic sites. For this reason, surgical/pathologic assessment of the regional lymph nodes is strongly advocated for all patients with corpus uteri cancer. This is also the recommendation of FIGO.

Fractional curettage is not adequate to establish cervical involvement or to distinguish between Stages I and II. That distinction can best be made by histologic verification of clinically suspicious cervical involvement or histopathologic examination of the removed uterus.

The pT, pN, and pM categories correspond to the T, N, and M categories and are used to designate cases where adequate pathologic specimens are available for accurate stage groupings. When there are insufficient surgical-pathologic findings, the clinical cT, cN, cM categories should be used on the basis of clinical evaluation.

DEFINITION OF TNM

The definitions of the T categories correspond to the stages accepted by FIGO. FIGO stages are further subdivided by histologic grade of tumor—for example, Stage IC G2. Both systems are included for comparison.

Primary Tumor (T) (Surgical-Pathologic findings)

TNM Categories	FIGO Stages	
TX		Primary tumor cannot be assessed
T0		No evidence of primary tumor
Tis	0	Carcinoma *in situ*
T1	I	Tumor confined to corpus uteri
T1a	IA	Tumor limited to endometrium
T1b	IB	Tumor invades less than one-half of the myometrium
T1c	IC	Tumor invades one-half or more of the myometrium
T2	II	Tumor invades cervix but does not extend beyond uterus
T2a	IIA	Tumor limited to the glandular epithelium of the endocervix. There is no evidence of connective tissue stromal invasion
T2b	IIB	Invasion of the stromal connective tissue of the cervix
T3	III	Local and/or regional spread as defined below
T3a	IIIA	Tumor involves serosa and/or adnexa (direct extension or metastasis) and/or cancer cells in ascites or peritoneal washings
T3b	IIIB	Vaginal involvement (direct extension or metastasis)
T4	IVA	Tumor invades bladder mucosa and/or bowel mucosa (bullous edema is not sufficient to classify a tumor as T4)

Regional Lymph Nodes (N)

NX		Regional lymph nodes cannot be assessed
N0		No regional lymph node metastasis
N1	IIIC	Regional lymph node metastasis to pelvic and/or para-aortic nodes

Distant Metastasis (M)

MX		Distant metastasis cannot be assessed
M0		No distant metastasis
M1	IVB	Distant metastasis (includes metastasis to abdominal lymph nodes other than para-aortic, and/or inguinal lymph nodes; excludes metastasis to vagina, pelvic serosa, or adnexa)

STAGE GROUPING

Stage 0	Tis	N0	M0
Stage I	T1	N0	M0
Stage IA	T1a	N0	M0
Stage IB	T1b	N0	M0
Stage IC	T1c	N0	M0
Stage II	T2	N0	M0
Stage IIA	T2a	N0	M0
Stage IIB	T2b	N0	M0
Stage III	T3	N0	M0
Stage IIIA	T3a	N0	M0
Stage IIIB	T3b	N0	M0
Stage IIIC	T1	N1	M0
	T2	N1	M0
	T3	N1	M0
Stage IVA	T4	Any N	M0
Stage IVB	Any T	Any N	M1

HISTOPATHOLOGIC TYPE

Endometrioid carcinomas
Villoglandular adenocarcinoma
Adenocarcinoma with benign squamous elements, squamous metaplasia, or squamous differentiation (adenoacanthoma).
Adenosquamous carcinoma (mixed adenocarcinoma and squamous cell carcinoma)
Mucinous adenocarcinoma
Serous adenocarcinoma (papillary serous)
Clear cell adenocarcinoma
Squamous cell carcinoma
Undifferentiated carcinoma
Malignant mixed mesodermal tumors

Sarcomas of the uterus should not be included.

HISTOLOGIC GRADE (G)

GX   Grade cannot be assessed
G1   Well differentiated
G2   Moderately differentiated
G3–4   Poorly differentiated or undifferentiated

Histopathology—Degree of Differentiation. Cases of carcinoma of the corpus uteri should be grouped according to the degree of differentiation of the adenocarcinoma as follows:

G1   5% or less of a non-squamous or non-morular solid growth pattern
G2   6% to 50% of a non-squamous or non-morular solid growth pattern
G3   More than 50% of a non-squamous or non-morular solid growth pattern

Notes on Pathologic Grading

1. Notable nuclear atypia, inappropriate for the architectural grade, raises the grade to 3.
2. Serous, clear cell, and mixed mesodermal tumors are *high risk* and considered Grade 3.
3. Adenocarcinomas with benign squamous elements (squamous metaplasia) are graded according to the nuclear grade of the glandular component.

PROGNOSTIC FACTORS

The presence or absence of metastatic disease in the regional lymph nodes is the most important prognostic factor in carcinomas clinically confined to the uterus. The AJCC strongly advocates the use of surgical/pathologic assessment of nodal status whenever possible. Palpation of regional nodes is well recognized to be much less accurate than pathologic evaluation of the nodes.

Historically, the factors of grade of the tumor and depth of myometrial invasion have been recognized as important prognostic factors. In surgically staged patients, using multivariate analysis, these factors are surrogates for the probability of nodal metastasis. Preoperative endometrial biopsy does not accurately correlate with tumor grade and depth of myometrial invasion.

The presence or absence of lymphovascular space involvement of the myometrium is important in most, but not all, series. When present, lymphovascular space involvement increases the probability of metastatic involvement of the regional lymph nodes.

The importance of tumor cells in peritoneal "washings" and the presence of metastatic foci in adnexal structures may have an adverse impact on prognosis, but they remain controversial and require further study.

Serous papillary and clear cell adenocarcinomas have a higher incidence of extrauterine disease at detection than endometrioid adenocarcinomas. The risk of extrauterine disease does not correlate with the depth of myometrial invasion, because widespread abdominal mestastases can be found even when there is no myometrial invasion. For this reason, they are classified as Grade 3 tumors.

In malignancies with squamous elements, the aggressiveness of the tumor seems to be related to the degree of differentiation of the glandular component rather than the squamous element. Clinicopathologic and immunohistochemical studies support classifying malignant mixed mesodermal tumors as high-grade (G3) malignancies of epithelial origin rather than as sarcomas with mixed epithelial and mesenchymal differentiation, as in earlier classification systems.

The data regarding the impact of DNA ploidy, estrogen and progesterone receptor status, and tumor suppressor gene and oncogene expression are not sufficiently mature to incorporate into the stage grouping at this time.

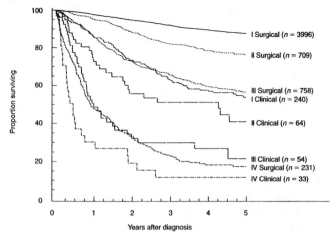

FIG. 29.1. Carcinoma of the corpus uteri, patients treated 1993–1995. Survival by mode of staging, $n = 6085$. (Reprinted with permission from Creasman W, Odicino F, Maisonneuve P et al: Carcinoma of the corpus uteri. FIGO Annual Report. J Epid Biostat 6:45–86, 2001.)

OUTCOMES RESULTS

The significance of clinical compared with surgical/pathologic staging is shown in Figure 29.1. The prognosis for patients with clinical Stage I disease is similar to that for women with surgical Stage III, and those with clinical Stage III cancers have the same prognosis as patients with surgical Stage IV lesions. These findings also emphasize the importance of clearly separating patients who are staged clinically from those who have more accurate surgical/pathologic staging recommended by AJCC and FIGO.

BIBLIOGRAPHY

Cirisano FD, Robboy SF, Dodge RK, et al: The outcome of stage I–II clinically and surgically staged papillary serous and clear cell endometrial cancers when compared with endometrioid carcinoma. Gynecol Oncol 77:55–65, 2000

Colombi RP: Sarcomatoid carcinomas of the female genital tract (malignant mixed mullerian tumors). Semin Diagn Pathol 10:169–175, 1993

Creasman W, Odicino F, Maisonneuve P, et al: Carcinoma of the corpus uteri: FIGO Annual Report. J Epidemiol Biostat 6:45–86, 2001

Creutzberg CL, van Patten LE, Koper PC, et al: Surgery and postop radiotherapy vs surgery alone for patients with stage I endometrial carcinoma: multicenter randomized trial. PORTEC Study Group. Lancet 355:1404–1411, 2000

Gershenson DM (Ed.): Guidelines for referral to a gynecologic oncologist: rationale and benefits. Gyn Oncology 78:S1–13, 2000

Marth C, Windbichler G, Petru E, et al: Parity as an independent prognostic factor in malignant mixed mesodermal tumors of the endometrium. Gynecol Oncol 64:121–125, 1997

Wheeler DT, Bell KA, Kurman RJ, et al: Minimal uterine serous carcinoma: diagnosis and clinicopathologic correlation. Am J Surg Pathol 24:797–806, 2000

Zaino RJ, Kurman RJ, Diana KL, et al: The utility of the revised International Federation of Gynecology and Obstetrics histologic grading of endometrial adenocarcinoma using a defined nuclear grading system. Cancer 75:81–86, 1995

Zerba MJ, Bristow R, Grumbine FC, et al: Inability of preoperative computed tomography scans to accurately predict the extent of myometrial invasion and extracorporal spread in endometrial cancer. Gynecol Oncol 78:67–70, 2000

HISTOLOGIES—CORPUS UTERI

8020/3	Carcinoma, undifferentiated, NOS
8070/3	Squamous cell carcinoma, NOS
8263/3	Villoglandular adenocarcinoma
8310/3	Clear cell adenocarcinoma, NOS
8380/3	Endometrioid adenocarcinoma, NOS
8383/3	Endometrioid adenocarcinoma, ciliated cell variant
8441/3	Serous cystadenocarcinoma, NOS
8460/3	Serous adenocarcinoma (papillary serous)
8480/3	Mucinous adenocarcinoma
8560/3	Adenosquamous carcinoma
8570/3	Adenocarcinoma with squamous metaplasia
8951/3	Malignant mixed mesodermal tumors

8

C56.9 Ovary

SUMMARY OF CHANGES

- The definition of TNM and the Stage Grouping for this chapter have not changed from the Fifth Edition.

ANATOMY

Primary Site. The ovaries are a pair of solid, flattened ovoids 2 to 4 cm in diameter that are connected by a peritoneal fold to the broad ligament and by the infundibulopelvic ligament to the lateral wall of the pelvis. They are attached medially to the uterus by the utero-ovarian ligament.

In some cases, an adenocarcinoma is primary in the peritoneum. The ovaries are not involved or are only involved with minimal surface implants. The clinical presentation, surgical therapy, chemotherapy, and prognosis of these peritoneal tumors mirror those of papillary serous carcinoma of the ovary. Patients who undergo prophylactic oophorectomy for a familial history of ovarian cancer appear to retain a 1 to 2% chance of developing peritoneal adenocarcinoma, which is histopathologically and clinically similar to primary ovarian cancer.

Regional Lymph Nodes. The lymphatic drainage occurs by the utero-ovarian and round ligament trunks and an external iliac accessory route into the following regional nodes:

External iliac
Internal iliac (hypogastric)
Obturator
Sacral
Common iliac
Para-aortic
Inguinal
Pelvic, NOS
Retroperitoneal, NOS

For pN0, histologic examination should include both pelvic and para-aortic lymph nodes.

Metastatic Sites. The peritoneum, including the omentum and the pelvic and abdominal visceral and parietal peritoneum, comprises common sites for seeding. Diaphragmatic and liver surface involvement are also common. However, to be consistent with FIGO staging, these implants within the abdominal cavity (T3) are not considered distant metastases. Primary peritoneal adenocarcinoma is always metastatic at diagnosis (M1).

Extraperitoneal sites, including parenchymal liver, lung, skeletal metastases, and supraclavicular and axillary nodes, are M1.

RULES FOR CLASSIFICATION

Ovarian cancer is surgically/pathologically staged. There should be histologic confirmation of the ovarian disease. Laparotomy and resection of the ovarian mass, as well as hysterectomy, form the basis for staging. Biopsies of all frequently involved sites, such as omentum, mesentery, diaphragm, peritoneal surfaces, pelvic nodes, and para-aortic nodes, are required for ideal staging of early disease. For example, in order to stage a patient confidently as Stage IA (T1 N0 M0), negative biopsies of all of the above sites should be obtained to exclude microscopic metastases. On the other hand, a single biopsy showing metastatic adenocarcinoma in the omentum is adequate to classify a patient as Stage IIIC, thus making other biopsies unnecessary from a staging standpoint. The final histologic and cytologic findings after surgery are to be considered in the staging. Operative findings prior to tumor debulking determine stage, which may be modified by histopathologic as well as clinical or radiologic evaluation (palpable supraclavicular node or pulmonary metastases on chest X-ray, for example).

Clinical Staging.   Although clinical studies similar to those for other sites may be used, surgical-pathologic evaluation of the abdomen and pelvis is necessary to establish a definitive diagnosis of ovarian cancer and rule out other primary malignancies (such as bowel, uterine, and pancreatic cancers or occasionally lymphoma) that may present with similar preoperative findings. A laparotomy is the most widely accepted procedure used for surgical-pathologic staging, but occasionally laparoscopy can be used. Occasionally, patients with advanced disease and/or women who are medically unsuitable candidates for surgery may be presumed to have ovarian cancer on the basis of cytology of ascites or pleural effusion showing typical adenocarcinoma, combined with imaging studies demonstrating enlarged ovaries. Such patients are usually considered as unstaged (TX), although positive cytology of a pleural effusion or supraclavicular lymph node occasionally allows designation of M1 or FIGO Stage IV disease.

Imaging studies are often done in conjunction with definitive abdominal-pelvic surgery, and chest X-ray, bone scans, computerized scanning (CT), or positron emission tomography (PET) may identify lung, bone, or brain metastases that should be considered in the final stage. Pleural effusions should be evaluated with cytology.

As with all gynecologic cancers, the final stage should be established at the time of initial treatment. It should not be modified or changed on the basis of subsequent findings.

Second-look laparotomies and laparoscopy after initial chemotherapy are being evaluated because of the limitation of routine examinations in detecting early recurrence. Findings related to these procedures do not change the patient's original stage.

Pathologic Staging.   Laparotomy and biopsy of all suspected sites of involvement provide the basis for staging. Histologic and cytologic data are required. This is the preferred method of staging for ovarian cancer. The operative note and/or the pathology report should describe the location and size of metastatic lesions and the primary tumors for optimal staging. In addition, the determination of tumor size outside of the pelvis must be noted and documented in the operative report. This is reported in centimeters and represents the largest implant, whether resected or not at the time of surgical exploration.

DEFINITION OF TNM

The definitions of the T categories correspond to the stages accepted by the Fédération Internationale de Gynécologie et d'Obstétrique (FIGO). Both systems are included for comparison.

Primary Tumor (T)

TNM Categories	FIGO Stages	
TX		Primary tumor cannot be assessed
T0		No evidence of primary tumor
T1	I	Tumor limited to ovaries (one or both)
T1a	IA	Tumor limited to one ovary; capsule intact, no tumor on ovarian surface. No malignant cells in ascites or peritoneal washings*
T1b	IB	Tumor limited to both ovaries; capsules intact, no tumor on ovarian surface. No malignant cells in ascites or peritoneal washings*
T1c	IC	Tumor limited to one or both ovaries with any of the following: capsule ruptured, tumor on ovarian surface, malignant cells in ascites or peritoneal washings
T2	II	Tumor involves one or both ovaries with pelvic extension and/or implants
T2a	IIA	Extension and/or implants on uterus and/or tube(s). No malignant cells in ascites or peritoneal washings
T2b	IIB	Extension to and/or implants on other pelvic tissues. No malignant cells in ascites or peritoneal washings
T2c	IIC	Pelvic extension and/or implants (T2a or T2b) with malignant cells in ascites or peritoneal washings
T3	III	Tumor involves one or both ovaries with microscopically confirmed peritoneal metastasis outside the pelvis
T3a	IIIA	Microscopic peritoneal metastasis beyond pelvis (no macroscopic tumor)
T3b	IIIB	Macroscopic peritoneal metastasis beyond pelvis 2 cm or less in greatest dimension
T3c	IIIC	Peritoneal metastasis beyond pelvis more than 2 cm in greatest dimension and/or regional lymph node metastasis

8

Note: The presence of non-malignant ascites is not classified. The presence of ascites does not affect staging unless malignant cells are present.

Note: Liver capsule metastasis T3/Stage III; liver parenchymal metastasis M1/Stage IV. Pleural effusion must have positive cytology for M1/Stage IV.

Regional Lymph Nodes (N)

NX		Regional lymph nodes cannot be assessed
N0		No regional lymph node metastasis
N1	IIIC	Regional lymph node metastasis

Distant Metastasis (M)

MX		Distant metastasis cannot be assessed
M0		No distant metastasis
M1	IV	Distant metastasis (excludes peritoneal metastasis)

pTNM Pathologic Classification.   The pT, pN, and pM categories correspond to the T, N, and M categories.

STAGE GROUPING			
Stage I	T1	N0	M0
Stage IA	T1a	N0	M0
Stage IB	T1b	N0	M0
Stage IC	T1c	N0	M0
Stage II	T2	N0	M0
Stage IIA	T2a	N0	M0
Stage IIB	T2b	N0	M0
Stage IIC	T2c	N0	M0
Stage III	T3	N0	M0
Stage IIIA	T3a	N0	M0
Stage IIIB	T3b	N0	M0
Stage IIIC	T3c	N0	M0
	Any T	N1	M0
Stage IV	Any T	Any N	M1

HISTOPATHOLOGIC TYPE

The American Joint Committee on Cancer (AJCC) endorses the histologic typing of malignant ovarian tumors as endorsed by the World Health Organization (WHO) and recommends that all ovarian epithelial tumors be subdivided according to a simplified version of this classification. The three main histologic types, which include nearly all ovarian cancers, are epithelial tumors, sex-cord stromal tumors, and germ cell tumors. Non-epithelial primary ovarian cancers may be staged using this classification but should be reported separately.

I. Epithelial tumors
   A. Serous tumors
      1. Benign serous cystadenoma
      2. Of borderline malignancy: Serous cystadenoma with proliferating activity of the epithelial cells and nuclear abnormalities, but with no infiltrative destructive growth (carcinomas of low potential malignancy)
      3. Serous cystadenocarcinoma
   B. Mucinous tumors
      1. Benign mucinous cystadenoma
      2. Of borderline malignancy: Mucinous cystadenoma with proliferating activity of the epithelial cells and nuclear abnormalities, but with no infiltrative destructive growth (carcinomas of low potential malignancy)
      3. Mucinous cystadenocarcinoma
   C. Endometrioid tumors
      1. Benign endometrioid cystadenoma
      2. Endometrioid tumors with proliferating activity of the epithelial cells and nuclear abnormalities, but with no infiltrative destructive growth (carcinomas of low potential malignancy)
      3. Endometrioid adenocarcinoma
   D. Clear cell tumors
      1. Benign clear cell tumors
      2. Clear cell tumors with proliferating activity of the epithelial cells and nuclear abnormalities, but with no infiltrative destructive growth (low potential malignancy)
      3. Clear cell cystadenocarcinoma
   E. Brenner (transitional cell tumors)
      1. Benign Brenner
      2. Borderline malignancy
      3. Malignant
      4. Transitional cell
   F. Squamous cell tumor
   G. Undifferentiated carcinoma
      1. A malignant tumor of epithelial structure that is too poorly differentiated to be placed in any other group
   H. Mixed epithelial tumor
      1. Tumors composed of two or more of the five major cell types of common epithelial tumors (types should be specified)

Cases with intraperitoneal carcinoma in which the ovaries appear to be incidentally involved and not the primary origin should be labeled as extraovarian peritoneal carcinoma. They are usually staged with the ovarian staging classification. Because the peritoneum is essentially always involved throughout the abdomen, the peritoneal tumors are usually within the Stage III (T3) or Stage IV (M1) categories.

HISTOLOGIC GRADE (G)

GX   Grade cannot be assessed
GB   Borderline malignancy
G1   Well differentiated
G2   Moderately differentiated
G3–4 Poorly differentiated or undifferentiated

PROGNOSTIC FACTORS

Histology and grade are important prognostic factors. Women with borderline tumors (low malignant potential) have an excellent prognosis, even when extraovarian disease is found. In patients with invasive ovarian cancer, well-differentiated lesions have a better prognosis than poorly differentiated tumors, stage for stage. Histologic type is also extremely important, because some stromal tumors (theca cell, granulosa) have an excellent prognosis, whereas epithelial tumors in general have a less favorable outcome. For this reason, epithelial cell types are generally reported together, and sex-cord stromal tumors and germ cell tumors are reported separately. Tumor cell type also helps to guide the type of chemotherapy that is recommended.

In advanced disease, the most important prognostic factor is the residual disease after the initial surgical management. Even with advanced stage, patients with no gross residual after the surgical debulking have a considerably better prognosis than those with minimal or extensive residual. Not only is the size of the residual important, but the number of sites of residual tumor also appears to be important (tumor volume).

The tumor marker CA-125 is useful for following the response to therapy in patients with epithelial ovarian cancer who have elevated levels of this marker. The rate of regression during chemotherapy treatment may have prognostic significance. Women with germ cell tumors may also have elevated serum tumor markers—alpha fetoprotein (AFP) or human chorionic gonadotropin (β-hCG). Other factors, such as growth factors and oncogene amplification, are currently under investigation.

OUTCOMES RESULTS

Epithelial carcinoma accounts for approximately 80% of all patients with cancer of the ovary. Because of the difficulty of diagnosing this cancer at an early stage, the overall prognosis of women with epithelial ovarian cancer is poor, despite the fact that patients with early stage disease have a favorable outlook. The prognostic significance of stage is shown in Figure 30.1.

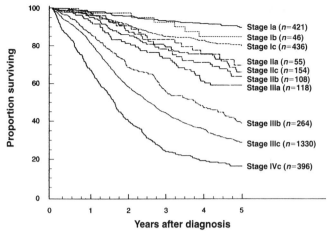

Fig 30.1. Carcinoma of the ovary, patient treated in 1993–1995. Survival by
FIGO stage, obviously malignant, n = 3328. From Heintz APM, Odicino F,
Maisonneuve P, et al: Carcinoma of the ovary. FIGO Annual Report. J Epid
Biostat 6:107–138, 2001.

BIBLIOGRAPHY

Friedlander ML: Prognostic factors in ovarian cancer. Semin Oncol 25:305–
314, 1998

Heintz APM, Odicino F, Maisonneuve P, et al: Carcinoma of the ovary. FIGO
Annual Report. J Epid Biostat 6:107–138, 2001

Leblanc E, Querleu D, Narducci F, et al: Surgical staging of early invasive epithelial ovarian tumors. Semin Surg Oncol 19:36–41, 2000

Manek S, Wells M: Pathology of borderline ovarian tumours. Clin Oncol 11:73–
77, 1999

Silverberg SG: Histopathologic grading of ovarian carcinoma: a review and
proposal. Intl J Gynecol Pathol 19:7–15, 2000

Trope C: Prognostic factors in ovarian cancer. Cancer Treat Res 95:287–352,
1998

HISTOLOGIES—OVARY

8020/3	Undifferentiated carcinoma
8070/3	Squamous cell tumor
8140/2	Adenocarcinoma *in situ,* NOS
8140/3	Adenocarcinoma, NOS
8310/3	Clear cell adenocarcinoma, NOS
8323/3	Mixed epithelial tumor
8380/0	Benign endometrioid cystadenoma
8380/1	Endometrioid cystadenoma of low malignant potential
8380/3	Endometrioid adenocarcinoma, NOS
8381/1	Endometrioid adenofibroma of borderline malignancy
8381/3	Endometrioid adenofibroma, malignant
8382/3	Endometrioid adenocarcinoma, secretory variant

8383/3	Endometrioid adenocarcinoma, ciliated cell variant
8440/3	Cystadenocarcinoma, NOS
8441/0	Benign serous adenoma
8441/3	Serous cystadenocarcinoma, NOS
8442/1	Serous cystadenoma of low malignant potential
8444/1	Clear cell cystadenoma of low malignant potential
8450/3	Clear cell cystadenocarcinoma
8460/3	Papillary serous cystadenocarcinoma
8461/3	Serous surface papillary carcinoma
8470/0	Benign mucinous cystadenoma
8470/2	Mucinous cystadenocarcinoma, non-invasive
8470/3	Mucinous cystadenocarcinoma, NOS
8472/1	Mucinous cystadenoma of low malignant potential
8480/3	Mucinous adenocarcinoma
8480/6	Pseudomyxoma peritonei
8481/3	Mucin-producing adenocarcinoma
8482/3	Mucinous adenocarcinoma, endocervical type
8490/3	Signet ring cell carcinoma
8560/3	Adenosquamous carcinoma
8562/3	Epithelial-myoepithelial carcinoma
8570/3	Adenocarcinoma with squamous metaplasia
8600/3	Thecoma, malignant
8620/3	Granulosa cell tumor, malignant
8630/3	Androblastoma, malignant
8631/3	Sertoli-Leydig cell tumor, poorly differentiated
8634/3	Sertoli-Leydig cell tumor, poorly differentiated, with heterologous elements
8640/3	Sertoli cell carcinoma
8650/3	Leydig cell tumor, malignant
8670/3	Steroid cell tumor, malignant
8930/3	Endometrial stromal sarcoma, NOS
8931/3	Endometrial stromal sarcoma, low grade
8933/3	Adenosarcoma
8935/3	Stromal sarcoma, NOS
8950/3	Mullerian mixed tumor
8951/3	Mesodermal mixed tumor
9000/0	Benign Brenner tumor
9000/1	Brenner tumor of borderline malignancy
9000/3	Brenner tumor, malignant
9014/3	Serous adenocarcinofibroma
9015/3	Mucinous adenocarcinofibroma
9050/3	Mesothelioma, malignant
9051/3	Fibrous mesothelioma, malignant
9052/3	Epithelioid mesothelioma, malignant
9053/3	Mesothelioma, biphasic, malignant
9060/3	Dysgerminoma
9064/3	Germinoma
9065/3	Germ cell tumor, nonseminomatous
9070/3	Embryonal carcinoma, NOS
9071/3	Yolk sac tumor
9072/3	Polyembryoma
9080/3	Teratoma, malignant, NOS
9081/3	Teratocarcinoma
9082/3	Malignant teratoma, undifferentiated

9083/3	Malignant teratoma, intermediate
9084/3	Teratoma with malignant transformation
9085/3	Mixed germ cell tumor
9090/3	Struma ovarii, malignant
9100/3	Choriocarcinoma, NOS
9101/3	Choriocarcinoma combined with other germ cell elements
9102/3	Malignant teratoma, trophoblastic
9105/3	Trophoblastic tumor, epithelioid
9110/3	Mesonephroma, malignant

8

31

Fallopian Tube

C57.0 Fallopian tube

SUMMARY OF CHANGES

- The definition of TNM and the Stage Grouping for this chapter have not changed from the Fifth Edition.

ANATOMY

Primary Site.   The fallopian tube extends from the posterior superior aspect of the uterine fundus laterally and anteriorly to the ovary. Its length is approximately 10 cm. The medial end arises in the cornual portion of the uterine cavity, and the lateral end opens to the peritoneal cavity.

Carcinoma of the fallopian tube is almost always an adenocarcinoma arising from an *in situ* lesion of the tubal mucosa. It invades locally into the muscular wall of the tube and then into the peritubal soft tissue or adjacent organs such as the uterus or ovary, or through the serosa of the tube into the peritoneal cavity. Metastatic tumor implants can be found throughout the peritoneal cavity. The tumor may obstruct the tubal lumen and present as a ruptured or unruptured hydrosalpinx or hematosalpinx.

Regional Nodes.   Carcinoma of the fallopian tube can also metastasize to the regional lymph nodes, which include

Common iliac
Internal iliac (hypogastric)
Obturator
Presacral
Para-aortic
Inguinal
Pelvic lymph nodes, NOS

Adequate evaluation of the regional lymph nodes usually includes aortic and pelvic nodes.

Distant Metastases.   Surface implants within the pelvic cavity and the abdominal cavity are common, but these are classified as T2 and T3 disease, respectively. Parenchymal liver metastases and extraperitoneal sites, including lung and skeletal metastases, are M1.

RULES FOR CLASSIFICATION

There should be histologic confirmation of primary disease with complete evaluation of the abdomen and pelvis as outlined in the staging of ovarian malignancy (See Chapter 30). In many patients, the diagnosis may be unsuspected until the fallopian tube is examined histopathologically. Tumors may involve one or both fallopian tubes, and complete assessment of both adnexal areas affects the staging of the disease.

Clinical Staging.   Perioperative imaging studies, including chest X-ray, computerized tomography scans, and magnetic resonance imaging, may identify distant metastases. Staging may be modified by imaging studies or clinical findings obtained prior to the initiation of treatment.

Pathologic Staging.   Laparotomy with resection of tubal masses, usually including hysterectomy and bilateral oophorectomy, form the basis for the operative management of fallopian tube carcinoma. Widespread intra-abdominal disease is common; therefore, adequate evaluation of potentially early stage lesions requires multiple biopsies of commonly involved sites, such as omentum, pelvic peritoneum, mesentery, bowel serosa, diaphragm, and regional nodes, in order to rule out microscopic metastases to any of these sites.

Cytologic studies of ascites (if present) or of pelvic and abdominal peritoneal washings (if no ascites are present) should be included in the staging. The surgical-pathologic findings form the basis for staging. Staging is based on the findings at the time the abdomen is opened, not on the residual disease after debulking.

It may be preferable to classify a patient as TX (primary tumor cannot be assessed) if inadequate staging biopsies and/or a lack of peritoneal cytology make it inaccurate to classify the patient with confidence as early stage (Stage T3a/IIIA has not been excluded by adequate staging biopsies).

DEFINITION OF TNM

Primary Tumor (T)

TNM Categories	FIGO Stages	
TX		Primary tumor cannot be assessed
T0		No evidence of primary tumor
Tis	0	Carcinoma *in situ* (limited to tubal mucosa)
T1	I	Tumor limited to the fallopian tube(s)
T1a	IA	Tumor limited to one tube, without penetrating the serosal surface; no ascites
T1b	IB	Tumor limited to both tubes, without penetrating the serosal surface; no ascites
T1c	IC	Tumor limited to one or both tubes with extension onto or through the tubal serosa, or with malignant cells in ascites or peritoneal washings
T2	II	Tumor involves one or both fallopian tubes with pelvic extension
T2a	IIA	Extension and/or metastasis to the uterus and/or ovaries
T2b	IIB	Extension to other pelvic structures
T2c	IIC	Pelvic extension with malignant cells in ascites or peritoneal washings

T3	III	Tumor involves one or both fallopian tubes, with peritoneal implants outside the pelvis
T3a	IIIA	Microscopic peritoneal metastasis outside the pelvis
T3b	IIIB	Macroscopic peritoneal metastasis outside the pelvis 2 cm or less in greatest dimension
T3c	IIIC	Peritoneal metastasis more than 2 cm in diameter

Note: Liver capsule metastasis is T3/Stage III; liver parenchymal metastasis M1/Stage IV. Pleural effusion must have positive cytology for M1/Stage IV.

Regional Lymph Nodes (N)

NX		Regional lymph nodes cannot be assessed
N0		No regional lymph node metastasis
N1	IIIC	Regional lymph node metastasis

Distant Metastasis (M)

MX		Distant metastasis cannot be assessed
M0		No distant metastasis
M1	IV	Distant metastasis (excludes metastasis within the peritoneal cavity)

STAGE GROUPING

Stage 0	Tis	N0	M0
Stage I	T1	N0	M0
Stage IA	T1a	N0	M0
Stage IB	T1b	N0	M0
Stage IC	T1c	N0	M0
Stage II	T2	N0	M0
Stage IIA	T2a	N0	M0
Stage IIB	T2b	N0	M0
Stage IIC	T2c	N0	M0
Stage III	T3	N0	M0
Stage IIIA	T3a	N0	M0
Stage IIIB	T3b	N0	M0
Stage IIIC	T3c	N0	M0
	Any T	N1	M0
Stage IV	Any T	Any N	M1

HISTOPATHOLOGIC TYPES

Adenocarcinoma is the most frequently seen histology.

HISTOLOGIC GRADE (G)

GX   Grade cannot be assessed
G1   Well differentiated
G2   Moderately differentiated

G3   Poorly differentiated
G4   Undifferentiated

PROGNOSTIC FACTORS

The surgical-pathologic stage is the most significant prognostic characteristic. Tumor differentiation is an important prognostic characteristic in all stages of disease. In patients with localized tumors, depth of invasion into the tubal musculature and rupture of the tube have prognostic importance. With advanced disease, the volume of residual tumor after surgical debulking appears to be related to prognosis.

OUTCOMES RESULTS

This is a very uncommon tumor. It is usually treated with surgery followed by chemotherapy. The 5-year survival in early disease is approximately 70%, but surgical staging is often inadequate. At 5 years, the overall survival for patients with advanced disease is about 20%.

BIBLIOGRAPHY

Alvarado-Cabrero I, Young RH, Vamvakas EC, et al: Carcinoma of the fallopian tube: a clinicopathological study of 105 cases with observations on staging and prognostic factors. Gynecol Oncol 72:367–379, 1999

Baekelandt M, Nesbakken AJ, Kristensen GB, et al: Carcinoma of the fallopian tube: clinicopathologic study of 151 patients treated at the Norwegian Radium Hospital. Cancer 89:2076–2084, 2000

Heintz APM, Odicino F, Maisonneuve P, et al: Carcinoma of the fallopian tube. FIGO Annual Report. J Epid Biostat 6:87–103, 2001

Nikrui N, Duska LR: Fallopian tube carcinoma. Surg Oncol Clin North Am 7:363–373, 1998

HISTOLOGIES—FALLOPIAN TUBE

8010/2	Carcinoma *in situ*, NOS
8010/3	Carcinoma, NOS
8140/2	Adenocarcinoma *in situ*, NOS
8140/3	Adenocarcinoma, NOS
8310/3	Clear cell adenocarcinoma, NOS
8380/3	Endometrioid adenocarcinoma, NOS
8381/3	Endometrioid adenofibroma, malignant
8382/3	Endometrioid adenocarcinoma, secretory variant
8383/3	Endometrioid adenocarcinoma, ciliated cell variant
8440/3	Cystadenocarcinoma, NOS
8441/3	Serous cystadenocarcinoma, NOS
8460/3	Papillary serous cystadenocarcinoma
8461/3	Serous surface papillary carcinoma
8470/2	Mucinous cystadenocarcinoma, non-invasive
8470/3	Mucinous cystadenocarcinoma, NOS
8480/3	Mucinous adenocarcinoma
8481/3	Mucin-producing adenocarcinoma

8482/3 Mucinous adenocarcinoma, endocervical type
8490/3 Signet ring cell carcinoma
8560/3 Adenosquamous carcinoma
8562/3 Epithelial-myoepithelial carcinoma
8570/3 Adenocarcinoma with squamous metaplasia

32

Gestational Trophoblastic Tumors

C58.9 Placenta

INTRODUCTION

Gestational trophoblastic tumors are uncommon (1 in 1,000 pregnancies) malignancies that arise from the placenta. Usually as a result of a genetic accident in the developing egg, the maternal chromosomes are lost, and the paternal chromosomes duplicate (46xx). The resulting tumor is known as a *complete* hydatidiform mole: There are no fetal parts, the tumor is composed of dilated, avascular, "grape-like" vesicles that may grow as large as, or larger than, the normal pregnancy that it replaces. There is obviously no heartbeat detected, and the patient may have vaginal bleeding similar to a miscarriage. Many times, the diagnosis is not made until a dilatation and curettage is done and the tissue is examined pathologically. In some patients, fetal parts will be found in association with mild proliferative trophoblastic (placental) tissue. Such patients have a *partial* hydatidiform mole, which has a 69xxx or 69xxy chromosomal complement resulting from twice the normal number of paternal chromosomes. Both of these tumors usually follow a benign course, resolving completely after evacuation by dilatation and suction or curettage, but approximately 20% of complete moles and 5% of partial moles persist locally or metastasize and thus require chemotherapy.

Much less frequently (about 1 in 20,000 pregnancies in the United States), a highly malignant, rapidly growing metastatic form of gestational trophoblastic disease called choriocarcinoma is encountered. This solid, anaplastic, vascular, and aggressively proliferative tumor is easily recognized microscopically and may present with symptoms of vaginal bleeding (as with a hydatidiform mole). However, metastatic lesions may be the first sign of this lesion, which can follow any pregnancy event, including an incomplete abortion or a full-term pregnancy.

The trophoblastic tissue that makes up these tumors produces a serum tumor marker, beta-human chorionic gonadotropin (β-hCG), which is very helpful in the diagnosis and monitoring of therapy in these patients.

Gestational trophoblastic tumors are very responsive to chemotherapy, with cure rates approaching 100%.

ANATOMY

Because of the responsiveness of this tumor to treatment and the accuracy of the serum tumor marker hCG in reflecting the status of disease, the traditional anatomic staging system used in most solid tumors has little prognostic significance. Trophoblastic tumors not associated with pregnancy (ovarian teratomas) are not included in this classification.

Primary Site. By definition, gestational trophoblastic tumors arise from placental tissue in the uterus. Although most of these tumors are non-invasive and are removed by dilatation and suction evacuation, local invasion of the myometrium can occur. When this is diagnosed on a hysterectomy specimen (rarely done these days), it may be reported as an *invasive* hydatidiform mole.

Regional lymph nodes. Nodal involvement in gestational trophoblastic tumors is rare but has a very poor prognosis when diagnosed. There is no regional nodal designation in the staging of these tumors. Nodal metastases should be classified as metastatic (M1) disease.

Metastatic sites. This is a highly vascular tumor that results in frequent, widespread metastases when these lesions become malignant. The cervix and vagina are common pelvic sites of metastases (T2), and the lungs are often involved by distant metastases (M1a). Other, less frequently encountered metastatic sites include kidney, gastrointestinal tract, and spleen (M1b). The liver and brain are occasionally involved and may harbor metastatic sites that are difficult to treat with chemotherapy.

RULES FOR CLASSIFICATION

Gestational trophoblastic tumors have a very high cure rate, and as a result, the ultimate goal of staging is to identify patients who are likely to respond to less intensive chemotherapeutic protocols and distinguish these individuals from patients who will require more intensive chemotherapy in order to achieve remission. In 1991, the International Federation of Gynecology and Obstetrics (FIGO) added non-anatomic risk factors to the traditional staging system. Further modifications have been made in an attempt to merge several prognostic classification systems. The current staging classification is still evolving.

Indications for Treatment. The following criteria are suggested for the diagnosis of trophoblastic tumors requiring chemotherapy:

- Three or more values of hCG showing no significant change (a plateau) over 4 weeks, or

---

- Rise of hCG of 10% or greater for 2 values over 3 weeks or longer, or
- Persistence of elevated hCG 6 months after evacuation of molar pregnancy, or
- Histologic diagnosis of choriocarcinoma

Diagnosis of Metastasis

- For the diagnosis of lung metastasis, chest X-ray is appropriate and should be used to count metastases for risk scoring. Lung CT scan may be used.
- For the diagnosis of intra-abdominal metastasis, CT scanning is preferred, although many institutions still use ultrasound to detect liver metastasis.
- For the diagnosis of brain metastasis, MRI is superior to CT scan, even with 1-cm cuts.

Prognostic Index Scores. The score on the Prognostic Scoring Index is used to substage patients (Table 32.1). Each stage is anatomically defined, but substage A (low risk) and B (high risk) are assigned on the basis of a non-anatomic risk factor scoring system. The prognostic scores are 0, 1, 2, and 4 for the individual risk factors. The current prognostic scoring system eliminates the ABO blood group risk factors that were featured in the WHO scoring system and upgrades the risk factor for liver metastasis from 2 to 4, the highest category.

Low risk is a score of 7 or less, and high risk is a score of 8 or greater.

8

DEFINITION OF TNM

Primary Tumor (T)

TNM Categories	FIGO Stages	
TX		Primary tumor cannot be assessed
T0		No evidence of primary tumor
T1	I	Tumor confined to uterus
T2	II	Tumor extends to other genital structures (ovary, tube, vagina, broad ligaments) by metastasis or direct extension

Distant Metastasis (M)

MX		Metastasis cannot be assessed
M0		No distant metastasis
M1		Distant metastasis
M1a	III	Lung metastasis
M1b	IV	All other distant metastasis

TABLE 32.1. Prognostic Scoring Index

Prognostic Factor	Risk Score			
	0	1	2	4
Age	<40	≥40		
Antecedent Pregnancy	Hydatidiform mole	Abortion	Term pregnancy	
Interval months from index pregnancy	<4	4–<7	7–12	>12
Pretreatment hCG (IU/ml)	$<10^3$	$≥10^3$–$<10^4$	10^4–$<10^5$	$≥10^5$
Largest tumor size, including uterus	<3 cm	3–<5 cm	≥5 cm	
Site of metastases	Lung	Spleen, kidney	Gastrointestinal tract	Brain, liver
Number of metastases identified		1–4	5–8	>8
Previous failed chemotherapy			Single drug	Two or more drugs
Total Score				

Low risk is a score of 7 or less. High risk is a score of 8 or greater.

STAGE GROUPING			
Stage	T	M	Risk Factors
Stage I	T1	M0	Unknown
Stage IA	T1	M0	Low risk
Stage IB	T1	M0	High risk
Stage II	T2	M0	Unknown
Stage IIA	T2	M0	Low risk
Stage IIB	T2	M0	High risk
Stage III	Any T	M1a	Unknown
Stage IIIA	Any T	M1a	Low risk
Stage IIIB	Any T	M1a	High risk
Stage IV	Any T	M1b	Unknown
Stage IVA	Any T	M1b	Low risk
Stage IVB	Any T	M1b	High risk

HISTOPATHOLOGIC TYPE

Hydatidiform mole
   Complete
   Partial
Invasive hydatidiform mole
Choriocarcinoma
Placental site trophoblastic tumors

8

OUTCOMES RESULTS

Gestational trophoblastic tumors may require only uterine evacuation for treatment, but even when chemotherapy is required, cure rates approach 100%. Prognostic factors are listed in the Prognostic Scoring Index. Patients with low-risk disease are usually treated with single-agent chemotherapy, whereas combined, multiple-agent chemotherapy usually results in a cure for high-risk patients.

BIBLIOGRAPHY

Horn LC, Bilek K: Histologic classification and staging of gestational tropho-blastic disease. Gen Diagn Pathol 143: 87–101, 1997

Lage JM: Protocol for the examination of specimens from patients with gestational trophoblastic malignancies: a basis for checklists. Cancer Committee, College of American Pathologists. Arch Pathol Lab Med 123: 50–54, 1999

Ngan HYS, Odicino F, Maisonneuve P, et al: Gestational trophoblastic diseases. FIGO Annual Report. J Epidem Biostat 6: 175–184, 2001

HISTOLOGIES—GESTATIONAL TROPHOBLASTIC TUMORS

9100/0	Hydatidiform mole, NOS
9100/1	Invasive hydatidiform mole
9100/3	Choriocarcinoma, NOS
9101/3	Choriocarcinoma combined with other germ cell elements
9102/3	Malignant teratoma, trophoblastic
9103/0	Partial hydatidiform mole
9104/1	Placental site trophoblastic tumor
9105/3	Trophoblastic tumor, epithelioid

PART IX
Genitourinary Sites

33

Penis

(Melanomas are not included.)

C60.0 Prepuce
C60.1 Glans penis

C60.2 Body of penis
C60.8 Overlapping lesion of
         penis

C60.9 Penis, NOS

SUMMARY OF CHANGES

· The definition of TNM and the Stage Grouping for this chapter have not
  changed from the Fifth Edition.

INTRODUCTION

Cancers of the penis are rare in the United States, although the incidence
varies in different countries of the world. Most are squamous cell carcinomas that arise in the skin or on the glans penis. Prognosis is favorable
provided that the lymph nodes are not involved. Melanomas can also occur. The staging classification, however, applies to carcinomas. Melanomas
are staged in Chapter 24. Some cancers of the penis may be described as
verrucous. Similarly, basaloid tumors are recognized as a subtype of squamous carcinoma. These are included under this classification. An *in situ*
lesion is also included and by definition should be coded as an *in situ*
carcinoma of the penis.

ANATOMY

Primary Site.   The penis is composed of three cylindrical masses of cav-
ernous tissue bound together by fibrous tissue. Two masses are lateral and
are known as the corpora cavernosa penis. The corpus spongiosum penis
is a median mass and contains the greater part of the urethra. The penis
is attached to the front and the sides of the pubic arch. The skin covering
the penis is thin and loosely connected with the deeper parts of the organ.
This skin at the root of the penis is continuous with that over the scrotum
and perineum. Distally, the skin becomes folded upon itself to form the
prepuce, or foreskin. Circumcision has been associated with a decreased
incidence of cancer of the penis.

Regional Lymph Nodes.   The regional lymph nodes are:

Single superficial inguinal (femoral)
Multiple or bilateral superficial inguinal (femoral)
Deep inguinal: Rosenmuller's or Cloquet's node

External iliac
Internal iliac (hypogastric)
Pelvic nodes, NOS

Metastatic Sites. Lung, liver, and bone are most often involved.

RULES FOR CLASSIFICATION

Clinical Staging. Clinical examination, endoscopy where possible, and histologic confirmation are required. Imaging techniques are indicated for metastatic disease detection.

Pathologic Staging. Complete resection of the primary site with appropriate margins is required. Where regional lymph node involvement is suspected, lymphadenectomy is usually indicated.

The definitions of Primary Tumor (T) for Ta, T1, T2, T3 and T4 are illustrated in Figures 33.1–33.5.

DEFINITION OF TNM

Primary Tumor (T)
TX   Primary tumor cannot be assessed
T0   No evidence of primary tumor
Tis   Carcinoma *in situ*
Ta   Non-invasive verrucous carcinoma
T1   Tumor invades subepithelial connective tissue
T2   Tumor invades corpus spongiosum or cavernosum
T3   Tumor invades urethra or prostate
T4   Tumor invades other adjacent structures

Regional Lymph Nodes (N)
NX   Regional lymph nodes cannot be assessed
N0   No regional lymph node metastasis
N1   Metastasis in a single superficial, inguinal lymph node
N2   Metastasis in multiple or bilateral superficial inguinal lymph nodes
N3   Metastasis in deep inguinal or pelvic lymph node(s) unilateral or bilateral

Distant Metastasis (M)
MX   Distant metastasis cannot be assessed
M0   No distant metastasis
M1   Distant metastasis

Additional Descriptor
The **m suffix** indicates the presence of multiple primary tumors and is recorded in parentheses—e.g., pTa(m)N0M0.

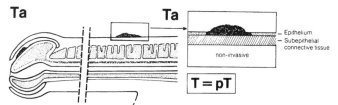

FIG. 33.1. Ta: Non-invasive verrucous carcinoma.

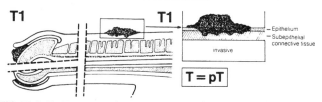

FIG. 33.2. T1: Tumor invading subepithelial connective tissue.

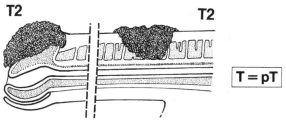

FIG. 33.3. T2: Tumor invading corpus spongiosum or cavernosum.

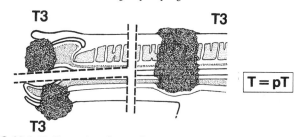

FIG. 33.4. T3: Tumor invading urethra or prostate.

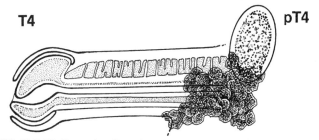

FIG. 33.5. T4: Tumor invading other adjacent structures.

STAGE GROUPING

Stage 0	Tis	N0	M0
	Ta	N0	M0
Stage I	T1	N0	M0
Stage II	T1	N1	M0
	T2	N0	M0
	T2	N1	M0
Stage III	T1	N2	M0
	T2	N2	M0
	T3	N0	M0
	T3	N1	M0
	T3	N2	M0
Stage IV	T4	Any N	M0
	Any T	N3	M0
	Any T	Any N	M1

HISTOPATHOLOGIC TYPE

Cell types are limited to carcinomas.

HISTOLOGIC GRADE (G)

GX   Grade cannot be assessed
G1   Well differentiated
G2   Moderately differentiated
G3–4   Poorly differentiated or undifferentiated

BIBLIOGRAPHY

Assimos DG, Jarow JP: Role of laparoscopic pelvic lymph node dissection in the management of patients with penile cancer and inguinal adenopathy. J Endocrinol 8:365–369, 1994

Aynaud O, Ionesco M, Barrasso R: Penile intraepithelial neoplasia: specific clinical features correlate with histologic and virologic findings. Cancer 74:1762–1767, 1994

Cubilla AL, Reuter VE, Gregoire L, et al: Basaloid squamous cell carcinoma: A distinctive human papilloma virus–related penile neoplasm. Am J Surg Path 22:755–761, 1998

Lopes A, Hidalgo GS, Kowalski LP, et al: Prognostic factors in carcinoma of the penis: multivariate analysis of 145 patients treated with amputation and lymphadenectomy. J Urology 156:1637–1642, 1996

Lubke WL, Thompson IM: The case for inguinal lymph node dissection in the treatment of T2–T4 N0 penile cancer. Semin Urol 11:80–84, 1993

Parra RO: Accurate staging of carcinoma of the penis in men with nonpalpable inguinal lymph nodes by modified inguinal lymphadenectomy. J Urol 155:560–563, 1996

Ravi R. Correlation between the extent of nodal involvement and survival following groin dissection for carcinoma of the penis. British Journal of Urology 72(5 Pt 2):817–819, 1993

Scappini P, Piscioloi F, Pusiol T, et al: Penile cancer: aspiration biopsy cytology for staging. Cancer 58:1526–1533, 1986

Villavicencio H, Rubio-Briones J, Regalado R, Chechile G, Algaba F, Palou J: Grade, local stage and growth pattern as prognostic factors in carcinoma of the penis. European Urology 32(4):442–447, 1997

Wajsman Z, Gamarra M, Park JJ, et al: Transabdominal fine needle aspiration of retroperitoneal lymph nodes in staging of genitourinary tract cancer (correlation with node dissection findings). J Urol 128:1238–1240, 1982

Wajsman Z, et al: Fine needle aspiration of metastatic lesions and regional lymph nodes in genitourinary cancer. Urology 19:356, 1982

HISTOLOGIES—PENIS

8010/2	Carcinoma *in situ*, NOS
8010/3	Carcinoma, NOS
8051/3	Verrucous carcinoma, NOS
8070/2	Squamous cell carcinoma *in situ*, NOS
8070/3	Squamous cell carcinoma, NOS
8081/2	Bowen disease
8090/3	Basal cell carcinoma
8140/2	Adenocarcinoma *in situ*, NOS
8140/3	Adenocarcinoma, NOS
8560/3	Adenosquamous carcinoma

9

34

Prostate

(Sarcomas and transitional cell carcinomas are not included.)

C61.9 Prostate gland

SUMMARY OF CHANGES

- T2 lesions have been divided to include T2a, T2b, and T2c once again. These are the same subcategories found in the Fourth Edition of the manual.

- Gleason score is emphasized as the grading system of choice and using the terms *well differentiated*, *moderately differentiated*, and *poorly differentiated* for grading is not recommended.

INTRODUCTION

Prostate cancer is the most common cancer in men, with increasing incidence in older age groups. Prostate cancer has a tendency to metastasize to bone. Earlier detection is possible with a blood test, prostate-specific antigen (PSA), and diagnosis is generally made using transrectal ultrasound (TRUS) guided biopsy.

ANATOMY

Primary Site.   Adenocarcinoma of the prostate frequently arises within the peripheral zone of the gland, where it may be amenable to detection by digital rectal examination (DRE). A less common site of origin is the anteromedial prostate, the transition zone, which is remote from the rectal surface and is the site of origin of benign nodular hyperplasia. The central zone, which makes up most of the base of the prostate, seldom gives rise to cancer but is often invaded by the spread of large cancers. Pathologically, cancers of the prostate are often multifocal.

There is agreement that the incidence of both clinical and latent carcinoma increases with age. However, this cancer is rarely diagnosed clinically in men under 40 years of age. There are substantial limitations in the ability of both DRE and TRUS to define precisely the size or local extent of disease; DRE is currently the most common modality used to define the local stage. Heterogeneity within the Tlc category resulting from inherent limitations of either DRE or imaging to quantify the cancer may be balanced by the inclusion of other prognostic factors, such as histologic grade, PSA level, and possibly extent of cancer on needle biopsies that contain cancer. Diagnosis of clinically suspicious areas of the prostate can be confirmed histologically by needle biopsy. Less commonly, prostate cancer may be diagnosed by inspection of the resected tissue from a transurethral resection of the prostate (TURP) for obstructive voiding symptoms.

The histologic grade of the prostate cancer is important for prognosis. The histopathologic grading of these tumors can be complex because of the morphologic heterogeneity so often encountered in surgical specimens. Either a histologic or a pattern type of grading method can be used. The Gleason score for assessing the histologic pattern of prostate cancer is preferred.

Regional Lymph Nodes.   The regional lymph nodes are the nodes of the true pelvis, which essentially are the pelvic nodes below the bifurcation of the common iliac arteries. They include the following groups:

Pelvic, NOS
Hypogastric
Obturator
Iliac (internal, external, or NOS)
Sacral (lateral, presacral, promontory [Gerota's], or NOS)

Laterality does not affect the "N" classification.

Distant Lymph Nodes.   Distant lymph nodes lie outside the confines of the true pelvis. They can be imaged using ultrasound, computed tomography, magnetic resonance imaging, or lymphangiography. Although enlarged lymph nodes can occasionally be visualized, because of a stage migration associated with PSA screening, very few patients will be found to have nodal disease, so false-positive and false-negative results are common when imaging tests are employed. In lieu of imaging, risk tables are generally used to determine individual patient risk of nodal involvement. Involvement of distant lymph nodes is classified as M1a. The distant lymph nodes include:

Aortic (para-aortic lumbar)
Common iliac
Inguinal, deep
Superficial inguinal (femoral)
Supraclavicular
Cervical
Scalene
Retroperitoneal, NOS

The significance of regional lymph node metastasis, pN, in staging prostate cancer lies in the presence of metastatic foci present within the lymph nodes.

Metastatic Sites.   Osteoblastic metastases are the most common non-nodal site of prostate cancer metastasis. In addition, this tumor frequently spreads to distant lymph nodes. Lung and liver metastases are usually identified late in the course of the disease.

RULES FOR CLASSIFICATION

Clinical Staging. Primary tumor assessment includes digital rectal examination of the prostate and histologic or cytologic confirmation of prostate carcinoma. All information available before the first definitive treatment may be used for clinical staging. Imaging techniques may be valuable in some cases; TRUS is the most commonly used imaging tool, but it has a poor ability to identify tumor location and extent. Tumor that is found in one or both lobes by needle biopsy, but is not palpable or visible by imaging, is classified as T1c. Considerable uncertainty exists about the ability of imaging to define the extent of a non-palpable lesion (see the definition of T1c below). For research purposes, investigators should specify whether clinical staging into the T1c category is based on DRE only or on DRE plus TRUS. In general, most patients diagnosed in an environment of ubiquitous PSA screening will be at a low risk of positive nodes or metastases, and the risk of false-positive imaging studies in asymptomatic patients has exceeded the frequency of true-positive or true-negative studies in several reports. For this reason, in patients with Gleason scores less than 7–8 and PSA values < 20 ng/ml, imaging studies may not always be helpful in accurate staging.

Since publication of the Fifth Edition of the *AJCC Cancer Staging Manual*, review of the results of clinical series of patients with T2 tumors has demonstrated that recurrence-free survival following treatment was significantly different if the Fourth Edition system of T2a, T2b, and T2c stratification was used. Therefore, to enhance the characterization of palpable tumors, the Sixth Edition has reincorporated the three clinical stages T2a (palpable tumor confined to less than one-half of one lobe), T2b (palpable tumor involving more than half of one lobe but not both lobes), and T2c (tumor involving both lobes).

Pathologic Staging. In general, total prostatoseminal-vesiculectomy, including regional node specimen, and histologic confirmation are required for pathologic T classification. However, under certain circumstances, pathologic T classification can be determined with other means. For example, (1) positive biopsy of the rectum permits a pT4 classification without prostatoseminal-vesiculectomy, and (2) a biopsy revealing carcinoma in extraprostatic soft tissue permits a pT3 classification, as does a biopsy revealing adenocarcinoma infiltrating the seminal vesicles. However, there is no pT1 category because there is insufficient tissue to assess the highest pT category. Margin positivity, potentially a consequence of surgical technique rather than anatomic extent of disease, should be specified along with pathologic stage. (Positive surgical margin should be indicated by an R1 descriptor [residual microscopic disease].)

In addition to pathologic stage, independent prognostic factors for survival have been identified for prostate cancer. These include age of patient, comorbid diseases, histologic grade, Gleason score, PSA, and percent free-PSA level, surgical margin status, and ploidy.

9

DEFINITION OF TNM

Primary Tumor (T)

Clinical

TX   Primary tumor cannot be assessed

T0   No evidence of primary tumor

T1   Clinically inapparent tumor neither palpable nor visible by imaging

T1a   Tumor incidental histologic finding in 5% or less of tissue resected

T1b   Tumor incidental histologic finding in more than 5% of tissue resected

T1c   Tumor identified by needle biopsy (e.g., because of elevated PSA)

T2   Tumor confined within prostate*

T2a   Tumor involves one-half of one lobe or less

T2b   Tumor involves more than one-half of one lobe but not both lobes

T2c   Tumor involves both lobes

T3   Tumor extends through the prostate capsule**

T3a   Extracapsular extension (unilateral or bilateral)

T3b   Tumor invades seminal vesicle(s)

T4   Tumor is fixed or invades adjacent structures other than seminal vesicles: bladder neck, external sphincter, rectum, levator muscles, and/or pelvic wall

Note: Tumor found in one or both lobes by needle biopsy, but not palpable or reliably visible by imaging, is classified as T1c.

**Note:* Invasion into the prostatic apex or into (but not beyond) the prostatic capsule is classified not as T3 but as T2.

Pathologic (pT)

pT2*   Organ confined

pT2a   Unilateral, involving one-half of one lobe or less

pT2b   Unilateral involving more than one-half of one lobe but not both lobes

pT2c   Bilateral disease

pT3   Extraprostatic extension

pT3a   Extraprostatic extension**

pT3b   Seminal vesicle invasion

pT4   Invasion of bladder, rectum

Note: There is no pathologic T1 classification.

**Note: Positive surgical margin should be indicated by an R1 descriptor (residual microscopic disease).

Regional Lymph Nodes (N)

Clinical

NX   Regional lymph nodes were not assessed

N0   No regional lymph node metastasis

N1   Metastasis in regional lymph node(s)

Pathologic

pNX   Regional nodes not sampled
pN0   No positive regional nodes
pN1   Metastases in regional node(s)

Distant Metastasis (M)*

MX   Distant metastasis cannot be assessed (not evaluated by any modality)
M0   No distant metastasis
M1   Distant metastasis
M1a   Non-regional lymph node(s)
M1b   Bone(s)
M1c   Other site(s) with or without bone disease

Note: When more than one site of metastasis is present, the most advanced category is used. pM1c is most advanced.

STAGE GROUPING				
Stage I	T1a	N0	M0	G1
Stage II	T1a	N0	M0	G2, 3–4
	T1b	N0	M0	Any G
	T1c	N0	M0	Any G
	T1	N0	M0	Any G
	T2	N0	M0	Any G
Stage III	T3	N0	M0	Any G
Stage IV	T4	N0	M0	Any G
	Any T	N1	M0	Any G
	Any T	Any N	M1	Any G

HISTOPATHOLOGIC TYPE

This classification applies to adenocarcinomas and squamous carcinomas, but not to sarcoma or transitional cell carcinoma of the prostate. Adjectives used to describe adenocarcinomas can include *mucinous, small cell, papillary, ductal,* and *neuroendocrine.* Transitional cell carcinoma of the prostate is classified as a urethral tumor (see Chapter 39). There should be histologic confirmation of the disease.

HISTOLOGIC GRADE (G)

Gleason score is considered to be the optimal method of grading, because this method takes into account the inherent heterogeneity of prostate cancer, and because it has been clearly shown that this method is of great prognostic value. A primary and a secondary pattern (the range of each is 1–5) are assigned and then summed to yield a total score. Scores of 2–10 are thus possible. (If a single focus of disease is seen, it should be reported as both scores. For example, if a single focus of Gleason 3 disease is seen, it is reported as $3 + 3$.)

GX   Grade cannot be assessed
G1   Well differentiated (slight anaplasia) (Gleason 2–4)
G2   Moderately differentiated (moderate anaplasia) (Gleason 5–6)
G3–4 Poorly differentiated/undifferentiated (marked anaplasia) (Gleason 7–10)

PROGNOSTIC FEATURES

Prostate-specific antigen, grade, and tumor stage all have a profound relationship with prognosis. An increasing number of molecular markers (such as ploidy, p53, and bcl-2) have been identified that predict stage at diagnosis and outcomes following therapy. A number of algorithms have been published that enable the merging of these data to predict local stage, risk of positive nodes, or risk of treatment failure.

Recent studies have demonstrated that Gleason score provides extremely important information about prognosis. In an analysis, conducted by the Radiation Therapy Oncology Group (RTOG), of nearly 1500 men treated on prospective randomized trials, Gleason score was the single most important predictor of death from prostate cancer. Combined with the AJCC stage, investigators demonstrated that four prognostic subgroups could be identified that allowed disease-specific survival to be predicted at 5, 10, and 15 years (See Fig. 34.1). Additional studies conducted by the

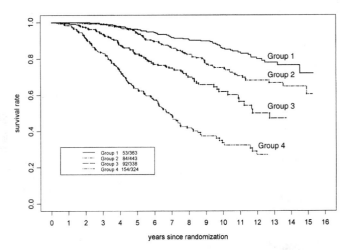

Group 1: Gleason Score (GS) = 2–6, T1–2 NX
Group 2: GS = 2–6, T3 NX or GS = 2–6, N+ or GS = 7, T1–2 NX
Group 3: GS = 7, T3 NX or GS = 7, N+ or GS = 8–10, T1–2 NX
Group 4: GS = 8–10, T3 NX or GS = 8–10, N+

FIG. 34.1. Four prognostic groups predicting long-term survival from prostate cancer following radiotherapy alone on Radiation Therapy Oncology Group clinical trials. (Reprinted from Roach M, Lu J, Pilepich M, et al. Int J Rad Onc Bio Phys 47(3):609–615, 2000, with permission from Elsevier Science.)

RTOG also demonstrated that a pretreatment PSA > 20 ng/ml predicts a greater likelihood of distant failure and a greater need for hormonal therapy. A recent validation study confirmed that a PSA > 20 ng/ml was associated with a greater risk of prostate cancer death. Thus, in addition to the AJCC clinical stage, pretreatment PSA and Gleason score provide important prognostic information that might affect decisions regarding therapy. Other clinical features, such as the number of positive biopsies and the presence of perineural invasion, may provide additional prognostic information. However, long-term confirmatory, multi-institutional studies demonstrating the independent impact of these factors on survival from prostate cancer are not yet available.

OUTCOMES BY STAGE, GRADE, AND PSA

A number of endpoints are useful in assessing disease outcomes. Biochemical (or PSA)-free recurrence indicates the likelihood that a patient treated for prostate cancer remains free of recurrent disease as manifested by a rising PSA. Prostate cancer-specific survival and overall survival are also useful endpoints.

BIBLIOGRAPHY

Aihara M, Wheeler TM, Ohori M, et al: Heterogeneity of prostate cancer in radical prostatectomy specimens. Urology 43:60–67, 1994

Albertsen PC, Fryback DG, Storer BE, et al: Long-term survival among men with conservatively treated localized prostate cancer. JAMA 274:626–631, 1995

Albertsen PC, Hanley JA, Harlan LC, Gilliland FD, Hamilton A, Liff JM, Stanford JL, Stephenson RA: The positive yield of imaging studies in the evaluation of men with newly diagnosed prostate cancer: a population-based analysis. J Urol 163(4):1138–1143, 2000

Albertsen PC, Hanley JA, Gleason DF, Barry MJ: Competing risk analysis of men aged 55 to 74 years at diagnosis managed conservatively for clinically localized prostate cancer. JAMA 280(11):975–980, 1998

Bazinet M, Meshref AW, Trudel C, Aronson S, et al: Prospective evaluation of prostate-specific antigen density and systematic biopsies for early detection of prostatic carcinoma. Urology 43:44–52, 1994

Carroll P, Coley C, McLeod D, Schellhammer P, Sweat G, Wasson J, Zietman A, Thompson I: Prostate-specific antigen best practice policy. Part II: Prostate cancer staging and post-treatment follow-up. Urology 57:225–229, 2001

Carvalhal GF, Smith DS, Mager DE, Ramos C, Catalona WJ: Digital rectal examination for detecting prostate cancer at prostate-specific antigen levels of 4 ng/ml or less. J Urol 161(3):835–839, 1999

Catalona WJ, Hudson MA, Scardino PT, et al: Selection of optimal prostate-specific antigen cutoffs for early detection of prostate cancer: receiver operating characteristic curves. J Urol 152:2037–2042, 1994

Catalona WJ, Smith DS: Cancer recurrence and survival rates after anatomic radical retropubic prostatectomy for prostate cancer: intermediate-term results. J Urol 160(6 Pt 2):2428–2434, 1998

Chodak GW, Thisted RA, Gerber GS, et al: Results of conservative management of clinically localized prostate cancer. N Engl J Med 330:242–248, 1994

9

Epstein JI, Chan DW, Sokoll LJ, Walsh PC, Cox JL, Rittenhouse H, Wolfert R, Carter HB: Nonpalpable stage T1c prostate cancer: prediction of insignificant disease using free/total prostate-specific antigen levels and needle biopsy findings. J Urol 160(6 Pt 2):2407–2411, 1998

Epstein JI, Partin, AW, Sauvageot, J, and Walsh, PC: Prediction of progression following radical prostatectomy: a multivariate analysis of 721 men with long-term follow-up. Amer J Surg Path, 20:286, 1996

Epstein JI, Pizov G, Walsh PC: Correlation of pathologic findings with progression after radical retropubic prostatectomy. Cancer 71:3582–3593, 1993

Ferguson JK, Bostwick DG, Suman V, et al: Prostate-specific antigen detected prostate cancer: pathological characteristics of ultrasound visible versus ultrasound invisible tumors. Eur Urol 27:8–12, 1995

Grignon DJ, Hammond EH: College of American Pathologists Conference XXVI on clinical relevance of prognostic markers in solid tumors. Arch Pathol Lab Med 119, December 1995

Han M, Walsh PC, Partin AW, Rodriguez R: Ability of the 1992 and 1997 American Joint Committee on Cancer staging systems for prostate cancer to predict progression-free survival after radical prostatectomy for Stage T2 disease. J Urol 164(1):89–92, 2000

Henson DE, Hutter RV, Farrow G: Practice protocol for the examination of specimens removed from patients with carcinoma of the prostate gland. Arch Pathol Lab Med 118:779–783, 1994

Humphrey PA, Frazier HA, Vollmer RT, et al: Stratification of pathologic features in radical prostatectomy specimens that are predictive of elevated initial postoperative serum prostate-specific antigen levels. Cancer 71:1822–1827, 1992

McNeal JE, Villers AA, Redwine EA, et al: Histologic differentiation, cancer volume, and pelvic lymph node metastasis in adenocarcinoma of the prostate. Cancer 66:1225–1233, 1990

Miller GJ: New developments in grading prostate cancer. Semin Urol 8:9–18, 1990

Montie JE: Staging of prostate cancer: current TNM classifications and future prospects for prognostic factors. Cancer Supplement 75:1814–1818, 1995

Optenberg SA, Clark JY, Brawer MK, Thompson IM, Stein CR, Friedrichs P. Development of a decision-making tool to predict risk of prostate cancer: The Cancer of the Prostate Risk Index (CAPRI) Test. Urology 50:665–672, 1997

Partin AW, Oesterling JE: The clinical usefulness of prostate-specific antigen: update 1994. J Urol 152:1358–1368, 1994

Pinover WH, Hanlon A, Lee WR, et al: Prostate carcinoma patients upstaged by imaging and treated with irradiation—an outcome-based analysis. Cancer 77(7):1334–1341, 1996

Pound CR, Partin AW, Eisenberger MA, Chan DW, Pearson JD, Walsh PC: Natural history of progression after PSA elevation following radical prostatectomy. JAMA. 281(17):1591–1597, 1999

Ramos CG, Carvalhal GF, Smith DS, Mager DE, Catalona WJ: Clinical and pathological characteristics, and recurrence rates of Stage T1c versus T2a or T2b prostate cancer. J Urol 161(5):1525–1529, 1999

Rifkin MD, Zerhouni EA, Gatsonis CA, Quint LE, et al: Comparison of magnetic resonance imaging and ultrasonography in staging early prostate cancer: results of a multi-institutional cooperative trial. N Engl J Med 323:621–625, 1990

Simon R, Altman DG: Statistical aspects of prognostic factor studies in oncology. Br J Cancer 69:979–985, 1994

Smith DS, Catalona WJ: Interexaminer variability of digital rectal examination in detecting prostate cancer. Urology 45:70–74, 1995

Southwick PC, Catalona WJ, Partin AW, Slawin KM, Brawer MK, Flanigan RC, Patel A, Richie JP, Walsh PC, Scardino PT, Lange PH, Gasior GH, Parson RE, Loveland KG: Prediction of post-radical prostatectomy pathological outcome for Stage T1c prostate cancer with percent free prostate specific antigen: a prospective multicenter clinical trial. J Urol 162(4):1346–1351, 1999

Terris MK, McNeal JE, Freiha FS, et al: Efficacy of transrectal ultrasound-guided seminal vesicle biopsies in the detection of seminal vesicle invasion by prostate cancer. J Urol 149:1035–1039, 1993

Zagars GK, von Eschenbach AC: Prostate-specific antigen—an important marker for prostate cancer treated by external beam radiation therapy. Cancer 72:538–548, 1993

Zincke H, Bergstrahl EJ, Blute ML, et al: Radical prostatectomy for clinically localized prostate cancer: long-term results of 1,143 patients from a single institution. J Clin Oncol 12:2254–2263, 1994

HISTOLOGIES—PROSTATE

8041/3	Small cell carcinoma, NOS
8070/3	Squamous cell carcinoma, NOS
8074/3	Squamous cell carcinoma, spindle cell
8082/3	Lymphoepithelial carcinoma
8098/3	Adenoid basal carcinoma
8120/3	Transitional cell carcinoma, NOS
8140/2	Adenocarcinoma *in situ,* NOS
8140/3	Adenocarcinoma, NOS
8148/2	Glandular intraepithelial neoplasia, grade III
8200/3	Adenoid cystic carcinoma
8240/3	Carcinoid tumor, NOS
8246/3	Neuroendocrine carcinoma, NOS
8260/3	Papillary adenocarcinoma
8480/3	Mucinous adenocarcinoma
8490/3	Signet ring cell carcinoma
8500/3	Infiltrating duct carcinoma, NOS
8560/3	Adenosquamous carcinoma

9

35

Testis

C62.0 Undescended testis   C62.1 Descended testis   C62.9 Testis, NOS

SUMMARY OF CHANGES

- The definition of TNM and the Stage Grouping for this chapter have not changed from the Fifth Edition.

INTRODUCTION

Cancers of the testis are usually found in young adults and account for less than 1% of all malignancies in males. However, during the 20th century, the incidence has more than doubled. Cryptorchidism is a predisposing condition, and other associations include atypical germ cells and multiple atypical nevi. Germ cell tumors of the testis are categorized into two main histologic types: seminomas and non-seminomas. The latter group is composed of either individual or combinations of histologic subtypes, including embryonal carcinoma, teratoma, choriocarcinoma, and yolk sac tumor. The presence of serum markers, including alpha-fetoprotein (AFP), human chorionic gonadotropin (hCG), and lactate dehydrogenase (LDH), is frequent in this disease. Staging and prognostication are based on determination of the extent of disease and assessment of serum tumor markers. Cancer of the testis is highly curable, even in cases with advanced, metastatic disease.

ANATOMY

Primary Site. The testes are composed of convoluted seminiferous tubules with a stroma containing functional endocrine interstitial cells. Both are encased in a dense capsule, the tunica albuginea, with fibrous septa extending into the testes and separating them into lobules. The tubules converge and exit at the mediastinum of the testis into the rete testis and efferent ducts, which join a single duct. This duct—the epididymis—coils outside the upper and lower poles of the testicle and then joins the vas deferens, a muscular conduit that accompanies the vessels and lymphatic channels of the spermatic cord. The major route for local extension of cancer is through the lymphatic channels. The tumor emerges from the mediastinum of the testis and courses through the spermatic cord. Occasionally, the epididymis is invaded early, and then the external iliac nodes may become involved. If there has been previous scrotal or inguinal surgery or if invasion of the scrotal wall is found (though this is rare), then the lymphatic spread may be to inguinal nodes.

Regional Lymph Nodes.   The following nodes are considered regional:

Interaortocaval
Para-aortic (Periaortic)
Paracaval
Preaortic
Precaval
Retroaortic
Retrocaval

The intrapelvic, external iliac, and inguinal nodes are considered regional only after scrotal or inguinal surgery prior to the presentation of the testis tumor. All nodes outside the regional nodes are distant. Nodes along the spermatic vein are considered regional.

Metastatic Sites.   Distant spread of testicular tumors occurs most commonly to the lymph nodes, followed by metastases to the lung, liver, bone, and other visceral sites. Stage is dependent on the extent of disease and on the determination of serum tumor markers. Extent of disease includes assessment for involvement and size of regional lymph nodes, evidence of disease in non-regional lymph nodes, and metastases to pulmonary and non-pulmonary visceral sites. The stage is subdivided on the basis of the presence and degree of elevation of serum tumor markers. Serum tumor markers are measured immediately after orchiectomy and, if elevated, should be measured serially after orchiectomy to determine whether normal decay curves are followed. The physiological half-life of AFP is 5–7 days, and the half-life of HCG is 24–48 hours. The presence of prolonged half-life times implies the presence of residual disease after orchiectomy. It should be noted that in some cases, tumor marker release may occur (for example, in response to chemotherapy or handling of a primary tumor intraoperatively) and may cause artificial elevation of circulating tumor marker levels. The serum level of lactate dehydrogenase (LDH) has prognostic value in patients with metastatic disease and is included for staging.

RULES FOR CLASSIFICATION

Clinical Staging.   Staging of testis tumors includes determination of the T, N, M, and S categories. Clinical examination and histologic assessment are required for clinical staging. Radiographic assessment of the chest, abdomen, and pelvis is necessary to determine the N and M status of disease. Serum tumor markers, including AFP, hCG, and LDH, should be obtained to complete the status of the serum tumor markers (S).

Pathologic Staging.   Histologic evaluation of the radical orchiectomy specimen must be used for the pT classification. The gross size of the tumor should be recorded. Careful gross examination should determine whether the tumor is intra- or extratesticular. If intratesticular, it should be determined whether the tumor extends through the tunica albuginea and whether it invades the epididymis and/or spermatic cord. Tissue sections should document these findings. The tumor should be sampled extensively, including all grossly diverse areas (hemorrhagic, mucoid, solid, cystic, etc.). The junction of tumor and non-neoplastic testis and at least one section remote from the tumor should be obtained to determine whether intratubular germ cell neoplasia (carcinoma *in situ*) is present. These sections will allow assessment of either the presence or absence of vascular invasion. If possible, most tissue sections should include overlying tunica albuginea. Small tumors (2 cm or less) may be submitted *in toto*. In larger tumors, a sufficient amount of tissue should be sampled, perhaps one section for each 1 or 2 cm of maximum tumor diameter.

The specimens from a defined node-bearing area (such as retroperitoneal lymph node dissection) must be used for the pN classification. Retroperitoneal lymph node dissection should be oriented by the surgeon. All lymph nodes should be dissected, and the diameters of the largest nodes should be recorded, along with the number of lymph nodes involved by tumor. Extranodal soft tissue extension of disease should be noted, if present. It is important to examine carefully and liberally sample the specimen, including cystic, fibrotic, hemorrhagic, necrotic, and solid areas. Laterality does not affect the N classification. In post-treatment specimens, it may be difficult to distinguish individual lymph nodes. The definitions for Primary Tumor (T) for pT1, pT2, and pT3 are illustrated in Figures 35.1, 35.2, and 35.3.

DEFINITION OF TNM

Primary Tumor (T)

The extent of primary tumor is usually classified after radical orchiectomy, and for this reason, a *pathologic* stage is assigned.

*pTX	Primary tumor cannot be assessed
pT0	No evidence of primary tumor (e.g., histologic scar in testis)
pTis	Intratubular germ cell neoplasia (carcinoma *in situ*)
PT1	Tumor limited to the testis and epididymis without vascular/lymphatic invasion; tumor may invade into the tunica albuginea but not the tunica vaginalis
pT2	Tumor limited to the testis and epididymis with vascular/lymphatic invasion, or tumor extending through the tunica albuginea with involvement of the tunica vaginalis
PT3	Tumor invades the spermatic cord with or without vascular/lymphatic invasion
pT4	Tumor invades the scrotum with or without vascular/lymphatic invasion

Note: Except for pTis and pT4, extent of primary tumor is classified by radical orchiectomy. TX may be used for other categories in the absence of radical orchiectomy.

Regional Lymph Nodes (N)

Clinical

NX   Regional lymph nodes cannot be assessed

N0   No regional lymph node metastasis

N1   Metastasis with a lymph node mass 2 cm or less in greatest dimension; or multiple lymph nodes, none more than 2 cm in greatest dimension

N2   Metastasis with a lymph node mass more than 2 cm but not more than 5 cm in greatest dimension; or multiple lymph nodes, any one mass greater than 2 cm but not more than 5 cm in greatest dimension

N3   Metastasis with a lymph node mass more than 5 cm in greatest dimension

Pathologic (pN)

pNX   Regional lymph nodes cannot be assessed

pN0   No regional lymph node metastasis

pNl   Metastasis with a lymph node mass 2 cm or less in greatest dimension and less than or equal to 5 nodes positive, none more than 2 cm in greatest dimension

pN2   Metastasis with a lymph node mass more than 2 cm but not more than 5 cm in greatest dimension; or more than 5 nodes positive, none more than 5 cm; or evidence of extranodal extension of tumor

pN3   Metastasis with a lymph node mass more than 5 cm in greatest dimension

Distant Metastasis (M)

MX   Distant metastasis cannot be assessed

M0   No distant metastasis

M1   Distant metastasis

Mla   Non-regional nodal or pulmonary metastasis

Mlb   Distant metastasis other than to non-regional lymph nodes and lungs

Serum Tumor Markers (S)

SX   Marker studies not available or not performed

S0   Marker study levels within normal limits

S1   LDH $< 1.5 \times$ N* **AND**
hCG (mIu/ml) < 5000 **AND**
AFP (ng/ml) < 1000

S2   LDH $1.5–10 \times$ N **OR**
hCG (mIu/ml) 5000–50,000 **OR**
AFP (ng/ml) 1000–10,000

S3   LDH $> 10 \times$ N **OR**
hCG (mIu/ml) $> 50,000$ **OR**
AFP (ng/ml) $> 10,000$

*N indicates the upper limit of normal for the LDH assay.

STAGE GROUPING

Stage 0	pTis	N0	M0	S0
Stage I	pT1–4	N0	M0	SX
Stage IA	pT1	N0	M0	S0
Stage IB	pT2	N0	M0	S0
	pT3	N0	M0	S0
	pT4	N0	M0	S0
Stage IS	Any pT/Tx	N0	M0	S1–3
Stage II	Any pT/Tx	N1–3	M0	SX
Stage IIA	Any pT/Tx	N1	M0	S0
	Any pT/Tx	N1	M0	S1
Stage IIB	Any pT/Tx	N2	M0	S0
	Any pT/Tx	N2	M0	S1
Stage IIC	Any pT/Tx	N3	M0	S0
	Any pT/Tx	N3	M0	S1
Stage III	Any pT/Tx	Any N	M1	SX
Stage IIIA	Any pT/Tx	Any N	M1a	S0
	Any pT/Tx	Any N	M1a	S1
Stage IIIB	Any pT/Tx	N1–3	M0	S2
	Any pT/Tx	Any N	M1a	S2
Stage IIIC	Any pT/Tx	N1–3	M0	S3
	Any pT/Tx	Any N	M1a	S3
	Any pT/Tx	Any N	M1b	Any S

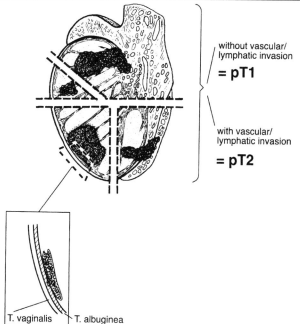

FIG. 35.1. Illustration of pT1 and pT2 showing tumor without and with vascular/lymphatic invasion.

HISTOPATHOLOGIC TYPE

Following the guidelines of the *World Health Organization Histological Classification of Tumors*, germ cell tumors may be either seminomatous or non-seminomatous. Seminomas may be classic type or with syncytiotro-

pT2

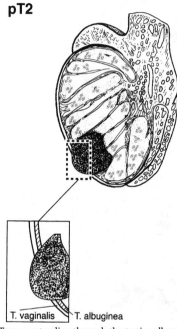

FIG. 35.2. pT2 Tumor extending through the tunica albuginea with involvement of the tunica vaginalis.

pT3

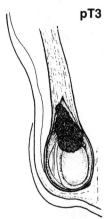

FIG. 35.3. pT3 Tumor invades the spermatic cord.

phoblasts. A distinct variant is spermatocytic seminoma, which is characteristically found in older patients, is often associated with intratumoral calcification, and tends not to metastasize. Non-seminomatous germ cell tumors may be pure (embryonal carcinoma, yolk sac tumor, teratoma, choriocarcinoma) or mixed. Mixtures of these types (including seminoma) should be noted, starting with the most prevalent component and ending with the least represented. Similarly, gonadal stromal. tumors should be classified according to the *World Health Organization Histological Classification of Tumours.*

BIBLIOGRAPHY

Bajorin D, Katz A, Chan E, et al: Comparison of criteria for assigning germ cell tumor patients to "good risk" and "poor risk" studies. J Clin Oncol 4:786–792, 1986

Birch R, Williams S, Cone A, et al: Prognostic factors for favorable outcome in disseminated germ cell tumors. J Clin Oncol 4:400–407, 1986

Boyer M, Raghavan D: Toxicity of treatment of germ cell tumors. Semin Oncol 19:128–142, 1992

Einhorn LH: Testicular cancer as a model for a curable neoplasm: the Richard and Hinda Rosenthal Foundation Award Lecture. Cancer Res., 41:3274–3280, 1981

Freedman LS, Parkinson MC, Jones WG, et al: Histopathology in the prediction of relapse of patients with Stage I testicular teratoma treated by orchiectomy alone. Lancet 2:294–298, 1987

Hoskin P, Dilly S, Easton D, et al: Prognostic factors in Stage I non-seminomatous germ cell tumors managed by orchiectomy and surveillance: implications for adjuvant chemotherapy. J Clin Oncol 4:1031–1036, 1986

International Germ Cell Cancer Collaborative Group: International germ cell consensus classification: a prognostic factor–based staging system for metastatic germ cell cancers. J Clin Oncol 15:594–603, 1997

Mead GM, Stenning SP, Parkinson MC, et al: The Second Medical Research Council study of prognostic factors in nonseminomatous germ cell tumors. J Clin Oncol 10:85–94, 1992

Peckham MJ, Barrett A, McElwain TJ et al: Nonseminoma germ cell tumours (malignant teratoma) of the testis: results of treatment and an analysis of prognostic factors. Br J Urol 53:162–172, 1981

Raghavan D, Colls B, Levi J, et al: Surveillance for Stage I non-seminomatous germ cell tumours of the testis: the optimal protocol has not yet been defined. Br J Urol 61:522–526, 1988

Williams SD, Birch R, Einhorn LH, et al: Treatment of disseminated germ-cell tumors with cisplatin, bleomycin and either vinblastine or etoposide. N Engl J Med 317:1433–1438, 1987

HISTOLOGIES—TESTIS

8590/1	Sex cord–gonadal stromal tumor, NOS
8592/1	Sex cord–gonadal stromal tumor, mixed forms
8620/1	Granulosa cell tumor, adult type
8640/3	Sertoli cell carcinoma
8650/1	Leydig cell tumor, NOS
9061/3	Seminoma, NOS
9063/3	Spermatocytic seminoma
9064/2	Intratubular malignant germ cells

HISTOLOGIES—TESTIS (CONT.)

9065/3	Germ cell tumor, non-seminomatous
9070/3	Embryonal carcinoma, NOS
9071/3	Yolk sac tumor
9081/3	Teratocarcinoma
9085/3	Mixed germ cell tumor
9100/3	Choriocarcinoma, NOS
9101/3	Choriocarcinoma combined with other germ cell elements

36

Kidney

(Sarcomas and adenomas are not included.)

C64.9 Kidney, NOS

SUMMARY OF CHANGES

- T1 lesions have been divided into T1a and T1b.

- T1a is defined as tumors 4 cm or less in greatest dimension, limited to the kidney.

- T1b is defined as tumors greater than 4 cm but not more than 7 cm in greatest dimension, limited to the kidney.

INTRODUCTION

Cancers of the kidney are relatively rare, accounting for less than 3% of all malignancies. Nearly all malignant tumors are carcinomas arising from the renal tubular epithelium or, less frequently, from the renal pelvis (see Chapter 37). These tumors are more common in males. Pain and hematuria are usually the presenting features, but a majority of kidney tumors are now being detected incidentally in asymptomatic individuals. These carcinomas have a tendency to extend into the renal vein and even into the vena cava. Staging depends on the size of the primary tumor, invasion of the adjacent structures, and vascular extension.

Since publication of the Fifth Edition of the *AJCC Cancer Staging Manual*, the evidence has become compelling that the T1 category should be subdivided into stages T1a and T1b, the former being tumors of 4 cm or less and the latter being tumors of 4–7 cm. The rationale is twofold: (1) the recurrence and survival difference between the two and (2) the current practice of applying partial nephrectomy for solitary tumors 4 cm or less in diameter. In the case of partial nephrectomy for tumors < 4 cm in diameter, evidence suggests that survival outcomes are equivalent to outcomes with radical nephrectomy (Lee CT et al. 2000). In a group of 485 patients undergoing nephron-sparing surgery for renal cell carcinoma and with a mean post-operative follow-up of 47 months, the authors segregated patients into four groups based on tumor size: 1—less than 2.5 cm; 2—2.5 to 4.0 cm; 3—4 to 7 cm; 4—more than 7 cm (Hafez KS et al. 1999). The authors found no difference in survival between groups 1 and 2, but survival was significantly greater in groups 1 and 2 than in both groups 3 and 4. Similar findings were reported in a second series of 394 patients (Lerner SE et al. 1996).

ANATOMY

Primary Site. Encased by a fibrous capsule and surrounded by perirenal fat, the kidney consists of the cortex (glomeruli, convoluted tubules) and the medulla (Henle's loops, pyramids of converging tubules). Each papilla opens into the minor calices; these in turn unite in the major calices and drain into the renal pelvis. At the hilus are the pelvis, ureter, and renal artery and vein. Gerota's fascia overlies the psoas and quadratus lumborum.

Regional Lymph Nodes.   The regional lymph nodes are:

Renal hilar
Paracaval
Aortic (para-aortic, periaortic, lateral aortic)
Retroperitoneal, NOS

Metastatic Sites.   Common metastatic sites include bone, liver, lung, brain, and distant lymph nodes.

RULES FOR CLASSIFICATION

The classification applies only to the renal cell carcinomas. Adenoma is excluded. There should be histologic confirmation of the disease. Refer to the list of histopathologic types below.

Clinical Staging.   Clinical examination, abdominal computed tomography scanning, and appropriate imaging techniques are required for assessment of the primary tumor and its extensions, both local and distant. Evaluation for distant metastases should be done by laboratory biochemical studies, chest X-rays, and, if clinically indicated, isotopic studies.

Pathologic Staging.   Histologic examination and confirmation of extent are recommended. Resection of the primary tumor, kidney, Gerota's fascia, perinephric fat, renal vein, and appropriate lymph nodes is recommended. Partial nephrectomy seems to be an acceptable treatment for T1a tumors with outcomes comparable to those with radical nephrectomy for this tumor stage. Laterality does not affect the N classification.

Specimen Handling.   It is recommended that the pathologic specimen be processed in such a fashion as to allow full pathologic assessment. Perinephric fat should be left intact and sectioned in such a manner so as to evaluate invasion of this structure. For specimens from partial nephrectomy, margins must be evaluated from at least two sections and should include the renal sinus for central tumors. For patients in whom an assessment of multiple tumors is required, thin sections will be needed (0.5–1.0 cm).

Figures 36.1 and 36.2 illustrate the definition of T1 and T2.

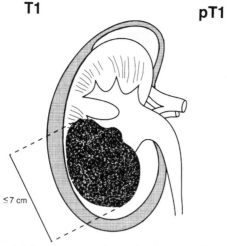

FIG. 36.1. T1 is defined as a tumor 7 cm or less in greatest dimension and limited to the kidney.

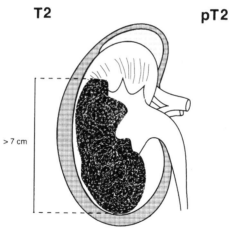

FIG. 36.2. T2 is defined as a tumor more than 7 cm in greatest dimension and limited to the kidney.

DEFINITION OF TNM

Primary Tumor (T)

TX   Primary tumor cannot be assessed
T0   No evidence of primary tumor
T1   Tumor 7 cm or less in greatest dimension, limited to the kidney
T1a   Tumor 4 cm or less in greatest dimension, limited to the kidney

T1b   Tumor more than 4 cm but not more than 7 cm in greatest dimension, limited to the kidney

T2   Tumor more than 7 cm in greatest dimension, limited to the kidney

T3   Tumor extends into major veins or invades adrenal gland or perinephric tissues but not beyond Gerota's fascia

T3a   Tumor directly invades adrenal gland or perirenal and/or renal sinus fat but not beyond Gerota's fascia

T3b   Tumor grossly extends into the renal vein or its segmental (muscle-containing) branches, or vena cava below the diaphragm

T3c   Tumor grossly extends into vena cava above diaphragm or invades the wall of the vena cava

T4   Tumor invades beyond Gerota's fascia

Regional Lymph Nodes (N)*

NX   Regional lymph nodes cannot be assessed

N0   No regional lymph node metastases

N1   Metastases in a single regional lymph node

N2   Metastasis in more than one regional lymph node

*Laterality does not affect the N classification.

Note: If a lymph node dissection is performed, then pathologic evaluation would ordinarily include at least eight nodes.

Distant Metastasis (M)

MX   Distant metastasis cannot be assessed

M0   No distant metastasis

M1   Distant metastasis

STAGE GROUPING

Stage I	T1	N0	M0
Stage II	T2	N0	M0
Stage III	T1	N1	M0
	T2	N1	M0
	T3	N0	M0
	T3	N1	M0
	T3a	N0	M0
	T3a	N1	M0
	T3b	N0	M0
	T3b	N1	M0
	T3c	N0	M0
	T3c	N1	M0
Stage IV	T4	N0	M0
	T4	N1	M0
	Any T	N2	M0
	Any T	Any N	M1

HISTOPATHOLOGIC TYPE

The predominant cancer is adenocarcinoma; subtypes are clear cell and granular cell carcinoma. The use of the following grading system is recommended when feasible. Sarcomas and adenomas are not included. The histopathologic types are

Conventional (clear cell) renal carcinoma
Papillary renal cell carcinoma
Chromophobe renal carcinoma
Collecting duct carcinoma

HISTOLOGIC GRADE (G)

GX   Grade cannot be assessed
G1   Well differentiated
G2   Moderately differentiated
G3–4   Poorly differentiated or undifferentiated

BIBLIOGRAPHY

Glazer AA, Novick AC: Long-term follow-up after surgical treatment for renal cell carcinoma extending into the right atrium. J Urol 155:448–450, 1996

Guinan PD, Vogelzang NJ, Freingen AM, et al: Renal cell carcinoma: tumor size, stage, and survival. J Urol 153:901–903, 1995

Hafez KS, Fergany AF, Novick AC: Nephron sparing surgery for localized renal cell carcinoma: impact of tumor size on patient survival, tumor recurrence and TNM staging. J Urol 162(6):1930–1933, 1999

Hermanek P, Schrott KM: Evaluation of the new tumor, nodes, and metastases classification of renal cell carcinoma. J Urol 144:238–242, 1990

Javidan J, Stricker HJ, Tamboli P, et al: Prognostic significance of the 1997 TNM classification of renal cell carcinoma. J Urol 162(4):1277–1281, 1999

Lee CT, Katz J, Shi W, Gthaler HT, Reuter VE, Russo P: Surgical management of renal tumors 4 cm or less in a contemporary cohort. J Urol 163:730–736, 2000

Lerner SE, Hawkins CA, Blute ML, Grabner A, Wollan PC, Eickholt JT, Zincke H: Disease outcome in patients with low stage renal cell carcinoma treated with nephron sparing or radical surgery. J Urol 155:1868–1873, 1996

McDonald JR, Priestley JT: Malignant tumors of the kidney: surgical and prognostic significance of tumor thrombosis of the renal vein. Surg Gynecol Obstet 77:295, 1983

Mostafi FK, et al: Histological typing of kidney tumors. WHO international histological classification of tumours. Geneva: World Health Organization, 1981

Targonski PV, Frank W, Stuhldreher D, et al: Value of tumor size in predicting survival from renal cell carcinoma among tumors, nodes, and metastases Stage I and Stage II patients. J Urol 152:1389–1392, 1994

Tsui KH, Shvarts O, Smith RB, Figlin RA, deKernion JB, Belldegrun A: Prognostic indicators for renal cell carcinoma: a multivariate analysis of 643 patients using the revised 1997 TNM staging criteria. J Urol 163(4):1090–1095, 2000

9

8032/3	Spindle cell carcinoma, NOS
8041/3	Small cell carcinoma, NOS
8140/3	Adenocarcinoma, NOS
8240/3	Carcinoid tumor, NOS
8260/3	Papillary adenocarcinoma, NOS
8290/3	Oxyphilic adenoma
8290/3	Oxyphilic adenocarcinoma
8310/3	Clear cell adenocarcinoma, NOS
8312/3	Renal cell carcinoma, NOS
8317/3	Renal cell carcinoma, chromophobe type
8318/3	Renal cell carcinoma, sarcomatoid
8319/3	Collecting duct carcinoma
8320/3	Granular cell carcinoma
8960/3	Nephroblastoma, NOS
8963/3	Malignant rhabdoid tumor
8966/2	Renomedullary interstitial cell tumor

37

Renal Pelvis and Ureter

C65.9 Renal pelvis   C66.9 Ureter

SUMMARY OF CHANGES

- The definition of TNM and the Stage Grouping for this chapter have not changed from the Fifth Edition.

INTRODUCTION

Urothelial (transitional cell) carcinoma may occur at any site within the upper urinary collecting system from the renal calyx to the ureterovesical junction. The tumors occur most commonly in adults and are rare before 40 years of age. There is a two- to threefold increase in incidence in men compared with women. The lesions are often multiple and are more common in patients with a history of urothelial carcinoma of the bladder. A number of analgesics (such as phenacetin) have also been associated with this disease. Local staging depends on the depth of invasion. A common staging system is used regardless of tumor location within the upper urinary collecting system, except for category T3, which differs between the pelvis or calyceal system and the ureter.

ANATOMY

Primary Site.   The renal pelvis and ureter form a single unit that is continuous with the collecting ducts of the renal pyramids and comprises the minor and major calyces, which are continuous with the renal pelvis. The ureteropelvic junction is variable in position and location but serves as a "landmark" that separates the renal pelvis and the ureter, which continues caudad and traverses the wall of the urinary bladder as the intramural ureter opening in the trigone of the bladder at the ureteral orifice. The renal pelvis and ureter are composed of the following layers: epithelium, subepithelial connective tissue, and muscularis, which is continuous with a connective tissue adventitial layer. It is in this outer layer that the major blood supply and lymphatics are found.

The intrarenal portion of the renal pelvis is surrounded by renal parenchyma; the extrarenal pelvis, by perihilar fat. The ureter courses through the retroperitoneum adjacent to the parietal peritoneum and rests on the retroperitoneal musculature above the pelvic vessels. As it crosses the vessels and enters the deep pelvis, the ureter is surrounded by pelvic fat until it traverses the bladder wall.

Regional Lymph Nodes.   The regional lymph nodes for the renal pelvis are:

Renal hilar
Paracaval

Aortic
Retroperitoneal, NOS

The regional lymph nodes for the ureter are:

Renal hilar
Iliac (common, internal [hypogastric], external)
Paracaval
Periureteral
Pelvic, NOS

Any amount of regional lymph node metastasis is a poor prognostic finding, and outcome is minimally influenced by the number, size, or location of the regional nodes that are involved.

Metastatic Sites.   Distant spread is most commonly to lung, bone, or liver.

RULES FOR CLASSIFICATION

Clinical Staging.   Primary tumor assessment includes radiographic imaging, usually by intravenous and/or retrograde pyelography. Computerized tomography scanning can be used to assess regional nodes. Ureteroscopic visualization of the tumor is desirable, and tissue biopsy through the ureteroscope may be performed if feasible. Urine cytology may help determine tumor grade if tissue is not available. Staging of tumors of the renal pelvis and ureter is not influenced by the presence of any concomitant bladder tumors that may be identified, although it may not be possible to identify the true source of the primary tumor in the presence of metastases if both upper- and lower-tract tumors are present. In that situation, the tumor of highest grade and/or stage is most likely to have contributed to the nodal or metastatic spread.

Pathologic Staging.   Pathologic staging depends on histologic determination of the extent of invasion by the primary tumor. Treatment frequently requires resection of the entire kidney, ureter, and a cuff of bladder surrounding the ureteral orifice. Appropriate regional nodes may be sampled. A more conservative surgical resection may be performed, especially with distal ureteral tumors or in the presence of compromised renal function.

Endoscopic resection through a ureteroscope or a percutaneous approach may be used in some circumstances. Submitted tissue may be insufficient for accurate histologic examination and pathologic staging. Laser or electrocautery coagulation or vaporization of the tumor may be performed, especially if the visible appearance is consistent with a low-grade and low-stage tumor. Under these circumstances, there may be no material available for histologic review.

Figures 37.1 and 37.2 illustrate the Primary Tumor (T) definition for Ta, T1, T2, and T3.

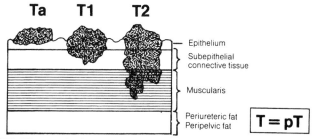

FIG. 37.1. Depth of invasion of Ta–T2 tumors.

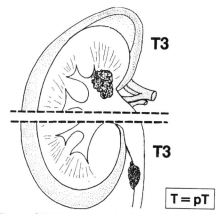

FIG. 37.2. Extent of T3 Tumor in renal pelvis and ureter.

DEFINITION OF TNM

Primary Tumor (T)

TX	Primary tumor cannot be assessed
T0	No evidence of primary tumor
Ta	Papillary non-invasive carcinoma
Tis	Carcinoma *in situ*
T1	Tumor invades subepithelial connective tissue
T2	Tumor invades the muscularis
T3	(For renal pelvis only) Tumor invades beyond muscularis into peripelvic fat or the renal parenchyma
T3	(For ureter only) Tumor invades beyond muscularis into periureteric fat
T4	Tumor invades adjacent organs, or through the kidney into the perinephric fat.

Regional Lymph Nodes (N)*

NX	Regional lymph nodes cannot be assessed
N0	No regional lymph node metastasis
N1	Metastasis in a single lymph node, 2 cm or less in greatest dimension

N2   Metastasis in a single lymph node, more than 2 cm but not more than 5 cm in greatest dimension; or multiple lymph nodes, none more than 5 cm in greatest dimension

N3   Metastasis in a lymph node, more than 5 cm in greatest dimension

Note: Laterality does not affect the N classification

Distant Metastasis (M)

MX   Distant metastasis cannot be assessed
M0   No distant metastasis
M1   Distant metastasis

STAGE GROUPING

Stage 0a	Ta	N0	M0
Stage 0is	Tis	N0	M0
Stage I	T1	N0	M0
Stage II	T2	N0	M0
Stage III	T3	N0	M0
Stage IV	T4	N0	M0
	Any T	N1	M0
	Any T	N2	M0
	Any T	N3	M0
	Any T	Any N	M1

HISTOPATHOLOGIC TYPE

The histologic types are

Urothelial (transitional cell) carcinoma
Squamous cell carcinoma
Epidermoid carcinoma
Adenocarcinoma

HISTOLOGIC GRADE

GX   Grade cannot be assessed
G1   Well differentiated
G2   Moderately differentiated
G3–4   Poorly differentiated or undifferentiated

BIBLIOGRAPHY

al-Abadi H, Nagel R: Transitional cell carcinoma of the renal pelvis and ureter: prognostic relevance of nuclear deoxyribonucleic acid ploidy studied by slide cytometry: an 8-year survival time study. J Urol 148(l):31–37, 1992

Anderstrom C, Johansson SL, Pettersson S, et al: Carcinoma of the ureter: a clinicopathologic study of 49 cases. J Urol 142(2 Pt 1):280–283, 1989

Balaji KC, McGuire M, Grotas J, et al: Upper tract recurrences following radical cystectomy: an analysis of prognostic factors, recurrence pattern and stage at presentation. J Urol 162:1603–1606, 1999

Borgmann V, al-Abadi H, Nagel R: Prognostic relevance of DNA ploidy and proliferative activity in urothelial carcinoma of the renal pelvis and ureter: a study on a follow-up period of 6 years. Urol Int 47(l):7–11, 1991

Corrado F, Ferri C, Mannini D, et al: Transitional cell carcinoma of the upper urinary tract: evaluation of prognostic factors by histopathology and flow cytometric analysis. J Urol 145(6):1159–1163, 1991

Grasso M, Fraiman M, Levine M: Ureteropyeloscopic diagnosis and treatment of upper urinary tract urothelial malignancies. Urology 54:240–246, 1999

Hall MC, Womack S, Sagalowsky AI, et al: Prognostic factors, recurrence, and survival in transitional cell carcinoma of the upper urinary tract: a 30-year experience in 252 patients. Urology 52:594–601, 1998

Herr HW: Extravesical tumor relapse in patients with superficial bladder tumors. J Clin Oncol 16:1099–1102, 1998

Hisataki T, Miyao N, Masumori N, et al: Risk factors for the development of bladder cancer after upper tract urothelial cancer. Urology 55:663–667, 2000

Huben RP, Mounzer AM, Murphy GP: Tumor grade and stage as prognostic variables in upper urothelial tumors. Cancer 62(9):2016–2020, 1988

Hurle R, Losa A, Manzetti A, Lembo A: Upper urinary tract tumors developing after treatment of superficial bladder cancer: 7-year follow-up of 591 consecutive patients. Urology 53:1144–1148, 1999

Jabbour ME, Desgrandchamps F, Cazin S, et al: Percutaneous management of grade II upper urinary tract transitional cell carcinoma: the long-term outcome. J Urol 163:1105–1107, 2000

Jinza S, Iki M, Noguchi S, et al: Nucleolar organizer regions: a new prognostic factor for upper tract urothelial cancer. J Urol 154(5):1688–1692, 1995

Millan-Rodriguez F, Chechile-Toniolo G, Salvador-Bayarri J, et al: Upper urinary tract tumors after primary superficial bladder tumors: prognostic factors and risk groups. J Urol 164:1183–1187, 2000

Scolieri MJ, Paik ML, Brown SL, Resnick MI: Limitations of computed tomography in the preoperative staging of upper tract urothelial carcinoma. Urology 56:930–930, 2000

Williams RD: Tumors of the kidney, ureter, and bladder. West J Med 56(5):523–534, 1992

9

HISTOLOGIES—RENAL PELVIS AND URETER

8010/2	Carcinoma *in situ*, NOS
8010/3	Carcinoma, NOS
8070/2	Squamous cell carcinoma *in situ*
8070/3	Squamous cell carcinoma, NOS
8120/2	Transitional cell carcinoma *in situ*
8120/3	Transitional cell carcinoma, NOS
8130/2	Papillary transitional cell carcinoma, non-invasive
8130/3	Papillary transitional cell carcinoma
8140/3	Adenocarcinoma, NOS

38

Urinary Bladder

C67.0 Trigone of bladder
C67.1 Dome of bladder
C67.2 Lateral wall of bladder

C67.3 Anterior wall of bladder
C67.4 Posterior wall of bladder
C67.5 Bladder neck
C67.6 Ureteric orifice

C67.7 Urachus
C67.8 Overlapping lesion of bladder
C67.9 Bladder, NOS

SUMMARY OF CHANGES

• The definition of TNM and the Stage Grouping for this chapter have not changed from the Fifth Edition.

INTRODUCTION

Bladder cancer is one of the most common malignancies in Western society, and it occurs more commonly in males. Predisposing factors include smoking, exposure to chemicals such as phenacetin and dyes, and schistosomiasis. It has also been suggested that the incidence of this disease correlates inversely with fluid intake. Hematuria is the most common presenting feature. Bladder cancer can present as a low-grade papillary lesion, as an *in situ* lesion that can occupy large areas of the mucosal surface, or as an infiltrative cancer that rapidly extends through the bladder wall and can thereafter metastasize. The papillary and *in situ* lesions may be associated with a malignant course, with sudden invasion of the bladder wall. The most common histologic variant is urothelial (transitional cell) carcinoma, although this may exhibit features of glandular or squamous differentiation. In less than 10% of cases, pure adenocarcinoma or squamous carcinoma of the bladder may occur, and less frequently, sarcoma, lymphoma, small cell anaplastic carcinoma, pheochromocytoma, or choriocarcinoma. Squamous carcinoma is associated with schistosomiasis and smoking.

9

ANATOMY

Primary Site. The urinary bladder consists of three layers: the epithelium and the subepithelial connective tissue, the muscularis, and the perivesical fat (peritoneum covering the superior surface and upper part). In the male, the bladder adjoins the rectum and seminal vesicle posteriorly, the prostate inferiorly, and the pubis and peritoneum anteriorly. In the female, the vagina is located posteriorly and the uterus superiorly. The bladder is located extraperitoneally.

Regional Lymph Nodes. The regional lymph nodes are the nodes of the true pelvis, which essentially are the pelvic nodes below the bifurcation of the common iliac arteries. The significance of regional lymph node metastasis in staging bladder cancer lies in the number and size, not in whether metastasis is unilateral or contralateral. One of the major prognostic determinants of ultimate cure is whether the tumor is confined to the bladder, and a major adverse prognostic feature is the presence of *any* lymph nodal metastases.

Regional nodes include:

Hypogastric
Obturator
Iliac (internal, external, NOS)
Perivesical
Pelvic, NOS
Sacral (lateral, sacral promontory [Gerota's])
Presacral

The common iliac nodes are considered sites of distant metastasis and should be coded as M1.

Metastatic Sites.   Distant spread is most commonly to lymph nodes, lung, bone, and liver.

RULES FOR CLASSIFICATION

Clinical Staging.   Primary tumor assessment includes bimanual examination under anesthesia before and after endoscopic surgery (biopsy or transurethral resection) and histologic verification of the presence or absence of tumor when indicated. Bimanual examination following endoscopic surgery is an indicator of clinical stage. The finding of bladder wall thickening, a mobile mass, or a fixed mass suggests the presence of T3a, T3b, and T4b disease, respectively. The suffix "m" is added to denote multiple tumors. The suffix "is" is added to any T to indicate associated carcinoma *in situ*. Appropriate imaging techniques for lymph node evaluation should be used. When indicated, evaluation for distant metastases includes imaging of the chest, biochemical studies, and isotopic studies to detect common metastatic sites. Computed tomography or other modalities may subsequently be used to supply information concerning minimal requirements for staging. Evidence suggests that MRI may be another useful modality for staging locally advanced bladder cancer. As yet, the role of positron emission tomography (PET) scanning in the staging and management of bladder cancer has not been defined. The primary tumor may be superficial or invasive and can be partially or totally resected with sufficient tissue from the tumor base for evaluation of full depth of tumor invasion. Visually adjacent cystoscopically normal mucosa should be considered for biopsy, and in most cases, multiple biopsies should be taken from other sites to rule out a field effect; urinary cytology and pyelography are important. It should be recalled that bladder cancer may occur in association with malignancies of the ureters, renal pelvis, or urethra. The definitions for Primary Tumor (T) are illustrated in Figure 38.1.

Pathologic Staging.   Microscopic examination and confirmation of extent are required. Total cystectomy and lymph node dissection generally are required for this staging. Laterality does not affect the N classification.

DEFINITION OF TNM

Primary Tumor (T)

TX	Primary tumor cannot be assessed
T0	No evidence of primary tumor
Ta	Non-invasive papillary carcinoma
Tis	Carcinoma *in situ:* "flat tumor"
T1	Tumor invades subepithelial connective tissue
T2	Tumor invades muscle
pT2a	Tumor invades superficial muscle (inner half)
pT2b	Tumor invades deep muscle (outer half)
T3	Tumor invades perivesical tissue
pT3a	microscopically
pT3b	macroscopically (extravesical mass)
T4	Tumor invades any of the following: prostate, uterus, vagina, pelvic wall, abdominal wall
T4a	Tumor invades prostate, uterus, vagina
T4b	Tumor invades pelvic wall, abdominal wall

Regional Lymph Nodes (N)

Regional lymph nodes are those within the true pelvis; all others are distant lymph nodes.

NX	Regional lymph nodes cannot be assessed
N0	No regional lymph node metastasis
N1	Metastasis in a single lymph node, 2 cm or less in greatest dimension
N2	Metastasis in a single lymph node, more than 2 cm but not more than 5 cm in greatest dimension; or multiple lymph nodes, none more than 5 cm in greatest dimension
N3	Metastasis in a lymph node, more than 5 cm in greatest dimension

Distant Metastasis (M)

MX	Distant metastasis cannot be assessed
M0	No distant metastasis
M1	Distant metastasis

9

STAGE GROUPING

Stage 0a	Ta	N0	M0
Stage 0is	Tis	N0	M0
Stage I	T1	N0	M0
Stage II	T2a	N0	M0
	T2b	N0	M0
Stage III	T3a	N0	M0
	T3b	N0	M0
	T4a	N0	M0
Stage IV	T4b	N0	M0
	Any T	N1	M0
	Any T	N2	M0
	Any T	N3	M0
	Any T	Any N	M1

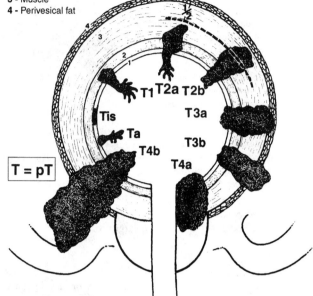

1 - Epithelium
2 - Subepithelial connective tissue
3 - Muscle
4 - Perivesical fat

T1 T2a T2b
T3a
Tis
Ta
T3b
T4b
T4a

T = pT

FIG. 38.1. Extent of primary bladder cancer.

HISTOPATHOLOGIC TYPE

The histologic types are:

Urothelial (transitional cell) carcinoma
   In situ
      Papillary
      Flat
      With squamous metaplasia
      With glandular metaplasia
      With squamous and glandular metaplasia
Squamous cell carcinoma
Adenocarcinoma
Undifferentiated carcinoma

The predominant cancer is urothelial (transitional cell) carcinoma.

HISTOLOGIC GRADE (G)

GX   Grade cannot be assessed
G1   Well differentiated
G2   Moderately differentiated
G3–4 Poorly differentiated or undifferentiated

PROGNOSTIC FACTORS

For primary tumors, the major established prognostic factors are grade and stage, although other factors identified in some series include hydronephrosis, anemia, size, expression of blood group substances, expression of epidermal growth factor receptor, and mutation of P53 and upregulation of Rb and other oncogene expression. For metastatic disease, adverse prognostic factors include poor performance status, visceral metastases, and abnormal liver function tests. The expression, up-regulation, or mutation of known oncogenes, such as P53, Rb, P21, and others, are under intense investigation in order to define which are the most important prognostic indices. To date, no consensus has been achieved, and conflicting data regarding the prognostic significance of P53 have been published. However, it does seem clear that two distinct molecular events are associated with the genesis of bladder cancer. Loss of heterozygosity of chromosome 9 is associated with the genesis of superficial bladder cancer, whereas loss of heterozygosity of chromosome 17, with mutation of the P53 suppressor gene, appears to be associated with the evolution of invasive disease and/or metastatic disease. Ploidy has been investigated as a prognostic factor. In superficial disease, an aneuploid DNA content is associated with shorter disease-free survival and with an increased chance of progression to a higher stage; however, in invasive and metastatic disease, the majority of cases are aneuploid, thus reducing the role of aneuploid DNA content as a discriminant of outcome.

BIBLIOGRAPHY

Barentsz JO, Jager GJ, Witjes JA, Ruijs JH: Primary staging of urinary bladder carcinoma: the role of MRI and a comparison with CT. Eur Radiol 6(2):129–133, 1996

Brown JL, Russell PJ, Philips J, Wotherspoon J, Raghavan, D: Clonal analysis of a bladder cancer cell line: an experimental model of tumour heterogeneity. Br J Cancer 61:369–376, 1990

Cote RJ, Esrig D, Groshen S, et al: p53 and treatment of bladder cancer. Nature 385:123–124, 1997

deVere White RW, Olsson CA, Deitch AD: Flow cytometry: role in monitoring transitional cell carcinoma of bladder. Urology 28:15–20, 1986

Esrig D, Elmajian D, Groshen S, et al: Accumulation of nuclear p53 and tumor progression in bladder cancer. N Engl J Med 331:1259–1264, 1994

Geller NL, Sternberg CN, Penenberg D, Scher H, Yagoda A: Prognostic factors for survival of patients with advanced urothelial tumors treated with methotrexate, vinblastine, doxorubicin, and cisplatin chemotherapy. Cancer 67:1525–1531, 1991

Greenlee RT, Hill-Harmon MB, Taylor M, Thun M: Cancer Statistics, 2001. CA Cancer J Clin 51:15–36, 2001

Herr HW: Staging invasive bladder tumors. J Surg Oncol 51:217–220, 1992

Herr HW, Lamm DL, Denis L: Management of superficial bladder cancer. In Raghavan D, Scher HI, Leibel SA, Lange PH (Eds.): Principles and practice of genitourinary oncology. Philadelphia: Lippincott-Raven, 273–280, 1997

Jewett HJ, Strong GH: Infiltrating carcinoma of the bladder: Relation of depth of penetration of the bladder wall to incidence of local extension and metastasis. J Urol 55:366–372, 1946

9

Johansson SL, Anderstrom CR: Primary adenocarcinoma of the urinary bladder and urachus. In Raghavan D, Brecher MI, Johnson DH, Meropol NJ, Moots PJ, Thigpen JT (Eds.): Textbook of uncommon cancer. Chichester, UK, NY: Wiley-Liss, 29–43, 1999

Koss LG: Tumors of the urinary bladder. In Atlas of tumor pathology, 2nd series, fascicle 11. Washington, DC: Armed Forces Institute of Pathology, 1975.

Loehrer PJ, Einhorn LH, Elson PJ, et al: A randomized comparison of cisplatin alone or in combination with methotrexate, vinblastine, and doxorubicin in patients with metastatic urothelial carcinoma: a cooperative group study. J Clin Oncol 10:1066–1073, 1992

Michaud DS, Spiegelman D, Clinton SK, et al: Fluid intake and the risk of bladder cancer in men. New Engl J Med 340:1390–1397, 1999

Neal DE, Marsh C, Bennett MK, et al: Epidermal-growth-factor receptors in human bladder cancer: comparison of invasive and superficial tumours. Lancet 1:366–368, 1985

Pagano F, Bassi P, Ferrante GL, et al: Is stage pT4 (D1) reliable in assessing transitional cell carcinoma involvement of the prostate in patients with a concurrent bladder cancer? A necessary distinction for contiguous or non-contiguous involvement. J Urology 155:244–247, 1996

Pagano F, Guazzieri S, Artibani W, et al: Prognosis of bladder cancer. III. The value of radical cystectomy in the management of invasive bladder cancer. Eur Urol 15:166–170, 1988

Raghavan D, Shipley WU, Garnick MB, et al: Biology and management of bladder cancer. N Engl J Med 322:1129–1133, 1990

Sarkis AS, Dalbagni G, Cordon-Cardo C, et al: Association of p53 nuclear overexpression and tumor progression in carcinoma *in situ* of the bladder. J Urol 152:388–392, 1994

Saxman SB, Propert K, Einhorn LH, et al: Long-term follow-up of phase III intergroup study of cisplatin alone or in combination with methotrexate, vinblastine, and doxorubicin in patients with metastatic urothelial carcinoma: a cooperative group study. J Clin Oncol 15:2564–2569, 1997

Shipley WU, Prout GR Jr, Kaufman DS, Peronne TL: Invasive bladder carcinoma: the importance of initial transurethral surgery and other significant prognostic factors for improved survival with full-dose irradiation. Cancer 60:514, 1987

Siemiatycki J, Dewar R, Nadon L, et al: Occupational risk factors for bladder cancer: results from a case-control study in Montréal, Québec, Canada. Am J Epidemiol 140:1061–1080, 1994

Spruck CH III, Ohneseit PF, Gonzalez-Zulueta M, et al: Two molecular pathways to transitional cell carcinoma of the bladder. Cancer Res 54:784–788, 1994

Stein JP, Ginsberg DA, Grossfeld GD, et al: Effect of p21[WAF1/CIP1] expression on tumor progression in bladder cancer. J Natl Cancer Inst 90:1072–1079, 1998

Stein JP, Lieskovsky G, Cote R, et al: Radical cystectomy in the treatment of high grade, invasive bladder cancer: long-term results in 1054 patients. J Clin Oncol 2001, 19(X):66

Sternberg CN, Swanson DA: Non-transitional cell bladder cancer. In Raghavan D, Scher HI, Leibel SA, Lange PH (Eds.): Principles and practice of genito-urinary oncology. Philadelphia: Lippincott-Raven, 315–330, 1997

Torti FM, Lum BL, Astron D, et al: Superficial bladder cancer: the primacy of grade in the development of invasive disease. J Clin Oncol 5:125, 1987

Wishnow KI, Levinson AK, Johnson DE: Stage B (P2/3aN0) transitional cell carcinoma of the bladder highly curable by radical cystectomy. Urology 39:12–16, 1992

HISTOLOGIES—BLADDER

8010/2	Carcinoma *in situ*, NOS
8010/3	Carcinoma, NOS
8020/3	Undifferentiated carcinoma, NOS
8051/3	Verrucous carcinoma, NOS
8070/2	Squamous cell carcinoma *in situ*, NOS
8070/3	Squamous cell carcinoma
8120/2	Transitional cell carcinoma *in situ*
8120/3	Transitional cell carcinoma, NOS
8130/2	Papillary transitional cell carcinoma, non-invasive
8130/3	Papillary transitional cell carcinoma
8131/3	Transitional cell carcinoma, micropapillary
8140/2	Adenocarcinoma *in situ*, NOS
8140/3	Adenocarcinoma, NOS
8255/3	Adenocarcinoma with mixed subtypes

9

C68.0 Urethra

SUMMARY OF CHANGES
- The definition of TNM and the Stage Grouping for this chapter have not changed from the Fifth Edition.

INTRODUCTION

Cancer of the urethra is a rare neoplasia that is found in both sexes but more common in females. The cancer may be associated in males with chronic stricture disease and in females with urethral diverticula. Tumors of the urethra may be of primary origin from the urethral epithelium or ducts, or they may be associated with multifocal urothelial neoplasia. Histologically, these tumors may represent the spectrum of epithelial neoplasms, including squamous, adenothelial, or urothelial (transitional cell) carcinoma. Prostatic urethral neoplasms arising from the prostatic urethral epithelium or from the periurethral portion of the prostatic ducts are considered urethral neoplasms as distinct from those arising elsewhere in the prostate (see Chapter 34).

ANATOMY

Primary Site. The male urethra consists of mucosa, submucosal stroma, and the surrounding corpus spongiosum. Histologically, the meatal and parameatal urethra are lined with squamous epithelium; the penile and bulbomembranous urethra with pseudostratified or stratified columnar epithelium, and the prostatic urethra with transitional epithelium. There are scattered islands of stratified squamous epithelium and glands of Littré liberally situated throughout the entire urethra distal to the prostate portion.

The epithelium of the female urethra is supported on subepithelial connective tissue. The periurethral glands of Skene are concentrated near the meatus but extend along the entire urethra. The urethra is surrounded by a longitudinal layer of smooth muscle continuous with the bladder. The urethra is contiguous to the vaginal wall. The distal two-thirds of the urethra is lined with squamous epithelium, the proximal one-third with transitional epithelium. The periurethral glands are lined with pseudostratified and stratified columnar epithelium.

Regional Lymph Nodes. The regional lymph nodes are:

Inguinal (superficial or deep)
Iliac (common, internal [hypogastric], obturator, external)

Presacral
Sacral, NOS
Pelvic, NOS

The significance of regional lymph node metastasis in staging urethral cancer lies in the number and size, not in whether unilateral or bilateral.

Metastatic Sites. Distant spread is most commonly to lung, liver, or bone.

RULES FOR CLASSIFICATION

Clinical Staging. Radiographic imaging, cystourethroscopy, palpation, and biopsy or cytology of the tumor prior to definitive treatment are desirable. The site of origin should be confirmed to exclude metastatic disease.

Pathologic Staging. The assignment of stage for non-prostatic urethral tumors is based on depth of invasion. Prostatic urethral tumor may arise from the prostatic epithelium or from the distal portions of the prostatic ducts and will be classified as prostatic urethral neoplasms. Other prostatic malignancies will be classified under prostate.

Figures 39.1 and 39.2 illustrate Primary Tumor (T) definitions for urethral malignancies and urothelial (transitional cell) carcinoma of the prostate.

DEFINITION OF TNM

Primary Tumor (T) (male and female)

TX   Primary tumor cannot be assessed
T0   No evidence of primary tumor
Ta   Non-invasive papillary, polypoid, or verrucous carcinoma
Tis   Carcinoma *in situ*
T1   Tumor invades subepithelial connective tissue
T2   Tumor invades any of the following: corpus spongiosum, prostate, periurethral muscle
T3   Tumor invades any of the following: corpus cavernosum, beyond prostatic capsule, anterior vagina, bladder neck
T4   Tumor invades other adjacent organs

Urothelial (Transitional Cell) Carcinoma of the Prostate

Tis   pu   Carcinoma *in situ*, involvement of the prostatic urethra
Tis   pd   Carcinoma *in situ*, involvement of the prostatic ducts
TI   Tumor invades subepithelial connective tissue
T2   Tumor invades any of the following: prostatic stroma, corpus spongiosum, periurethral muscle

T3	Tumor invades any of the following: corpus cavernosum, beyond prostatic capsule, bladder neck (extraprostatic extension)
T4	Tumor invades other adjacent organs (invasion of the bladder)

Regional Lymph Nodes (N)

NX	Regional lymph nodes cannot be assessed
N0	No regional lymph node metastasis
N1	Metastasis in a single lymph node 2 cm or less in greatest dimension
N2	Metastasis in a single node more than 2 cm in greatest dimension, or in multiple nodes

Distant Metastasis (M)

MX	Distant metastasis cannot be assessed
M0	No distant metastasis
M1	Distant metastasis

STAGE GROUPING

Stage 0a	Ta	N0	M0
Stage 0is	Tis	N0	M0
	Tis pu	N0	M0
	Tis pd	N0	M0
Stage I	T1	N0	M0
Stage II	T2	N0	M0
Stage III	T1	N1	M0
	T2	N1	M0
	T3	N0	M0
	T3	N1	M0
Stage IV	T4	N0	M0
	T4	N1	M0
	Any T	N2	M0
	Any T	Any N	M1

HISTOPATHOLOGIC TYPE

The classification applies to urothelial (transitional cell), squamous, and glandular carcinomas of the urethra and to urothelial (transitional cell) carcinomas of the prostate and prostatic urethra. There should be histologic or cytologic confirmation of the disease.

HISTOLOGIC GRADE (G)

GX	Grade cannot be assessed
G1	Well differentiated
G2	Moderately differentiated
G3–4	Poorly differentiated or undifferentiated

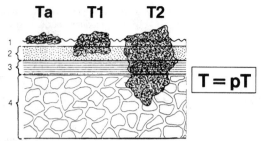

FIG. 39.1. Definition of Primary Tumor (T). 1–epithelium, 2–subepithelial connective tissue, 3–urethral muscle, 4–urogenital diaphragm.

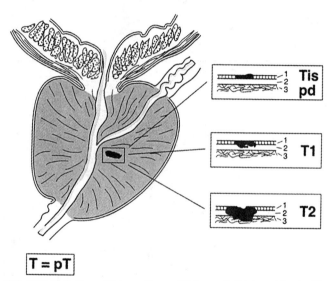

FIG. 39.2. Definition of Primary Tumor (T) for urothelial (transitional cell) carcinoma of the prostate. 1–Epithelium, 2–subepithelial connective tissue, 3–prostatic stroma.

BIBLIOGRAPHY

Amin MB, Young RH: Primary carcinomas of the urethra. Seminars in Diagnostic Pathology 14(2):147–60, 1997

Dalbagni G, Zhang ZF, Lacombe L, Herr HW: Female urethral carcinoma: an analysis of treatment outcome and a plea for a standardized management strategy. Br J Urol 82(6):835–841, 1998

Dalbagni G, Zhang ZF, Lacombe L, Herr HW: Male urethral carcinoma: analysis of treatment outcome. Urology 53(6):1126–1132, 1999

Davis JW, Schellhammer PF, Schlossberg SM: Conservative surgical therapy for penile and urethral carcinoma. Urology 53(2):386–392, 1999

Gheiler EL, Tefilli MV, Tiguert R, de Oliveira JG, Pontes JE, Wood DP Jr: Management of primary urethral cancer. Urology 52(3):487–493, 1998

Grigsby PW: Carcinoma of the urethra in women. International Journal of Radiation Oncology, Biology, Physics 41(3):535–541, 1998

Krieg R, Hoffman R: Current management of unusual genitourinary cancers. Part 2: Urethral cancer. Oncology 13(11):1511–1520, 1999

Levine RL: Urethral cancer. Cancer 45:1965–1972, 1980

Matzkin H, Soloway MS, Hardeman S: Transitional cell carcinoma of the prostate. J Urol 146:1207–1212, 1991

Micaily B, Dzeda MF, Miyamoto CT, Brady LW: Brachytherapy for cancer of the female urethra. Seminars in Surgical Oncology 13(3):208–214, 1997

Milosevic MF, Warde PR, Banerjee D, Gospodarowicz MK, McLean M, Catton PA, Catton CN: Urethral carcinoma in women: results of treatment with primary radiotherapy. Radiotherapy & Oncology 56(1):29–35, 2000

Rogers RE, Burns B: Carcinoma of the female urethra. Obstet Gynecol 33:54–57, 1969

Steele GS, Fielding JR, Renshaw A, Loughlin KR: Transitional cell carcinoma of the fossa navicularis. Urology 50(5):792–795 (review), 1997

Vernon HK, Wilkins RD: Primary carcinoma of the male urethra. Br J Urol 21:232–235, 1950

Wishnow KI, Ro JY: Importance of early treatment of transitional cell carcinoma of the bladder. J Urol 140:289, 1988

HISTOLOGIES—URETHRA

8010/2	Carcinoma *in situ*, NOS
8010/3	Carcinoma, NOS
8070/2	Squamous cell carcinoma, *in situ*
8070/3	Squamous cell carcinoma, NOS
8120/2	Transitional cell carcinoma *in situ*
8120/3	Transitional cell carcinoma, NOS
8130/2	Papillary transitional cell carcinoma, non-invasive
8130/3	Papillary transitional cell carcinoma
8140/3	Adenocarcinoma, NOS

9

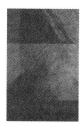

PART X
Ophthalmic Sites

10

40

Carcinoma of the Eyelid

C44.1 Eyelid

SUMMARY OF CHANGES
• A listing of site-specific categories is now included in T4.

INTRODUCTION

The tumors of the eyelid can be broadly categorized under epithelial tumors originating from the skin and conjunctival surfaces and glandular tumors originating from sebaceous, sweat, and apocrine glands as well as hair follicles. Lymphoproliferative and melanocytic malignancies and occasionally soft tissue sarcomas (Kaposi's sarcoma, fibrous histiocytoma, leiomyosarcoma, etc.) are also encountered.

ANATOMY

Primary Site.   The eyelid is covered externally by epidermis and internally by tarsal conjunctiva, which are continuous with the bulbar conjunctiva that covers the eyeball. Basal cell carcinoma and squamous cell carcinoma arise from the epidermal surface. Sebaceous carcinoma arises from the meibomian glands in the tarsus, the glands of Zeis at the lid margin, and the sebaceous glands of the caruncle. Other tumors arise from the skin appendages and mesenchymal tissues of the lid.

Regional Lymph Nodes.   The eyelids contain a network of lymphatics that can be divided primarily into pre- and post-tarsal plexuses, which are anastamosed. The lymphatics of the lateral two-thirds of the upper eyelid and the lateral one-third of the lower eyelid drain into the preauricular nodes. The remaining lymphatics of the eyelids drain into the submandibular lymph nodes.

If performed for pN, histologic examination of the regional lymphadenectomy specimen would ordinarily include one or more lymph nodes.

Local Invasion.   Malignancies of the eyelid may directly extend into the adjacent structures including the soft tissues of the orbit, the lacrimal gland, and the globe. Therefore, local tumor invasion (T4) should include extension to the bulbar conjunctiva, sclera and globe, soft tissues of the orbit, perineural space, bone/periosteum of the orbit, nasal cavity and paranasal sinuses, and central nervous system.

Metastatic Sites.   Eyelid malignancies metastasize to distant sites, including cervical, axillary, and mediastinal lymph nodes, as well as to lungs, liver, and other viscera.

10

RULES FOR CLASSIFICATION

There should be histopathologic identification of the neoplasm to permit classification of the tumor into a given histopathologic type, such as basal cell carcinoma, sebaceous carcinoma, or Merkel cell tumor. In addition to criteria used for identification of the tumor, other histopathologic prognostic criteria, including the type and differentiation of the tumor, tumor presence or absence at surgical margins, perineural invasion, and vascular invasion, should be noted.

Any histopathologically unverified case should be categorized separately. Any unspecified case (malignant sarcoma, type unspecified) must be categorized separately.

Clinical Staging.   The assessment of the malignancy should be based on inspection, palpation, biomicroscopic examination, ultrasonic biomicroscopy, and, when indicated, radiologic (ultrasonography, computed tomography, magnetic resonance imaging) examination of the orbit, nasal cavity and paranasal sinuses, and central nervous system.

Pathologic Staging.   The nature of the histopathologic specimen (fine-needle aspiration biopsy, excisional biopsy, lumpectomy, or total excision) should be noted. In total excision specimens, histopathologic study of the surgical margins is mandatory. If the specimen includes the globe, then conjunctival margins and the resection margin of the optic nerve need to be examined.

DEFINITION OF TNM

The following definitions apply to clinical and pathologic staging.

Primary Tumor (T)

TX   Primary tumor cannot be assessed
T0   No evidence of primary tumor
Tis   Carcinoma *in situ*
T1   Tumor of any size, not invading the tarsal plate or, at the eyelid margin, 5 mm or less in greatest dimension
T2   Tumor invades tarsal plate or, at the eyelid margin, more than 5 mm but not more than 10 mm in greatest dimension
T3   Tumor involves full eyelid thickness or, at the eyelid margin, more than 10 mm in greatest dimension
T4   Tumor invades adjacent structures, which include bulbar conjunctiva, sclera and globe, soft tissues of the orbit, perineural space, bone and periosteum of the orbit, nasal cavity and paranasal sinuses, and central nervous system

Regional Lymph Nodes (N)

NX   Regional lymph nodes cannot be assessed
N0   No regional lymph node metastasis
N1   Regional lymph node metastasis

Distant Metastasis (M)

MX   Distant metastasis cannot be assessed
M0   No distant metastasis
M1   Distant metastasis

STAGE GROUPING

No stage grouping is presently recommended.

HISTOPATHOLOGIC TYPE

Basal cell carcinoma
Squamous cell carcinoma
Sebaceous carcinoma
Merkel cell tumor
Skin appendage carcinoma
Sarcoma

HISTOLOGIC GRADE (G)

GX   Grade cannot be assessed
G1   Well differentiated
G2   Moderately differentiated
G3   Poorly differentiated
G4   Undifferentiated or differentiation is not applicable

BIBLIOGRAPHY

Doxanas MT, Iliff WJ, Iliff NT, et al: Squamous cell carcinoma of the eyelids. Ophthalmology 94:538–541, 1987

Farmer ER, Helwig EB: Metastatic basal cell carcinoma: A clinicopathologic study of seventeen cases. Cancer 46:748–757, 1980

Grossniklaus HE, McLean IW: Cutaneous melanoma of the eyelid. Clinicopathologic features. Ophthalmology 98:1867–1873, 1991

Rao NA, Hidayat AA, McLean IW, et al: Sebaceous carcinomas of the ocular adnexa: A clinicopathologic study of 104 cases, with five-year follow-up data. Hum Pathol 13:113–122, 1982

Reifler DM, Hornblass A: Squamous cell carcinoma of the eyelid. Surv Ophthalmol 30:349–365, 1986

Shields CL: Basal cell carcinoma of the eyelids. Int Ophthalmol Clin 33:1–4, 1993

HISTOLOGIES—CARCINOMA OF THE EYELID

8010/2   Carcinoma *in situ*, NOS
8010/3   Carcinoma, NOS
8013/3   Large cell neuroendocrine carcinoma
8015/3   Glassy cell carcinoma
8020/3   Carcinoma, undifferentiated, NOS
8021/3   Carcinoma, anaplastic, NOS
8032/3   Spindle cell carcinoma, NOS

8033/3	Pseudosarcomatous carcinoma
8070/2	Squamous cell carcinoma *in situ*, NOS
8070/3	Squamous cell carcinoma, NOS
8071/3	Squamous cell carcinoma, keratinizing, NOS
8074/3	Squamous cell carcinoma, spindle cell
8076/2	Squamous cell carcinoma *in situ* with questionable stromal invasion
8076/3	Squamous cell carcinoma, microinvasive
8077/2	Squamous intraepithelial neoplasia, grade III
8081/2	Bowen disease
8082/3	Lymphoepithelial carcinoma
8083/3	Basaloid squamous cell carcinoma
8084/3	Squamous cell carcinoma, clear cell type
8090/3	Basal cell carcinoma
8091/3	Multifocal superficial basal cell carcinoma
8094/3	Basosquamous carcinoma
8095/3	Metatypical carcinoma
8098/3	Adenoid basal carcinoma
8102/3	Trichilemmocarcinoma
8110/3	Pilomatrix carcinoma
8120/3	Transitional cell carcinoma, NOS
8121/3	Schneiderian carcinoma
8140/2	Adenocarcinoma *in situ*, NOS
8140/3	Adenocarcinoma, NOS
8141/3	Scirrhous adenocarcinoma
8147/3	Basal cell adenocarcinoma
8190/3	Trabecular adenocarcinoma
8200/3	Adenoid cystic carcinoma
8240/3	Carcinoid tumor, NOS
8241/3	Enterochromaffin cell carcinoid
8242/3	Enterochromaffin-like cell tumor, malignant
8246/3	Neuroendocrine carcinoma, NOS
8247/3	Merkel cell carcinoma
8249/3	Atypical carcinoid tumor
8260/3	Papillary adenocarcinoma, NOS
8390/3	Skin appendage carcinoma
8400/3	Sweat gland adenocarcinoma
8401/3	Apocrine adenocarcinoma
8402/3	Nodular hidradenoma, malignant
8403/3	Malignant eccrine spiradenoma
8407/3	Sclerosing sweat duct carcinoma
8408/3	Eccrine papillary adenocarcinoma
8409/3	Eccrine poroma, malignant
8410/3	Sebaceous adenocarcinoma
8413/3	Eccrine adenocarcinoma
8430/3	Mucoepidermoid carcinoma
8480/3	Mucinous adenocarcinoma
8550/3	Acinar cell carcinoma
8560/3	Adenosquamous carcinoma
8562/3	Epithelial-myoepithelial carcinoma
8570/3	Adenocarcinoma with squamous metaplasia
8940/3	Mixed tumor, malignant, NOS
8941/3	Carcinoma in pleomorphic adenoma

41

Carcinoma of the Conjunctiva

C69.0 Conjunctiva

ANATOMY

Primary Site.   The conjunctiva consists of stratified epithelium that contains mucus-secreting goblet cells; these cells are most numerous in the fornices. Palpebral conjunctiva lines the eyelid; bulbar conjunctiva covers the eyeball. Conjunctival epithelium merges with that of the cornea at the limbus. It is at this exposed site, particularly at the temporal limbus, that carcinoma is most likely to arise. Conjunctival intraepithelial neoplasia (C.I.N.) embraces all forms of intraepithelial dysplasia, including *in situ* squamous cell carcinoma.

Regional Lymph Nodes.   The regional lymph nodes are:

> Preauricular (parotid)
> Submandibular
> Cervical

For pN, histologic examination of a regional lymphadenectomy specimen, if performed, will include one or more regional lymph nodes.

Metastatic Sites.   Tumors of the conjunctiva, in addition to spreading by way of regional lymphatics, may also involve the eyelid proper, the eye, orbit, adjacent paranasal sinus structures, and the brain.

RULES FOR CLASSIFICATION

10

Clinical Staging.   The assessment of cancer is based on inspection, slit-lamp examination, palpation of the regional lymph nodes, and, when indicated, radiologic examination (including computed tomography and magnetic resonance imaging) and ultrasonographic examination of the orbit, paranasal sinuses, brain, and chest.

Pathologic Staging.   Complete resection of the primary site is indicated if possible. Cryotherapy and/or topical chemotherapy may be considered as adjunctive therapies. Extensive tumor involvement of orbital soft tissues requires exenteration. The specimen should be thoroughly sampled for histologic study of surgical margins, type of tumor, and grade of malignancy.

DEFINITION OF TNM

These definitions apply to both clinical and pathologic staging.

Primary Tumor (T)

TX	Primary tumor cannot be assessed
T0	No evidence of primary tumor
Tis	Carcinoma *in situ*
T1	Tumor 5 mm or less in greatest dimension
T2	Tumor more than 5 mm in greatest dimension, without invasion of adjacent structures
T3	Tumor invades adjacent structures, excluding the orbit
T4	Tumor invades the orbit with or without further extension
T4a	Tumor invades orbital soft tissues, without bone invasion
T4b	Tumor invades bone
T4c	Tumor invades adjacent paranasal sinuses
T4d	Tumor invades brain

Regional Lymph Nodes (N)

NX	Regional lymph nodes cannot be assessed
N0	No regional lymph node metastasis
N1	Regional lymph node metastasis

Distant Metastasis (M)

MX	Distant metastasis cannot be assessed
M0	No distant metastasis
M1	Distant metastasis

STAGE GROUPING

No stage grouping is presently recommended.

HISTOPATHOLOGIC TYPE

This classification applies only to carcinoma of the conjunctiva.

Conjunctival intraepithelial neoplasia (C.I.N.) including *in situ* squamous cell carcinoma.
Squamous cell carcinoma
Mucoepidermoid carcinoma
Basal cell carcinoma

HISTOLOGIC GRADE (G)

GX	Grade cannot be assessed
G1	Well differentiated
G2	Moderately differentiated
G3	Poorly differentiated
G4	Undifferentiated

BIBLIOGRAPHY

Brownstein S: Mucoepidermoid carcinoma of the conjunctiva with intraocular invasion. Ophthalmology 88:1226–1230, 1981

Buus DR, Tse DT, Folberg R: Microscopically controlled excision of conjunctival squamous cell carcinoma. Am J Ophthalmol 117:97–102, 1994

Campbell RJ: Tumors of eyelid, conjunctiva and cornea. In: Garner A, Klintworth GK (Eds). Pathobiology of ocular disease: A dynamic approach, 2nd ed, Part A, New York: Marcel Dekker, 1367–1403, 1994

Cohen BH, Green WR, Iliff NT, et al: Spindle cell carcinoma of the conjunctiva. Arch Ophthalmol 98:1809–1813, 1980

Lee GA, Hirst LW: Ocular surface squamous neoplasia. Surv Ophthalmol 39:429–450, 1995

Grossniklaus HE, Green WR, Luckenbach M, Chan CC: Conjunctival lesions in adults. A clinical and histopathologic review. Cornea 6:78–116, 1987

Grossniklaus HE, Martin DF, Solomon AR: Invasive conjunctival tumor with keratoacanthoma features. Am J Ophthalmol 109:736–738, 1990

Husain SE, Patrinely JR, Zimmerman LE, et al: Primary basal cell carcinoma of the limbal conjunctiva. Ophthalmology 100:1720–1722, 1993

Jakobiec FA, Folberg R, Iwamoto T: Clinicopathologic characteristics of premalignant and malignant melanocytic lesions of the conjunctiva. Ophthalmology 96:147–166, 1989

Johnson TE, Tabbara KF, Weatherhead RG, et al: Secondary squamous cell carcinoma of the orbit. Arch Ophthalmol 115:75–78, 1997

McLean IW, Burnier MN, Zimmerman LE, et al: Tumors of the conjunctiva In: Rosai J, Ed. Atlas of Tumor Pathology: Tumors of the Eye and Ocular Adnexa, Third series, fascicle 12, Washington DC: Armed Forces Institute of Pathology, 49–95, 1994

Rao NA, Font RL: Mucoepidermoid carcinoma of the conjunctiva: a clinicopathologic study of five cases. Cancer 38:1699–1709, 1976.

HISTOLOGIES—CARCINOMA OF THE CONJUNCTIVA

8010/2	Carcinoma *in situ*, NOS
8010/3	Carcinoma, NOS
8013/3	Large cell neuroendocrine carcinoma
8015/3	Glassy cell carcinoma
8020/3	Carcinoma, undifferentiated, NOS
8021/3	Carcinoma, anaplastic, NOS
8032/3	Spindle cell carcinoma, NOS
8033/3	Pseudosarcomatous carcinoma
8070/2	Squamous cell carcinoma *in situ*, NOS
8070/3	Squamous cell carcinoma, NOS
8071/3	Squamous cell carcinoma, keratinizing, NOS
8074/3	Squamous cell carcinoma, spindle cell
8076/2	Squamous cell carcinoma *in situ* with questionable stromal invasion
8076/3	Squamous cell carcinoma, microinvasive
8077/2	Squamous intraepithelial neoplasia, grade III
8081/2	Bowen disease
8082/3	Lymphoepithelial carcinoma
8083/3	Basaloid squamous cell carcinoma
8084/3	Squamous cell carcinoma, clear cell type
8090/3	Basal cell carcinoma
8091/3	Multifocal superficial basal cell carcinoma
8094/3	Basosquamous carcinoma
8095/3	Metatypical carcinoma

10

8098/3	Adenoid basal carcinoma
8120/3	Transitional cell carcinoma, NOS
8121/3	Schneiderian carcinoma
8140/2	Adenocarcinoma *in situ*, NOS
8140/3	Adenocarcinoma, NOS
8141/3	Scirrhous adenocarcinoma
8246/3	Neuroendocrine carcinoma, NOS
8247/3	Merkel cell carcinoma
8249/3	Atypical carcinoid tumor
8260/3	Papillary adenocarcinoma, NOS
8390/3	Skin appendage carcinoma
8400/3	Sweat gland adenocarcinoma
8401/3	Apocrine adenocarcinoma
8402/3	Nodular hidradenoma, malignant
8403/3	Malignant eccrine spiradenoma
8407/3	Sclerosing sweat duct carcinoma
8408/3	Eccrine papillary adenocarcinoma
8409/3	Eccrine poroma, malignant
8430/3	Mucoepidermoid carcinoma
8480/3	Mucinous adenocarcinoma
8550/3	Acinar cell carcinoma
8560/3	Adenosquamous carcinoma
8562/3	Epithelial-myoepithelial carcinoma
8570/3	Adenocarcinoma with squamous metaplasia
8940/3	Mixed tumor, malignant, NOS
8941/3	Carcinoma in pleomorphic adenoma

42

Malignant Melanoma of the Conjunctiva

C69.0 Conjunctiva

ANATOMY

Primary Site. Melanocytes have been noted to exist in the basal layer of the conjunctival epithelium. These melanocytes can be the source of acquired melanosis, malignant melanoma, and junctional and compound nevi. Melanocytic conjunctival tumors range from melanocytic hypertrophy and melanoma *in situ* to invasive malignant melanoma. Local clinically relevant classifications divide these tumors by conjunctival location, uni- or multifocality, and tumor thickness. Factors that influence both treatment and prognosis include local invasion, nodal spread, and distant metastasis.

Regional Lymph Nodes. The regional lymph nodes are:

Preauricular (parotid)
Submandibular
Cervical

For pN, histologic examination of a regional lymphadenectomy specimen will ordinarily include one or more regional lymph nodes.

Metastatic Sites. In addition to spread by lymphatics and the bloodstream, direct extension into the orbit, eyelids, and sinuses occurs.

RULES FOR CLASSIFICATION

The classification applies only to conjunctival melanoma. In general, there should be a histologic evaluation of the tumor.

Clinical Staging. The clinical assessment of a melanocytic conjunctival tumor is based on inspection, slit-lamp examination, and palpation of the regional lymph nodes. All conjunctival surfaces should be inspected (including eversion of the upper lid). Inspection of the ipsilateral sinuses is indicated if punctal involvement has been noted.

Radiologic evaluations to stage local disease may include computed tomography, magnetic resonance imaging, and/or ultrasonography of the orbits and sinuses. Complete metastatic surveys may include hematology screening as well as radiologic evaluations of the head, chest, and abdomen. Bone scans may be employed.

Pathologic Staging.   Complete resection of the primary site is indicated. Cryotherapy, chemotherapy, and radiation therapy have been employed when complete resection is not possible or have been employed as an adjunctive treatment. Histopathologic evaluations for negative peripheral and deep margins should be performed. To best judge the depth of penetration of the tumor, sections should be made perpendicular to the epithelial surface. Perpendicular sections can be facilitated if the surgeon places the specimen epithelial side superior on a moist filter paper. The role of sentinel node biopsy is unknown.

DEFINITION OF TNM

Clinical

Primary Tumor (T)

TX	Primary tumor cannot be assessed
T0	No evidence of primary tumor
T1	Tumor of the bulbar conjunctiva
T2	Tumor of the bulbar conjunctiva with corneal extension
T3	Tumor extending into the conjunctival fornix, palpebral conjunctiva, or caruncle
T4	Tumor invades the eyelid, globe, orbit, sinuses, or central nervous system

Regional Lymph Nodes (N)

NX	Regional lymph nodes cannot be assessed
N0	No regional lymph node metastasis
N1	Regional lymph node metastasis

Distant Metastasis (M)

MX	Distant metastasis cannot be assessed
M0	No distant metastasis
M1	Distant metastasis

Pathologic

Primary Tumor (pT)

pTX	Primary tumor cannot be assessed
pT0	No evidence of primary tumor
pT1	Tumor of the bulbar conjunctiva confined to the epithelium
pT2	Tumor of the bulbar conjunctiva not more than 0.8 mm in thickness with invasion of the substantia propria
pT3	Tumor of the bulbar conjunctiva more than 0.8 mm in thickness with invasion of the substantia propria or tumors involving the palpebral or caruncular conjunctiva
pT4	Tumor invades the eyelid, globe, orbit, sinuses, or central nervous system

Regional Lymph Nodes (pN)

pNX   Regional lymph nodes cannot be assessed
pN0   No regional lymph node metastasis
pN1   Regional lymph node metastasis present

Distant Metastasis (pM)

pMX   Distant metastasis cannot be assessed
pM0   No distant metastasis
pM1   Distant metastasis

STAGE GROUPING

No stage grouping is presently recommended.

HISTOPATHOLOGIC TYPE

This categorization applies only to melanoma of the conjunctiva.

HISTOLOGIC GRADE (G)

Histologic grade represents the origin of the primary tumor.

GX   Origin cannot be assessed
G0   Primary acquired melanosis without cellular atypia
G1   Conjunctival nevus
G2   Primary acquired melanosis with cellular atypia (epithelial disease only)
G3   *De novo* malignant melanoma

BIBLIOGRAPHY

Folberg R, McLean IW, Zimmerman LE: Primary acquired melanosis of the conjunctiva. Hum Pathol 16:129–135, 1985

Finger PT, Czechonska G, Liarikos S: Topical mitomycin C chemotherapy for conjunctival melanoma and PAM with atypia. Br J Ophthalmol 82:476–479, 1998

Paridaens AD, Minassian DC, McCartney AC, et al: Prognostic factors in primary malignant melanoma of the conjunctiva: a clinicopathologic study of 256 cases. Br J Ophthalmol 78:252–259, 1994

Seregard S: Conjunctival melanoma. Surv Ophthalmol 42:321–350, 1998

HISTOLOGIES—MALIGNANT MELANOMA OF THE CONJUNCTIVA

8720/2   Melanoma *in situ*
8720/3   Malignant melanoma, NOS
8723/3   Malignant melanoma, regressing
8730/3   Amelanotic melanoma
8740/3   Malignant melanoma in junctional nevus
8741/2   Precancerous melanosis, NOS

HISTOLOGIES—MALIGNANT MELANOMA OF THE CONJUNCTIVA (CONT.)

8741/3	Malignant melanoma in precancerous melanosis
8742/2	Lentigo maligna
8742/3	Lentigo maligna melanoma
8743/3	Superficial spreading melanoma
8744/3	Acral lentiginous melanoma, malignant
8745/3	Desmoplastic melanoma, malignant
8761/3	Malignant melanoma in giant pigmented nevus
8770/3	Mixed epithelioid and spindle cell melanoma
8771/3	Epithelioid cell melanoma
8772/3	Spindle cell melanoma

Malignant Melanoma of the Uvea

C69.3 Choroid   C69.4 Ciliary body and iris

SUMMARY OF CHANGES

Iris

- T1 lesions have been divided into T1a, T1b, and T1c.

- T1a is defined as tumor limited to the iris not more than 3 clock hours in size.

- T1b is defined as tumor limited to the iris more than 3 clock hours in size.

- T1c is defined as tumor limited to the iris with melanomalytic glaucoma.

- The definition of T2 lesions has been modified, and T2 has been divided by the addition T2a.

- T2 is defined as tumor confluent with or extending into the ciliary body and/or choroid.

- T2a is defined as tumor confluent with or extending into the ciliary body and/or choroid with melanomalytic glaucoma.

- The definition of T3 lesions has been modified, and T3 has been divided by the addition T3a.

- T3 is defined as tumor confluent with or extending into the ciliary body and/or choroid with extrascleral extension.

- T3a is defined as tumor confluent with or extending into the ciliary body with extrascleral extension and melanomalytic glaucoma.

Ciliary Body and Choroid

- The definition of T1 lesions has been modified, and T1 has been divided into T1a, T1b, and T1c.

- T1 is defined as tumor 10 mm or less in greatest diameter and 2.5 mm or less in greatest height (thickness).

- T1a is defined as tumor 10 mm or less in greatest diameter and 2.5 mm or less in greatest height (thickness) without extraocular extension.

- T1b is defined as tumor 10 mm or less in greatest diameter and 2.5 mm or less in greatest height (thickness) with microscopic extraocular extension.

- T1c is defined as tumor 10 mm or less in greatest diameter and 2.5 mm or less in greatest height (thickness) with macroscopic extraocular extension.

- The definition of T2 lesions has been modified, and T2 has been divided into T2a, T2b, and T2c.

- T2 is defined as tumor 10 mm to 16 mm in greatest basal diameter and between 2.5 and 10 mm in maximum height.

continued

10

ANATOMY

Primary Site.   The uvea (uveal tract) is the middle layer of the eye, situated between the cornea and sclera externally and the retina and its analogous tissues internally. The uveal tract is divided into three regions—iris, ciliary body, and choroid—and it is a highly vascular structure. The choroid primarily comprises blood vessels with little intervening stroma. Uveal melanomas are believed to arise from uveal melanocytes and are therefore of neural crest origin. Because there are no lymphatic channels within the eye, uveal melanomas are thought to metastasize exclusively hematogenously to visceral organs. In the rare event that uveal melanoma metastasizes to lymph nodes, it is typically after extraocular spread and invasion of conjunctival, adnexal, and/or orbital lymphatics.

Uveal melanomas arise most commonly in the choroid, less in the ciliary body, and least in the iris. Choroidal melanomas extend commonly through Bruch's membrane into the retina and vitreous, less commonly through the sclera into the orbit, and rarely into the optic nerve.

Intraocular location of a uveal melanoma can also affect a patient's prognosis for metastasis. Tumors confined to the iris carry the most favorable prognosis, followed by those in the choroids; ciliary involvement carries the least favorable prognosis. Tumor size (primarily largest tumor diameter) continues to be the dominant predictor for metastasis. It is currently impossible to distinguish clinically between a large nevus and a small uveal melanoma. Clinical findings of orange pigment, subretinal fluid, and thickness greater than 2 mm are more commonly associated with uveal melanomas than with nevi.

Pigmented iris tumors that demonstrate intrinsic vascularity, size greater than 3 clock hours and thickness greater than 1 mm, sector cataract, pigment dispersion (melanocytes and melanin granules or melanocytic tumor cells), secondary glaucoma, and extrascleral extension are more likely to be malignant melanomas than benign melanocytic proliferations. In general, small uveal melanocytic lesions are observed for growth prior to being clinically defined as uveal melanomas.

Regional Lymph Nodes.   This category applies only to extrascleral extension and conjunctival invasion. Regional lymphadenectomy will ordinarily include six or more regional lymph nodes. The regional lymph nodes are:

Preauricular
Submandibular
Cervical

Metastatic Sites. Uveal melanomas may metastasize hematogenously to various visceral organs. The liver is the most common site, and often the only site, of clinically detectable metastasis. Less common sites include the lung, pleura, subcutaneous tissues, bone, and brain.

RULES FOR CLASSIFICATION

Clinical Staging. The assessment of the tumor is based on clinical examination, including slit-lamp examination and direct and indirect ophthalmoscopy. Additional methods, such as ultrasonography, computerized stereometry, fluorescein angiography, and isotope examination, may enhance the accuracy of appraisal.

Pathologic Staging. Resection of the primary site by iridectomy, iridocyclectomy, eye wall resection, or enucleation is needed for complete pathologic staging. Assessment of the extent of the tumor, measured in clock hours of involvement, basal dimension, and height and margins of resection, is necessary. Resection or needle biopsy of enlarged regional lymph nodes or orbital masses is desirable.

DEFINITION OF TNM

These definitions apply to both clinical* and pathologic staging.

Primary Tumor

All Uveal Melanomas
TX   Primary tumor cannot be assessed
T0   No evidence of primary tumor

Iris
T1   Tumor limited to the iris
T1a   Tumor limited to the iris not more than 3 clock hours in size
T1b   Tumor limited to the iris more than 3 clock hours in size
T1c   Tumor limited to the iris with melanomalytic glaucoma
T2   Tumor confluent with or extending into the ciliary body and/or choroid
T2a   Tumor confluent with or extending into the ciliary body and/or choroid with melanomalytic glaucoma
T3   Tumor confluent with or extending into the ciliary body and/or choroid with scleral extension

10

T3a   Tumor confluent with or extending into the ciliary body with scleral extension and melanomalytic glaucoma

T4   Tumor with extraocular extension

Ciliary Body and Choroid

T1*   Tumor 10 mm or less in greatest diameter and 2.5 mm or less in greatest height (thickness)

T1a   Tumor 10 mm or less in greatest diameter and 2.5 mm or less in greatest height (thickness) without microscopic extraocular extension

T1b   Tumor 10 mm or less in greatest diameter and 2.5 mm or less in greatest height (thickness) with microscopic extraocular extension

T1c   Tumor 10 mm or less in greatest diameter and 2.5 mm or less in greatest height (thickness) with macroscopic extraocular extension

T2*   Tumor greater than 10 mm but not more than 16 mm in greatest basal diameter and between 2.5 and 10 mm in maximum height (thickness)

T2a   Tumor 10 mm to 16 mm in greatest basal diameter and between 2.5 and 10 mm in maximum height (thickness) without microscopic extraocular extension

T2b   Tumor 10 mm to 16 mm in greatest basal diameter and between 2.5 and 10 mm in maximum height (thickness) with microscopic extraocular extension

T2c   Tumor 10 mm to 16 mm in greatest basal diameter and between 2.5 and 10 mm in maximum height (thickness) with macroscopic extraocular extension

T3*   Tumor more than 16 mm in greatest diameter and/or greater than 10 mm in maximum height (thickness) without extraocular extension

T4   Tumor more than 16 mm in greatest diameter and/or greater than 10 mm in maximum height (thickness) with extraocular extension

Note: When basal dimension and apical height do not fit this classification, the largest tumor diameter should be used for classification. In clinical practice, the tumor base may be estimated in optic disc diameters (dd) (average: 1 dd = 1.5 mm). The height may be estimated in diopters (average: 3 diopters = 1 mm). Techniques such as ultrasonography, visualization, and photography are frequently used to provide more accurate measurements.

Regional Lymph Nodes (N)

NX   Regional lymph nodes cannot be assessed

N0   No regional lymph node metastasis

N1   Regional lymph node metastasis

Distant Metastasis (M)

MX   Distant metastasis cannot be assessed

M0   No distant metastasis

M1   Distant metastasis

STAGE GROUPING			
Stage I	T1	N0	M0
	T1a	N0	M0
	T1b	N0	M0
	T1c	N0	M0
Stage II	T2	N0	M0
	T2a	N0	M0
	T2b	N0	M0
	T2c	N0	M0
Stage III	T3	N0	M0
	T4	N0	M0
Stage IV	Any T	N1	M0
	Any T	Any N	M1

HISTOPATHOLOGIC TYPE

The histopathologic types are

Spindle cell melanoma
Mixed cell melanoma
Epithelioid cell melanoma

HISTOLOGIC GRADE (G)

GX   Grade cannot be assessed
G1   Spindle cell melanoma
G2   Mixed cell melanoma
G3   Epithelioid cell melanoma

BIBLIOGRAPHY

Factors predictive of growth and treatment of small choroidal melanoma: COMS Report No. 5. the Collaborative Ocular Melanoma Study Group. Arch Ophthalmol 115:1537–1544, 1997

Finger PT. Radiation therapy for choroidal melanoma. Surv Ophthalmol 42:215–232, 1997

Histopathologic characteristics of uveal melanomas in eyes enucleated from the Collaborative Ocular Melanoma Study. COMS Report No. 6. The Collaborative Ocular Melanoma Study Group. Am J Ophthalmol 125:745–766,1998

Markowitz JA, Hawkins BS, Diener-West M, et al: A review of mortality from choroidal melanoma. I. Quality of published reports, 1966 through 1988. Arch Ophthalmol 110:239–244. 1992

McLean IW. Uveal nevi and melanomas. In Spencer WH (Ed.): Ophthalmic pathology: an atlas and textbook. Philadelphia: Saunders, 2121–2217, 1996

McLean IW, Burnier MN, Zimmerman LE, et al: Tumors of the Ureal Tract. In: Rosai J. ed. Atlas of Tumor Pathology: Tumors of the Eye and Ocular adnexa, Third Series, Fascicle 12, Washington, DC: Armed Forces Institute of Pathology, 155–214, 1994

Moshfeghi DM, Moshfeghi AA, Finger PT: Enucleation. Surv Ophthalmol, 44:277–301, 2000

10

Packard RB: Pattern of mortality in choroidal malignant melanoma. Br J Ophthalmol 64:565–575, 1980

Seddon JM, Albert DM, Lavin PT, et al: A prognostic factor study of disease-free interval and survival following enucleation for uveal melanoma. Arch Ophthalmol 101:1894–1899, 1983

Shields CL, Shields JA, Shields MB, et al: Prevalence and mechanisms of secondary intraocular pressure elevation in eyes with intraocular tumors. Ophthalmology 94:839–846, 1987

HISTOLOGIES—MALIGNANT MELANOMA OF THE UVEA

8720/2	Melanoma *in situ*
8720/3	Malignant melanoma, NOS
8723/3	Malignant melanoma, regressing
8730/3	Amelanotic melanoma
8740/3	Malignant melanoma in junctional nevus
8741/2	Precancerous melanosis, NOS
8741/3	Malignant melanoma in precancerous melanosis
8742/2	Lentigo maligna
8742/3	Lentigo maligna melanoma
8743/3	Superficial spreading melanoma
8744/3	Acral lentiginous melanoma, malignant
8745/3	Desmoplastic melanoma, malignant
8761/3	Malignant melanoma in giant pigmented nevus
8770/3	Mixed epithelioid and spindle cell melanoma
8771/3	Epithelioid cell melanoma
8772/3	Spindle cell melanoma

Retinoblastoma

C69.2 Retina

ANATOMY

Primary Site.   The retina is composed of neurons and glial cells. The precursors of the neuronal elements give rise to retinoblastoma, whereas the glial cells give rise to astrocytomas, which are benign and extremely rare in the retina. The retina is limited internally by a membrane that separates it from the vitreous cavity. Externally, it is limited by the retinal pigment epithelium and Bruch's membrane, which separate it from the choroid and act as natural barriers to extension of retinal tumors into the choroid. The continuation of the retina with the optic nerve allows direct extension of retinoblastomas into the optic nerve and then to the subarachnoid space. Because the retina has no lymphatics, spread of retinal tumors is either by direct extension into adjacent structures or by distant metastasis through hematogenous routes.

Regional Lymph Nodes.   Because there are no intraocular lymphatics, this category of staging applies only to anterior extrascleral extension. The regional lymph nodes are preauricular (parotid), submandibular, and cervical.

Local Extension.   Local extension anteriorly can result in soft tissue involvement of the face or a mass protruding from between the lids. Posterior extension results in retinoblastoma extending into the orbit, paranasal sinuses, and/or brain.

Metastatic Sites.   Retinoblastoma can metastasize through hematogenous routes to various sites, most notably the bone marrow, skull, long bones, and brain.

RULES FOR CLASSIFICATION

Clinical Staging. All suspected cases of retinoblastoma should have a neural imaging scan. If it is possible to obtain only one imaging study, computerized tomography (CT) is recommended because detection of calcium in the eye on CT confirms the clinical suspicion of retinoblastoma. The request should include cuts through the pineal region of the brain. Magnetic resonance imaging is particularly useful if extension into either the extraocular space or the optic nerve is suspected or if there is a concern about the possible presence of a primitive neuroectodermal tumor (PNET) in the pineal region (trilateral retinoblastoma).

A staging examination under anesthesia should include ocular ultrasound and retinal drawings of each eye, with each identifiable tumor measured and numbered. Digital images of the retina may be very helpful. In bilateral cases, each eye must be classified separately. This classification does not apply to complete spontaneous regression of the tumor. Tumor size or the distance from the tumor to the disc or fovea is recorded in millimeters. These millimeter distances are measured by ultrasound, estimated by comparison with a normalized optic disc (1.5 mm), or deduced from the fact that the field of a 28-diopter condensing lens has a retinal diameter of 13 mm.

Pathologic Staging. If one eye is enucleated, pathologic staging of that eye provides information supplemental to the clinical staging. First, the pathology should provide histologic verification of the disease. All clinical and pathologic data from the resected specimen are to be used.

DEFINITION OF TNM

Clinical Classification (cTNM). The classification that follows was extensively revised from the last publication. In T1 eyes, the tumor is confined to the retina, the tissue of origin. The classification below reflects a decade's experience with the response to chemotherapy followed by focal consolidation. The likelihood of salvaging good vision and the eye goes down progressively from T1 through T2. There is a corresponding increase in the morbidity and intensity of therapy from T1 through T2.

Primary Tumor (T)

TX	Primary tumor cannot be assessed
T0	No evidence of primary tumor
T1	Tumor confined to the retina (no vitreous seeding or significant retinal detachment). No retinal detachment or subretinal fluid >5 mm from the base of the tumor
T1a	Any eye in which the largest tumor is less than or equal to 3 mm in height **and** no tumor is located closer than 1 DD (1.5 mm) to the optic nerve or fovea
T1b	All other eyes in which the tumor(s) are confined to the retina regardless of location or size (up to half the volume of the eye). No vitreous seeding. No retinal detachment or subretinal fluid >5 mm from the base of the tumor

T2	Tumor with contiguous spread to adjacent tissues or spaces (vitreous or subretinal space)
T2a	*Minimal tumor spread to vitreous and/or subretinal space.* Fine local or diffuse vitreous seeding and/or serous retinal detachment up to total detachment may be present, but **no** clumps, lumps, snowballs, or avascular masses **are allowed** in the vitreous or subretinal space. Calcium flecks in the vitreous or subretinal space are allowed. The tumor may fill up to 2/3 the volume of the eye.
T2b	*Massive tumor spread to the vitreous and/or subretinal space.* Vitreous seeding and/or subretinal implantation may consist of lumps, clumps, snowballs, or avascular tumor masses. Retinal detachment may be total. Tumor may fill up to 2/3 the volume of the eye.
T2c	Unsalvageable intraocular disease. Tumor fills more than 2/3 the eye **or** there is no possibility of visual rehabilitation **or** one or more of the following are present:

- Tumor-associated glaucoma, either neovascular or angle closure
- Anterior segment extension of tumor
- Ciliary body extension of tumor
- Hyphema (significant)
- Massive vitreous hemorrhage
- Tumor in contact with lens
- Orbital cellulitis-like clinical presentation (massive tumor necrosis)

T3	Invasion of the optic nerve and/or optic coats
T4	Extraocular tumor

Regional Lymph Nodes (N)

NX	Regional lymph nodes cannot be assessed
N0	No regional lymph node involvement
N1	Regional lymph node involvement (preauricular, submandibular, or cervical)
N2	Distant lymph node involvement

Distant Metastasis (M)

MX	Distant metastasis cannot be assessed
M0	No distant metastasis
M1	Metastasis to central nervous system and/or bone, bone marrow, or other sites

10

Pathologic Classification (pTNM). There is one major difference in the pathologic classification from the last edition. No differentiating pathologic separation is proposed for those eyes in which the tumor may vary in size but is confined to the retina, vitreous, or subretinal space.

Primary Tumor (pT)

pTX	Primary tumor cannot be assessed
pT0	No evidence of primary tumor
pT1	Tumor confined to the retina, vitreous, or subretinal space. No optic nerve or choroidal invasion
pT2	Minimal invasion of the optic nerve and/or optic coats

pT2a	Tumor invades optic nerve up to, but not through, the level of the lamina cribrosa
pT2b	Tumor invades choroid focally
pT2c	Tumor invades optic nerve up to, but not through, the level of the lamina cribrosa **and** invades the choroid focally
pT3	Significant invasion of the optic nerve and/or optic coats
pT3a	Tumor invades optic nerve through the level of the lamina cribrosa but not to the line of resection
pT3b	Tumor massively invades the choroid
pT3c	Tumor invades the optic nerve through the level of the lamina cribrosa but not to the line of resection **and** massively invades the choroid
pT4	Extraocular tumor extension that includes:
	Invasion of optic nerve to the line of resection
	Invasion of orbit through the sclera
	Extension both anteriorly or posteriorly into the orbit
	Extension into the brain
	Extension into the subarachnoidal space of the optic nerve
	Extension to the apex of the orbit
	Extension to, but not through, the chiasm
	Extension into the brain beyond the chiasm

Regional Lymph Nodes (pN)

pNX	Regional lymph nodes cannot be assessed
pN0	No regional lymph node metastasis
pN1	Regional lymph node metastasis

Distant Metastasis (pM)

pMX	Distant metastasis cannot be assessed
pM0	No distant metastasis
pM1	Distant metastasis
pM1a	Bone marrow
pM1b	Other sites

STAGE GROUPING

No stage grouping applies.

HISTOPATHOLOGIC TYPE

This classification applies only to retinoblastoma.

BIBLIOGRAPHY

Cohen MD, Bugaieski EM, Haliloglu M, Faught P, Siddiqui AR: Visual presentation of the staging of pediatric solid tumors. Radiographics 16:523–545, 1996

Dagher R, Helman L: Rhabdomyosarcoma: an overview. Oncologist 4:34–44, 1999

Ellsworth RM: The practical management of retinoblastoma. Tr Am Ophthalmol Soc 67:462–534, 1969

Fleming ID: Staging of pediatric cancers: problems in the development of a national system. Semin Surg Oncol 8:94–97, 1992

Warrier RP, Regueira O. Wilms' tumor. Pediatr Nephrol 6:358–364, 1992

HISTOLOGIES—RETINOBLASTOMA

9510/3	Retinoblastoma, NOS
9511/3	Retinoblastoma, differentiated
9512/3	Retinoblastoma, undifferentiated
9513/3	Retinoblastoma, diffuse

10

45

Carcinoma of the Lacrimal Gland

C69.5 Lacrimal gland

SUMMARY OF CHANGES
- The definition of TNM and the Stage Grouping for this chapter have not changed from the Fifth Edition.

INTRODUCTION

The retrospective study of 265 epithelial tumors of the lacrimal gland conducted by the Armed Forces Institute of Pathology has improved our understanding of the histologic classification and clinical behavior of epithelial tumors of the lacrimal gland. Our current understanding of lacrimal gland carcinoma is based on a solid foundation. The historic works of Forrest (1954) and Zimmerman (1962) alleviated confusion by applying to epithelial tumors of the lacrimal gland the histopathologic classification of salivary gland tumors. The histologic classification used is a modification of the World Health Organization (WHO) classification of salivary gland tumors.

ANATOMY

Primary Site.   In the normal, fully developed orbit, the lacrimal gland is clinically impalpable and is situated in the lacrimal fossa posterior to the superotemporal orbital rim. The gland is not truly encapsulated. The lacrimal gland is divided into the deep orbital and the superficial palpebral lobes by the levator aponeurosis.

Regional Lymph Nodes.   The regional lymph nodes include:

Preauricular (parotid)
Submandibular
Cervical

For pN, histologic examination of a regional lymphadenectomy specimen, if performed, will include one or more regional lymph nodes.

Metastatic Sites.   The lung is the most common metastatic site, followed by bone and remote viscera.

RULES FOR CLASSIFICATION

Clinical Staging.   A complete physical examination and imaging of the orbit should be performed. Computed tomography and/or magnetic resonance imaging can provide critical diagnostic and staging data.

Pathologic Staging.   Complete resection of the mass is indicated. The specimen should be thoroughly sampled for evaluation of surgical margins,

10

---

type of tumor, and the grade of malignancy. Perineural spread, most characteristic of adenoid cystic carcinoma, frequently results in an underestimation of the true extent of disease.

DEFINITION OF TNM

This classification applies to both clinical and pathologic staging of lacrimal gland carcinomas.

Primary Tumor (T)

TX Primary tumor cannot be assessed
T0 No evidence of primary tumor
T1 Tumor 2.5 cm or less in greatest dimension, limited to the lacrimal gland
T2 Tumor more than 2.5 cm but not more than 5 cm in greatest dimension, limited to the lacrimal gland
T3 Tumor invades the periosteum
T3a Tumor not more than 5 cm invades the periosteum of the lacrimal gland fossa
T3b Tumor more than 5 cm in greatest dimension with periosteal invasion
T4 Tumor invades the orbital soft tissues, optic nerve, or globe with or without bone invasion; tumor extends beyond the orbit to adjacent structures, including brain

Regional Lymph Nodes (N)

NX Regional lymph nodes cannot be assessed
N0 No regional lymph node metastasis
N1 Regional lymph node metastasis

Distant Metastasis (M)

MX Distant metastasis cannot be assessed
M0 No distant metastasis
M1 Distant metastasis

STAGE GROUPING

No stage grouping is presently recommended.

HISTOPATHOLOGIC TYPE

The major malignant primary epithelial tumors include the following:

Malignant mixed tumor (carcinoma arising in pleomorphic adenoma), which includes adenocarcinoma and adenoid cystic carcinoma arising in a pleomorphic adenoma (benign mixed tumor).
Adenoid cystic carcinoma, arising *de novo*
Adenocarcinoma, arising *de novo*
Mucoepidermoid carcinoma
Squamous cell carcinoma

HISTOLOGIC GRADE (G)

GX   Grade cannot be assessed
G1   Well differentiated
G2   Moderately differentiated: includes adenoid cystic carcinoma without basaloid (solid) pattern
G3   Poorly differentiated: includes adenoid cystic carcinoma with basaloid (solid) pattern
G4   Undifferentiated

BIBLIOGRAPHY

Font RL, Gamel JW: Epithelial tumors of the lacrimal gland: an analysis of 265 cases. In Jakobiec FA (Ed.): Ocular and adnexal tumors, Birmingham, AL: Aesculapius, chap 53, 1978

Forres, AW: Epithelial lacrimal gland tumors: pathology as a guide to prognosis. Trans Amer Acad Ophthalmol Otolaryngol 58:848–866, 1954

Henderson JW: Orbital tumors, 3rd ed. New York: Raven Press, 1994

Jakobiec FA, Bilyk JR, Font RL: Lacrimal gland tumors. In Spencer WH (Ed.): Ophthalmic pathology: an atlas and textbook, 4th ed, vol. 4. Philadelphia: Saunders; 2485–2525, 1996

McLean IW, Burnier MN, Zimmerman LE, et al: Tumors of the lacrimal gland and sac. In: Rosai J, ed. Atlas of Tumor Pathology: Tumors of the Eye and Ocular Adnexa, Third Series, Fascicle 12, Washington DC: Armed Forces Institute of Pathology, 215–232, 1994

Tellado MV, McLean IW, Specht CS, et al: Adenoid cystic carcinomas of the lacrimal gland in childhood and adolescence. Ophthalmology 104:1622–1625, 1997

Vangveeravong S, Katz SE, Rootman J, et al: Tumors arising in the palpebral lobe of the lacrimal gland. Ophthalmology 103:1606–1612, 1996

Zimmerman LE, Sanders TE, Ackerman LV: Epithelial tumors of the lacrimal gland: prognostic and therapeutic significance of histologic types. In: Zimmerman LE, ed. Tumors of the eye and adnexa, International Ophthalmology Clinics. Boston, MA: Little, Brown, 337–367, 1962

HISTOLOGIES—CARCINOMA OF THE LACRIMAL GLAND

8010/3	Carcinoma, NOS
8020/3	Carcinoma, undifferentiated, NOS
8021/3	Carcinoma, anaplastic, NOS
8070/3	Squamous cell carcinoma, NOS
8071/3	Squamous cell carcinoma, keratinizing, NOS
8072/3	Squamous cell carcinoma, large cell, nonkeratinizing, NOS
8073/3	Squamous cell carcinoma, small cell, nonkeratinizing
8074/3	Squamous cell carcinoma, spindle cell
8075/3	Squamous cell carcinoma, adenoid
8140/3	Adenocarcinoma, NOS
8200/3	Adenoid cystic carcinoma
8430/3	Mucoepidermoid carcinoma
8562/3	Epithelial-myoepithelial carcinoma
8940/3	Mixed tumor, malignant, NOS
8941/3	Carcinoma in pleomorphic adenoma

10

46

Sarcoma of the Orbit

C69.6 Orbit, NOS   C69.8 Overlappning lesion of eye and adnexa

---

SUMMARY OF CHANGES

• A listing of site-specific categories is now included in T4.

INTRODUCTION

The primary malignant neoplasms of the orbit include soft tissue sarcomas (rhabdomyosarcoma, osteogenic sarcoma, leiomyosarcoma, etc.), lympho-proliferative tumors (lymphoma, plasma cell tumors, etc.), and melano-cytic tumors.

ANATOMY

Primary Site.   The orbital sarcomas originate from striated muscle (rhab-domyosarcoma), smooth muscle (leiomyosarcoma), cartilage (chondrosar-coma), bone (osteogenic sarcoma), fibroconnective tissue (fibrosarcoma, fibrous histiocytoma), vascular tissues (angiosarcoma, hemangiopericy-toma), peripheral nerve (Schwannoma, paraganglioma), and optic nerve tissues (glioma, meningioma).

Regional Lymph Nodes.   Although there is no organized lymphatic net-work behind the orbital septum, the drainage of the orbit takes place into the submandibular, parotid, and cervical lymph nodes through vascular anastamosis. The venous drainage of the orbit is primarily into the cav-ernous sinus. For pN, the examination of a regional lymphadenectomy specimen would ordinarily include one or more lymph node(s).

Local Invasion.   The malignancy of the orbit may directly extend into adjacent structures. Therefore, local tumor invasion (T4) would include extension to involve the eyelid, globe, temporal fossa, nasal cavity and paranasal sinuses, and central nervous system.

10

Metastatic Sites.   Metastatic spread occurs by the blood-stream and lymphatics.

RULES FOR CLASSIFICATION

Clinical Staging.   Clinical classification should be based on the symptoms and signs related to loss of vision and visual field, degree of global dis-placement and loss of extraocular motility, and degree of compressive optic neuropathy. Diagnostic tests should include ultrasonography, computed tomography, magnetic resonance imaging, and other imaging procedures when indicated.

Pathologic Staging.   The nature of the histopathology specimen (fine-needle aspiration biopsy, excisional biopsy, lumpectomy, or total excision) should be noted. Pathologic classification is based on the specific histopathology of the tumor, its differentiation (grade), and the extent of removal (evaluation of its excisional margins). In total excision specimens, evaluation of the surgical margins should be mandatory.

DEFINITION OF TNM

Primary Tumor (T)

TX   Primary tumor cannot be assessed
T0   No evidence of primary tumor
T1   Tumor 15 mm or less in greatest dimension
T2   Tumor more than 15 mm in greatest dimension without invasion of globe or bony wall
T3   Tumor of any size with invasion of orbital tissues and/or bony walls
T4   Tumor invasion of globe or periorbital structure, such as eyelids, temporal fossa, nasal cavity and paranasal sinuses, and/or central nervous system

Regional Lymph Nodes (N)

NX   Regional lymph nodes cannot be assessed
N0   No regional lymph node metastasis
N1   Regional lymph node metastasis

Distant Metastasis (M)

MX   Distant metastasis cannot be assessed
M0   No distant metastasis
M1   Distant metastatsis

STAGE GROUPING

No stage grouping is presently recommended.

HISTOPATHOLOGIC TYPE

Malignancies of the orbit primarily include a broad spectrum of malignant soft tissue tumors.

HISTOLOGIC GRADE (G)

GX   Grade cannot be assessed
G1   Well differentiated
G2   Moderately differentiated
G3   Poorly differentiated
G4   Undifferentiated

BIBLIOGRAPHY

Antman KH, Eilber FR, Shiu MH: Soft tissue sarcomas: current trends in diagnosis and management. Curr Probl Cancer Nov/Dec:337–367, 1989

Dhir SP, Munjal VP, Jain IS, et al: Osteosarcoma of the orbit. J Pediatr Ophthalmol Strabismus 17:312–314, 1980

Font RL, Hidayat AA: Fibrous histiocytoma of the orbit. A clinicopathologic study of 150 cases. Hum Pathol 13:199–209, 1982

Jakobiec FA, Rini F, Char D, et al: Primary liposarcoma of the orbit. Problems in the diagnosis and management of five cases. Ophthalmology 96:180–191, 1989

Kaltreider SA, Sestro M, Lemke BN: Leimyosarcoma of the orbit. A case report and review of the literature. Ophthal Plast Reconstr Surg 3:35–41, 1987

Karcioglu ZA, Al-Rasheed W, Gray AJ: Second malignant neoplasms in retinoblastoma patients. Middle East J Ophthalmol 5:99–104, 1997

Lyons CJ, McNab AA, Garner A, Wright JE: Orbital malignant peripheral nerve sheath tumours. Br J Ophthalmol 73:731–738, 1989

Maurer HM, Berltangady M, Genha EA, et al: The Intergroup Rhabdomyosarcoma Study-I. A final report. Cancer 61:209–220, 1988

Rice CD, Brown HH: Primary orbital melanoma associated with orbital melanocytosis. Arch Ophthalmol 108:1130–1134, 1990

Rootman J: Diseases of the orbit: A multidisciplinary approach, 2nd (ed.). Philadelphia: Lippincott, in press.

Shields CL, Shields JA: Orbital rhabdomyosarcoma. In: Fraunfelder FT, Roy FH, (Eds.): Current Ocular Therapy. 5th ed. Philadelphia: WB Saunders, 2000

Shields JA, Bakewell B, Augusburger JJ, Flanagan JC: Classification and incidence of space-occupying lesions of the orbit: A survey of 645 biopsies. Arch Ophthalmol 102:1606–1611, 1984

HISTOLOGIES—SARCOMA OF THE ORBIT

8800/3	Sarcoma, NOS
8801/3	Spindle cell sarcoma
8802/3	Giant cell sarcoma
8803/3	Small cell sarcoma
8804/3	Epithelioid sarcoma
8805/3	Undifferentiated sarcoma
8806/3	Desmoplastic small round cell tumor
8810/3	Fibrosarcoma, NOS
8811/3	Fibromyxosarcoma
8812/3	Periosteal fibrosarcoma
8813/3	Fascial fibrosarcoma
8814/3	Infantile fibrosarcoma
8815/3	Solitary fibrous tumor, malignant
8830/3	Malignant fibrous histiocytoma
8840/3	Myxosarcoma
8850/3	Liposarcoma, NOS
8851/3	Liposarcoma, well differentiated
8852/3	Myxoid liposarcoma
8853/3	Round cell liposarcoma
8854/3	Pleomorphic liposarcoma
8855/3	Mixed liposarcoma
8857/3	Fibroblastic liposarcoma
8858/3	Dedifferentiated liposarcoma
8890/3	Leiomyosarcoma, NOS

10

8891/3	Epithelioid leiomyosarcoma
8896/3	Myxoid leiomyosarcoma
8900/3	Rhabdomyosarcoma, NOS
8901/3	Pleomorphic rhabdomyosarcoma, adult type
8902/3	Mixed type rhabdomyosarcoma
8910/3	Embryonal rhabdomyosarcoma, NOS
8912/3	Spindle cell rhabdomyosarcoma
8920/3	Alveolar rhabdomyosarcoma
8963/3	Malignant rhabdoid tumor
9040/3	Synovial sarcoma, NOS
9044/3	Clear cell sarcoma, NOS
9050/3	Mesothelioma, malignant
9120/3	Hemangiosarcoma
9130/3	Hemangioendothelioma, malignant
9133/3	Epithelioid hemangioendothelioma
9140/3	Kaposi's sarcoma
9150/3	Hemangiopericytoma, malignant
9180/3	Osteosarcoma, NOS
9181/3	Chondroblastic osteosarcoma
9182/3	Fibroblastic osteosarcoma
9184/3	Osteosarcoma in Paget disease of bone
9220/3	Chondrosarcoma, NOS
9231/3	Myxoid chondrosarcoma
9240/3	Mesenchymal chondrosarcoma
9243/3	Dedifferentiated chondrosarcoma
9250/3	Giant cell tumor of bone, malignant
9260/3	Ewing sarcoma
9370/3	Chordoma, NOS
9490/3	Ganglioneuroblastoma
9500/3	Neuroblastoma, NOS
9501/3	Medulloepithelioma, NOS
9502/3	Teratoid medulloepithelioma
9503/3	Neuroepithelioma, NOS

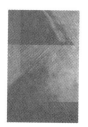

PART XI
Central Nervous System

47

Brain and Spinal Cord

Code	Location	Diagnosis
C70.0	Cerebral meninges	Meningioma
C71.0	Cerebrum	Astrocytoma
C71.1	Frontal lobe	Anaplastic astrocytoma
C71.2	Temporal lobe	Glioblastoma
C71.3	Parietal lobe	Oligodendroglioma
C71.4	Occipital lobe	Ganglioglioma
C71.5	Ventricle NOS	Ependymoma
C71.6	Cerebellum NOS	Central neurocytoma
C71.7	Brain stem	Pilocytic astrocytoma
C71.8	Overlapping lesion of brain	Medulloblastoma
C71.9	Brain NOS	Brain stem glioma
C72.0	Spinal cord	Any, if location is not specified
C72.1	Cauda equina	Any, involving more than one site
C72.2	Olfactory nerve	Astrocytoma, ependymoma
C72.3	Optic nerve	Ependymoma
C72.4	Acoustic/vestibular nerve	Esthesioneuroblastoma
C72.5	Cranial nerve, NOS	Optic glioma
C72.8	Overlapping lesion of brain and central nervous system	Vestibular schwannoma
C72.9	Nervous system, NOS	Schwannoma
C75.1	Pituitary gland	PNET, CNS lymphoma
C75.2	Craniopharyngeal duct	
C75.3	Pineal gland	

SUMMARY OF CHANGES

• Central Nervous System Tumors continue to have no TNM designation.

INTRODUCTION

Attempts at developing a TNM-based classification and staging system for tumors of the central nervous system (CNS) have largely been unsuccessful. Previous editions of this manual had proposed a system that was used with poor compliance and proved not to be particularly useful as a predictor of outcome in clinical trials for the management of patients with primary CNS tumors. The reasons for this are several and have to do with the fact that tumor size is significantly less relevant than tumor histology and the location of the tumor, so that the T classification is less pertinent than the biologic nature of the tumor tissue itself. Because the brain and spinal cord have no lymphatics, the N classification does not apply at all, as there are no lymph nodes that can be identified in either classification or staging. An M classification is not pertinent to the majority of neoplasms that affect the central nervous system, because most patients with tumors of the central nervous system do not live long enough to develop metastatic disease (except for some pediatric tumors that tend to "seed" through the cerebrospinal fluid spaces).

Many important studies have been done regarding the most common tumors affecting the brain and spinal cord, and a variety of prognostic factors have been identified. Unfortunately, these factors do not easily fall

11

into the usual categories that have traditionally been part of the American Joint Committee on Cancer (AJCC) TNM system.

For those reasons, it was the recommendation of the CNS Tumor Task Force that a formal classification and staging system not be attempted at this time. This chapter, however, will attempt to highlight what is known about prognostic factors in tumors of the central nervous system. (Table 47.1).

PROGNOSTIC FACTORS IN CNS TUMORS

Tumor Histology. The histology of tumors that affect the brain and spinal cord is by far the most important variable with regard to prognosis, and in many cases it determines the treatment modalities that are employed. The latest World Health Organization (WHO) classification system has combined tumor nomenclature with an associated grading system, so the actual histologic diagnosis directly correlates with the histologic grade of the tumor. This should clarify some of the inconsistencies that existed in the past when a number of different grading systems, each slightly different from the others, were used. The most common histologies for brain and spinal cord tumors are given in Table 47.2, along with the tumor grade for each different diagnostic category. *Note:* The histologic grade code used

TABLE 47.1. Prognostic factors in CNS tumors

Histology

    Pathologic grade and accuracy of diagnosis

    Presence and extent of necrosis

    Presence of gemistocytes

    Proliferative fraction

    Presence of oligodendroglial component

    Presence or absence of cells in mitosis

Age of patient

Functional neurologic status

    Karnofsky Performance Score

Symptom presentation and duration before diagnosis

    Presentation with seizure, long duration are favorable prognostic factors

Location of tumor

    Unifocal or multifocal

Primary or recurrent tumor

Extent of resection

    Biopsy, subtotal, radical removal

Metastatic spread

    CNS or extraneural

Patterns of enhancement on imaging studies

TABLE 47.2. Histologies for brain and spinal cord tumors: WHO classification of tumors of the nervous system

Tumors of Neuroepithelial Tissue		Neuronal and mixed neuronal-glial tumors	
Astrocytic tumors		Gangliocytoma	9492/0
Diffuse astrocytoma	9400/3[1]	Dysplastic gangliocytoma of cerebellum (Lhermitte-Duclos)	9493/0
Fibrillary astrocytoma	9420/3		
Protoplasmic astrocytoma	9410/3	Desmoplastic infantile astrocytoma/ ganglioglioma	9412/1
Gemistocytic astrocytoma	9411/3	Dysembryoplastic neuroepithelial tumor	9413/0
Anaplastic astrocytoma	9401/3	Ganglioglioma	9505/1
Glioblastoma	9440/3	Anaplastic ganglioglioma	9505/3
Giant cell glioblastoma	9441/3	Central neurocytoma	9506/1
Gliosarcoma	9442/3	Cerebellar liponeurocytoma	9506/1
Pilocytic astrocytoma	9421/3	Paraganglioma of the filum terminale	8680/1
Pleomorphic xanthoastrocytoma	9424/3		
Subependymal giant cell astrocytoma	9384/1	**Neuroblastic tumors**	
Oligodendroglial tumors		Olfactory neuroblastoma (aesthesioneuroblastoma)	9522/3
Oligodendroglioma	9450/3	Olfactory neuroepithelioma	9523/3
Anaplastic oligodendroglioma	9451/3	Neuroblastomas of the adrenal gland and sympathetic nervous system	9500/3
Mixed gliomas			
Oligoastrocytoma	9382/3		
Anaplastic oligoastrocytoma	9382/3	**Pineal parenchymal tumors**	
Ependymal tumors		Pineocytoma	9361/1
Ependymoma	9391/3	Pineoblastoma	9362/3
Cellular	9391/3	Pineal parenchymal tumor of intermediate differentiation	9362/3
Papillary	9393/3		
Clear cell	9391/3		
Tanycytic	9391/3	**Embryonal tumors**	
Anaplastic ependymoma	9392/3	Medulloepithelioma	9501/3
Myxopapillary ependymoma	9394/1	Ependymoblastoma	9392/3
Subependymoma	9383/1	Medulloblastoma	9470/3
Choroid plexus tumors		Desmoplastic medulloblastoma	9471/3
Choroid plexus papilloma	9390/0		
Choroid plexus carcinoma	9390/3	Large cell medulloblastoma	9474/3
Glial tumors of uncertain origin		Medullomyoblastoma	9472/3
Astroblastoma	9430/3		
Gliomatosis cerebri	9381/3	Melanotic medulloblastoma	9470/3
Chordoid glioma of the third ventricle	9444/1		

continued

11

TABLE 47.2. Histologies for brain and spinal cord tumors: WHO classification of tumors of the nervous system (continued)

Embryonal tumors (cont.)			Atypical	9539/1
Supratentorial primitive neuroectodermal tumor (PNET)	9473/3		Papillary	9538/3
			Rhabdoid	9538/3
Neuroblastoma	9500/3		Anaplastic meningioma	9530/3
Ganglioneuroblastoma	9490/3		**Mesenchymal, non-meningothelial tumors**	
Atypical teratoid/rhabdoid tumor	9508/3		Lipoma	8850/0
Tumors of Peripheral Nerves			Angiolipoma	8861/0
Schwannoma			Hibernoma	8880/0
(neurilemmoma, neurinoma)	9560/0		Liposarcoma (intracranial)	8850/3
Cellular	9560/0		Solitary fibrous tumor	8815/0
Plexiform	9560/0		Fibrosarcoma	8810/3
Melanotic	9560/0		Malignant fibrous histiocytoma	8830/3
Neurofibroma	9540/0		Leiomyoma	8890/0
Plexiform	9550/0		Leiomyosarcoma	8890/3
Perineurioma	9471/0		Rhabdomyoma	8900/0
Intraneural perineurioma	9571/0		Rhabdomyosarcoma	8900/3
Soft tissue perineurioma	9571/0		Chondroma	9220/0
Malignant peripheral nerve			Chondrosarcoma	9220/3
sheath tumor (MPNST)	9540/3		Osteoma	9180/0
Epithelioid	9540/3		Osteosarcoma	9180/3
MPNST with divergent mesenchymal and/or epithelial differentiation	9540/3		Osteochondroma	9210/0
			Hemangioma	9120/0
Melanotic	9540/3		Epithelioid hemangioendothelioma	9133/1
Melanotic psammomatous	9540/3		Hemangiopericytoma	9150/1
Tumors of the Meninges			Angiosarcoma	9120/3
			Kaposi sarcoma	9140/3
Tumors of meningothelial cells			**Primary melanocytic lesions**	
Meningioma	9530/0		Diffuse melanocytosis	8728/0
Meningothelial	9531/0		Meningeal melanocytoma	8728/1
Fibrous (fibroblastic)	9532/0		Malignant melanoma	8720/3
Transitional (mixed)	9537/0		Meningeal melanomatosis	8728/3
Psammomatous	9533/0		**Tumors of uncertain histogenesis**	
Angiomatous	9534/0		Hemangioblastoma	9161/1
Microcystic	9530/0		***Lymphomas & Haemopoietic Neoplasms***	
Secretory	9530/0			
Lymphoplasmacyte-rich	9530/0		Malignant lymphomas (not otherwise specified)	9590/3
Metaplastic	9530/0		Plasmacytoma	9731/3
Clear cell	9538/1		Granulocytic sarcoma	9930/3
Chordoid	9538/1			

continued

TABLE 47.2. Histologies for brain and spinal cord tumors: WHO classification of tumors of the nervous system (continued)

Germ Cell Tumors		Mixed germ cell tumor	9085/3
Germinoma	9064/3	*Tumors of the Sellar Region*	
Embryonal carcinoma	9070/3	Craniopharyngioma	9350/1
Yolk sac tumor	9071/3	Adamantinomatous	9351/1
Choriocarcinoma	9100/3	Papillary	9352/1
Teratoma	9080/1	Granular cell tumor	9582/0
Mature	9080/0	Metastatic Tumors	
Immature	9080/3		
Teratoma with malignant transformation	9084/3		

[1]Morphology code of the International Classification of Diseases for Oncology (ICD-O) and the Systematized Nomenclature of Medicine (SNOMED). Behavior is Coded /0 for benign tumors, /1 for low or uncertain malignant potential or borderline malignancy, /2 for *in situ* lesions, and /3 for malignant tumors.

Source: P. Kleihues and W. Cavenee (Eds.), World Health Organization Classification of Tumours: Pathology and Genetics. Tumours of the Nervous System (Lyon: International Agency for Research on Cancer, 2000).

for staging purposes is *not* the same code that is assigned as the differentiation code in the sixth digit of the ICD-O morphology code.

Age of the Patient. Most retrospective outcome studies of brain tumor therapy show that the age of the patient at the time of diagnosis is one of the most powerful predictors of outcome. This fact holds true for the gliomas, which are the most common primary brain tumors, and for most other tumors that affect the adult population, including most metastatic tumors to the brain. There are, however, some childhood tumors that have a very poor prognosis, are inherently high grade, and rapidly progress to a fatal outcome. Some metastatic tumors, such as melanoma, occur in younger patients and also violate this general statement with regard to the specific effect of age on prognosis.

Extent of Tumor Resection. In patients who are treated surgically for tumors of the central nervous system, the extent of resection is often directly correlated with the outcome. This is a less powerful predictor than tumor histology or age, but most retrospective studies confirm that extent of removal is positively correlated with survival. For this reason, documentation of whether a surgical tumor removal is "gross total," "subtotal," or "biopsy only," is useful in determining future therapy and prognosis. Any staging system to be developed for CNS tumors should take into account, in a systematic and clearly documented fashion, extent of removal or tumor residual.

Tumor Location. Because of the differential importance of various areas of the brain, the location of a given tumor affecting the brain can have a major impact on the functional outcome, survival, and nature of therapy.

The location codes available for tumors affecting the central nervous system in the ICD-O and ICD-10 manuals are generally satisfactory, and they offer the advantage of consistency to the records of patients with CNS tumors.

Functional Neurologic Status. Another important prognostic factor in most retrospective studies of CNS tumors is the functional neurologic status of the patient at the time of diagnosis. This traditionally has been estimated using the Karnofsky Performance Scale, which is reproducible, is well known by most investigators, and is in common use for stratification of patients entering clinical trials for the treatment of brain tumors. The outcome and prognosis of patients correlate fairly well with functional neurologic status, and once again, any staging system should include a validated and reliable measure of this parameter. Other measures of outcome, both cognitive and functional, are increasingly used in studies of CNS tumors.

Metastatic Spread. Tumors affecting the central nervous system rarely develop extraneural metastases, probably because of inherent biologic characteristics of these tumors, and also because the brain does not have a well-developed lymphatic drainage system. In addition, many patients with tumors of the central nervous system have a short life expectancy, which further limits the likelihood of metastatic spread. Certain tumors do spread through cerebrospinal fluid (CSF) pathways, and such spread has a major impact on survival. Dissemination through the CSF pathway is a hallmark of certain childhood tumors, many of which carry a poor prognosis; this phenomenon, however, is rarely seen in adult patients with the more common CNS tumors. Primary lymphomas of the central nervous system may spread along the craniospinal axis and sometimes exhibit intraocular dissemination. Although metastatic spread is of importance in certain instances, its overall impact in staging is relatively minor. The M category, however, should be part of any classification and staging system that is developed in the future for CNS tumors, and it should differentiate between extraneural metastasis and metastasis within the CNS and CSF pathways.

BRAIN TUMOR SURVIVAL DATA

Data are available from the SEER program for current survival statistics for "brain tumors," a category that includes malignant primary brain tumors (gliomas). For this relatively ill-defined group of patients, there are 17,200 new cases estimated for 2001. Five-year survivals are 30% in adults and 64% in children.

Excellent observational data for malignant gliomas (glioblastomas and malignant [grade 3] gliomas) are available from the Glioma Outcome Project, evaluating 788 patients accrued from 1997 through 2000. The 50% survival for glioblastoma multiforme (GBM) is 10.6 months, and the 96-week survival is 10%. For grade 3 gliomas, 70% have survived 96 weeks. Approximately 11% of the patients were enrolled in clinical trials.

TABLE 47.3. Prognostic biogenetic markers (under investigation)

Proliferation index—Ki-67(MIB-1), PCNA, bcl-2 expression, cyclin-D1 expression
DNA studies—flow cytometry, DNA index, BrdULI, comparative genomic hybridization
Activation of cellular oncogenes—ras, N-myc, C-myc, pescadillo
Inactivation of tumor suppressor genes—p53, p16(CDKN2A), Rb, PTEN, DMBT1, MDM2, NF2
Allelic loss / loss of heterozygosity (LOH)— chromosomes 10, 22q, 19q, 17p
Cytokine dysregulation—CDK4, EGFR, VEGF, PKC
Chromosomal aberrations—chromosomes 1, 9, 10, 11, 17, 19, and 22
Other molecular observations—telomerase activity and hTERT expression, DNA methyltransferase, double minutes, AgNOR instability

PROGNOSTIC BIOGENETIC MARKERS (UNDER INVESTIGATION)

The field of molecular neuropathology has provided us with a number of potential biogenetic markers that may be useful in staging CNS tumors and in making recommendations for therapy. The discovery of the pivotal role of oncogenes and of the loss of tumor suppressor genes in the tumorigenesis of CNS tumors has led to a flurry of activity that may prove quite fruitful in providing valid biologic markers in these difficult tumors. Table 47.3 provides a glimpse of some of the current markers and techniques under investigation. It is hoped that ways will be found to apply these methods of scientific analysis of tumor growth potential to predict survival more effectively than is possible today.

BIBLIOGRAPHY

Aldape K, Simmons M, Davis RL, et al: Discrepancies in diagnoses of neuro-epithelial neoplasms: the San Francisco Bay Area Gliomas Study. Cancer 88:2342–2349, 2000.

Anderson FA, et al: The Glioma Outcomes Project: a resource for measuring and improving glioma outcomes. Neurosurg Focus 4:1–5, 1998

Avgeropoulos NG, Batchelor TT: New treatment strategies for malignant gliomas. The Oncologist 4:209–224, 1999

Curran WJ, Scott CB, Horton J, et al: Recursive partitioning analysis of prognostic factors in three Radiation Therapy Oncology Group malignant glioma trials. J Natl Cancer Inst 85:704–710, 1993

Guthrie BL, Laws ER Jr: Prognostic factors in patients with brain tumors. In Morantz RA, Walsh JW (Eds.): Brain tumors. New York: Marcel Dekker; 799–808, 1994

Jelsma R, Bucy PC: Glioblastoma multiforme: its treatment and some factors affecting survival. Arch Neurol 20:161–171, 1969

Kaye AH, Laws ER Jr: Brain Tumors. 2nd edition, London: Churchill Livingstone, 2001

Kleihues P, Cavenee W (Eds.): World Health Organization classification of tumours: pathology and genetics. Tumours of the Nervous System. Lyon: International Agency for Research on Cancer, 2000

11

Salcman M: Survival in glioblastoma: historical perspective. Neurosurgery 7:435–439, 1980

Scanlon PW, Taylor WF: Radiotherapy of intracranial astrocytomas: analysis of 417 cases treated from 1960 through 1969. Neurosurgery 5:301–308, 1979

VandenBerg SR: Current diagnostic concepts of astrocytic tumors. J Neuropathol Exp Neurol 51:644–657, 1992

PART XII
Lymphoid
Neoplasms

Lymphoid Neoplasms

INTRODUCTION

Lymphoid malignancies are a diverse and sometimes confusing group of disorders. These malignancies share derivation from B-cells, T-cells, and NK-cells, but they have a wide range of presentations, clinical course, and response to therapy. The incidence of lymphoid malignancies is significant and increasing. Non-Hodgkin lymphomas occur in approximately 55,000 new individuals each year and have been increasing rapidly in incidence over the past several decades. Hodgkin lymphoma occurs in approximately 8,000 new individuals each year in the United States and seems stable in incidence. Approximately 13,000 new cases of multiple myeloma and up to 15,000 new cases of lymphoid leukemias occur annually in the United States.

PATHOLOGY

Lymphoid neoplasms include Hodgkin disease (Hodgkin lymphoma) and B-cell, T-cell, and NK-cell (natural killer cell) neoplasms (collectively known as non-Hodgkin lymphomas [NHL] and lymphoid leukemias). Traditionally, classifications have distinguished between "lymphomas"— neoplasms that typically present with an obvious tumor or mass of lymph nodes or extranodal sites—and "leukemias"—neoplasms that typically involve the bone marrow and peripheral blood, without tumor masses. However, we now know that many B- and T/NK-cell neoplasms may have both tissue masses *and* circulating cells, either in the same patient or from one patient to another. Thus it is artificial to call them different diseases, when in fact they are just different stages or phases of the same disease. For this reason, we now refer to these diseases as lymphoid neoplasms rather than as lymphomas or leukemias, reserving the latter terms for the specific clinical presentation. In the current classification of lymphoid neoplasms, diseases that typically produce tumor masses are called lymphomas, those that typically have only circulating cells are called leukemias, and those that often have both solid and circulating phases are designated lymphoma/leukemia. Finally, plasma cell neoplasms, including multiple myeloma and plasmacytoma, have typically not been considered "lymphomas," but plasma cells are part of the B-cell lineage, and thus these tumors are B-cell neoplasms, which are now included in the classification of lymphoid neoplasms.

Lymphoid neoplasms are malignancies of lymphoid cells. Lymphoid cells include lymphoblasts, lymphocytes, follicle center cells (centrocytes and centroblasts), immunoblasts, and plasma cells. These cells are responsible for immune responses to infections. Immune responses involve recognition by lymphocytes of foreign molecules, followed by proliferation and differentiation to generate either specific cytotoxic cells (T or NK—natural killer—cells) or antibodies (B-cells and plasma cells). Lymphoid cells are normally found in greatest numbers in lymph nodes and in other lymphoid tissues such as Waldeyer's ring (which includes the palatine and lingual tonsils and adenoids), the thymus, Peyer's patches of the small intestine, the spleen, and the bone marrow. Lymphocytes also circulate in the peripheral blood and are found in small numbers in almost every organ of the body, where they either wait to encounter antigens or carry out specific immune reactions. Lymphoid neoplasms may occur in any site to which lymphocytes normally travel. Because lymphocytes normally do travel—in contrast to epithelial cells, for example—it is often impossible to determine the "primary site" of a lymphoid neoplasm or to use a staging scheme that was developed for epithelial cancers, such as the TNM scheme.

For the purposes of coding and staging, lymph nodes, Waldeyer's ring, and spleen are considered *nodal* or *lymphatic* sites. *Extranodal* or *extralymphatic* sites include the bone marrow, the gastrointestinal tract, skin, bone, central nervous system, lung, gonads, ocular adnexae (conjunctiva, lachrymal glands, and orbital soft tissue), liver, kidneys, and uterus. Hodgkin lymphoma rarely presents in an extranodal site, but about 25% of non-Hodgkin lymphomas are extranodal at presentation. The frequency of extranodal presentation varies dramatically among different lymphomas, however, with some (mycosis fungoides and MALT lymphomas) being virtually always extranodal and some (follicular lymphoma, B-cell small lymphocytic lymphoma) seldom being extranodal, except for bone marrow involvement.

CLASSIFICATION OF LYMPHOID NEOPLASMS

Many different classification schemes have been proposed for lymphoid neoplasms, and this had led to much confusion on the part of both pathologists and oncologists. Until recently in the United States, a classification called the Working Formulation was used. This scheme had the advantage of being simple, with only 10 categories, and not requiring any special studies such as immunophenotyping or genetic studies. In addition, it provided simple clinical groupings for determining the approach to treatment (low, intermediate, and high clinical grades). Since it was introduced in 1982, advances in understanding of the immune system and of the lymphoid neoplasms have led to the recognition of many new categories of lymphoid neoplasms and the development of better methods for diagnosis and classification—as well as for treatment—and the Working Formulation has become obsolete. In 1994 the International Lymphoma Study Group (ILSG) introduced a new classification, called the Revised European–American Classification of Lymphoid Neoplasms (REAL), which incorporated both morphology, new information such as immunophenotype and genetic features, and clinical features, to define over 25 different categories of lymphoid neoplasms, including Hodgkin lymphoma. More recently, the World Health Organization (WHO) decided to update its Classification of Diseases of the Hematopoietic and Lymphoid Systems and has adopted the REAL classification for lymphoid neoplasms (the WHO classification also includes myeloid and histiocytic neoplasms). The REAL/WHO classification is now the standard for clinical trials in lymphoma (Table 48.1).

The REAL/WHO classification is a list of distinct disease entities, which are defined by a combination of morphology, immunophenotype, and genetic features and which have distinct clinical features. The relative importance of each of these features varies among diseases, and there is no one "gold standard." Morphology remains the first and most basic approach and is sufficient for both diagnosis and classification in many typical cases of lymphoma. Immunophenotyping and—particularly—molecular genetic studies are not needed in all cases, but they are very important in some diseases, are useful in difficult cases, and improve interobserver reproducibility. As mentioned above, the classification includes all lymphoid neoplasms: Hodgkin lymphoma, non-Hodgkin lymphomas, lymphoid leukemias, and plasma cell neoplasms. Both lymphomas and lymphoid leukemias are included, because both solid and circulating phases are present in many lymphoid neoplasms, and drawing a distinction between them is artificial. Thus, B-cell chronic lymphocytic leukemia and B-cell small lymphocytic lymphoma are simply different manifestations of the same neoplasm, as are lymphoblastic lymphomas and acute lymphoblastic leukemias. In addition, Hodgkin lymphoma and plasma cell myeloma are now recognized as lymphoid neoplasms of B-lineage and therefore belong in a compilation of lymphoid neoplasms.

Major Categories of Hodgkin Lymphoma

Nodular lymphocyte predominance Hodgkin lymphoma (NLPHL)
Classic Hodgkin lymphoma (CHL)
> Nodular sclerosis Hodgkin lymphoma (NSHL)
> Mixed cellularity Hodgkin lymphoma (MCHL)
> Lymphocyte rich classic Hodgkin lymphoma (LRCHL)
> Lymphocyte depletion Hodgkin lymphoma (LDHL)

T-cell Neoplasms. T-cell neoplasms, other than precursor T-lymphoblastic lymphoma/leukemia and mycosis fungoides, are uncommon in the United States and Europe, accounting for 10%–15% of all non-Hodgkin lymphomas (Table 48.1).

NON-HODGKIN LYMPHOMAS

All newly diagnosed patients with non-Hodgkin lymphomas should have formal documentation of the anatomic disease extent prior to the initial therapeutic intervention; that is, clinical stage must be assigned and recorded. Patients with recurrent disease should not have clinical stage assigned again at the time of relapse, although recording of the anatomic disease extent at the time of recurrence is recommended. The retreatment classification (see the section "General Rules of the TNM System") using "r-stage" may be used for this purpose. However, the clinical stage at diagnosis should not be confused with the "r-stage."

12

TABLE 48.1. WHO classification of lymphoid neoplasms

B-cell Neoplasms

Precursor B-cell neoplasm

- Precursor B-lymphoblastic leukemia/lymphoma (precursor B-cell acute lymphoblastic leukemia)

Mature (peripheral) B-cell neoplasms

- B-cell chronic lymphocytic leukemia/small lymphocytic lymphoma
- B-cell prolymphocytic leukemia
- Lymphoplasmacytic lymphoma
- Splenic marginal zone B-cell lymphoma (with or without villous lymphocytes)
- Hairy cell leukemia
- Plasma cell myeloma/plasmacytoma
- Extranodal marginal zone B-cell lymphoma of MALT type
- Nodal marginal zone B-cell lymphoma (with or without monocytoid B cells)
- Follicular lymphoma
- Mantle cell lymphoma
- Diffuse large B-cell lymphoma
- Burkitt lymphoma/Burkitt cell leukemia

T-cell and NK-cell Neoplasms

Precursor T-cell neoplasm

- Precursor T-lymphoblastic lymphoma/leukemia (precursor T-cell acute lymphoblastic leukemia)

Mature (peripheral) T/NK-cell neoplasms

- T-cell prolymphocytic leukemia
- T-cell granular lymphocytic leukemia
- Aggressive NK-cell leukemia
- Adult T-cell lymphoma/leukemia (HTLV1 +)
- Extranodal NK/T-cell lymphoma, nasal type
- Enteropathy-type T-cell lymphoma
- Hepatosplenic γδ T-cell lymphoma
- Subcutaneous panniculitis-like T-cell lymphoma
- Mycosis fungoides/Sezary syndrome
- Anaplastic large cell lymphoma, T/null cell, primary cutaneous type
- Peripheral T-cell lymphoma, not otherwise characterized
- Angioimmunoblastic T-cell lymphoma
- Anaplastic large cell lymphoma, T/null cell, primary systemic type

The current anatomic staging classification for non-Hodgkin lymphoma, known as the Ann Arbor classification, was originally developed for Hodgkin lymphoma, and its use was subsequently extended to non-Hodgkin lymphoma. The pattern of disease in Hodgkin lymphoma varies considerably from that encountered in non-Hodgkin lymphoma. Consequently, significant difficulties arose when the Ann Arbor classification was applied to non-Hodgkin lymphoma. However, the Ann Arbor classification has been used in Hodgkin lymphoma and non-Hodgkin lymphoma for over 30 years. It has been accepted as the best means of describing the anatomic disease extent and has been found useful as a universal system for a variety of lymphomas. The AJCC and UICC have adopted the Ann Arbor classification as the official system for classifying the anatomic extent of disease in Hodgkin lymphoma and non-Hodgkin lymphoma.

STAGING

Stage I: Involvement of a single lymph node region (I); or localized involvement of a single extralymphatic organ or site in the absence of any lymph node involvement (IE) (rare in Hodgkin lymphoma).

Stage II: Involvement of two or more lymph node regions on the same side of the diaphragm (II); or localized involvement of a single extralymphatic organ or site in association with regional lymph node involvement with or without involvement of other lymph node regions on the same side of the diaphragm (IIE). The number of regions involved may be indicated by a subscript, as in, for example, II_3.

Stage III: Involvement of lymph node regions on both sides of the diaphragm (III), which also may be accompanied by extralymphatic extension in association with adjacent lymph node involvement (IIIE) or by involvement of the spleen (IIIS) or both (IIIE,S).

Stage IV: Diffuse or disseminated involvement of one or more extralymphatic organs, with or without associated lymph node involvement; or isolated extralymphatic organ involvement in the absence of adjacent regional lymph node involvement, but in conjunction with disease in distant site(s). Any involvement of the liver or bone marrow, or nodular involvement of the lung(s). The location of Stage IV disease is identified further by specifying the site according to the notations listed on page 400.

Although anatomic disease extent is one prognostic factor in non-Hodgkin lymphoma, the prognostic factors that form the International Prognostic Index for non-Hodgkin lymphoma (Table 48.4) should be used for treatment decisions along with histologic subtype of lymphoma. Additional factors that have been reported to affect the outcome in preliminary studies include tumor bulk, beta-2 microglobulin, and S-phase fraction.

ANATOMY

The Ann Arbor staging system is further described in the section on Hodgkin lymphoma. It is proposed that for non-Hodgkin lymphoma, the E designation should indicate the presentation of lymphoma in extranodal sites and the lack of an E designation should indicate lymphomas presenting in lymph nodes.

Clinical Staging. Clinical staging includes the careful recording of medical history and physical examination; imaging of chest, abdomen, and

12

TABLE 48.2. Recommendation for the diagnostic evaluation of patients with lymphoma

A. Mandatory procedures
   1. Biopsy, with interpretation by a qualified pathologist
   2. History, with special attention to the presence and duration of fever, night sweats, and unexplained loss of 10% or more of body weight in the previous 6 months
   3. Physical examination
   4. Laboratory tests
      a. Complete blood cell count and platelet count
      b. Erythrocyte sedimentation rate
      c. Liver function tests
   5. Radiographic examinations
      a. Chest X-ray
      b. CT of chest, abdomen, and pelvis
      c. Gallium scan
   6. Bone marrow biopsy
B. Ancillary procedures
   1. Laparotomy and splenectomy if decisions regarding management are likely to be influenced
   2. Liver biopsy (needle), if there is a strong clinical indication of hepatic involvement
   3. Radioisotopic bone scans, in selected patients with bone pain
   4. CT of head and neck in extranodal or nodal presentation to define disease extent
   5. Gastroscopy and/or GI series in patients with GI presentations
   6. MRI spine in patients with suspected spinal involvement
   7. CSF cytology in patients with Stage IV disease and bone marrow involvement, testis involvement, or parameningeal involvement

pelvis; blood chemistry determination; complete blood count; and bone marrow biopsy (Table 48.2).

The basic staging investigation in non-Hodgkin lymphoma includes physical examination, complete blood count, LDH, liver function tests, chest X-ray, CT scan of abdomen and pelvis, and bone marrow biopsy. CT scans of the neck, thorax, abdomen, and pelvis are commonly obtained. In patients presenting with extranodal lymphoma, imaging of the presenting area with either CT or MRI is required to define local disease extent. In patients at high risk for occult CNS involvement, CSF cytology is performed. Gallium scan is commonly used to determine extent of disease and gallium avidity. Biopsies of any suspicious lesions may also be conducted as part of the initial clinical staging, especially if this would alter stage assignment. Bone marrow biopsy is a standard clinical staging investigation. However, liver biopsy is not required as part of clinical staging, unless abnormal liver function occurs in the presence of otherwise limited stage disease.

Pathologic Staging. The use of the term *pathologic staging* is reserved for patients who undergo staging laparotomy with an explicit intent to assess the presence of abdominal disease or to define histologic microscopic disease extent in the abdomen. Staging laparotomy and pathologic staging have been essentially abandoned as useful procedures.

Definition of Lymph Node Regions. The staging classification for non-Hodgkin lymphoma uses the term *lymph node region*. The lymph node regions were defined at the Rye symposium in 1965 and have been used in the Ann Arbor classification. They are not based on any physiological principles but, rather, have been agreed upon by convention. The currently accepted classification of core nodal regions is as follows: right cervical (including cervical, supraclavicular, occipital, and preauricular lymph nodes) nodes and left cervical nodes, right axillary, left axillary, right infraclavicular, and left infraclavicular lymph nodes, mediastinal lymph nodes, hilar lymph nodes, para-aortic lymph nodes, mesenteric lymph nodes, right pelvic lymph nodes, left pelvic lymph nodes, right inguinofemoral lymph nodes and left inguinofemoral lymph nodes. In addition to these core regions, non-Hodgkin lymphoma may involve epitochlear lymph nodes, popliteal lymph nodes, internal mammary lymph nodes, occipital lymph nodes, submental lymph nodes, preauricular lymph nodes, and many other small nodal areas.

Definition of Extranodal Involvement. Lymphomas presenting in extranodal sites should be staged using the E suffix. For example, lymphoma presenting in the thyroid gland with cervical lymph node involvement should be staged as IIE, lymphoma presenting only in cervical lymph nodes as Stage I. Frequently, extensive lymph node involvement is associated with extranodal extension of disease that may also directly invade other organs. Such extension may be described with an E suffix but should not be recorded as Stage IV. For example, mediastinal lymph nodes with lung extension should be classified as Stage IIE disease. Primary lung lymphoma with hilar and mediastinal lymph node involvement should be classified as Stage IIE.

By convention, any involvement of bone marrow, liver, pleura, or CSF calls for classification as Stage IV disease.

Mycosis fungoides is a primary cutaneous T-cell lymphoma with its own staging system. A TNM classification for mycosis fungoides has been in clinical use and should be maintained (Table 48.3).

ANATOMIC STAGING CRITERIA

12

Clinical Staging. *Lymph node involvement* is demonstrated by (a) clinical enlargement of node when alternative pathology may reasonably be ruled out (suspicious nodes should always be biopsied if treatment decisions are based on their involvement) and (b) enlargement on plain radiograph, CT, or lymphangiography. Nodes larger than 1.5 cm are considered abnormal.

TABLE 48.3. TNM(B) classification for mycosis fungoides

T1 Limited patch/plaque	(<10% of skin surface involved)
T2 Generalized patch/plaque	(≥10% of skin surface involved)
T3 Cutaneous tumors	(one or more)
T4 Generalized erythroderma	(with or without patches, plaques, or tumors)

N0 Lymph nodes clinically uninvolved

N1 Lymph nodes clinically enlarged, histologically uninvolved

N2 Lymph nodes clinically unenlarged, histologically involved

N3 Lymph nodes enlarged and histologically involved

M0 No visceral disease

M1 Visceral disease present

B0 No circulating atypical cells (<1000 Sezary cells [CD4 + CD7 −]/ml)

B1 Circulating atypical cells (≥1000 Sezary cells [CD4 + CD7 −]/ml)

Stage Classification of Mycosis Fungoides			
IA	T1	N0	M0
IB	T2	N0	M0
IIA	T1–2	N1	M0
IIB	T3	N0–1	M0
IIIA	T4	N0	M0
IIIB	T4	N1	M0
IVA	T1–4	N2–3	M0
IVB	T1–4	N0–3	M1

Spleen involvement is demonstrated by unequivocal palpable splenomegaly alone, by equivocal palpable splenomegaly with radiologic confirmation (ultrasound or CT), or by either enlargement or multiple focal defects that are neither cystic nor vascular (radiologic enlargement alone is inadequate).

Liver involvement is demonstrated by multiple focal defects that are neither cystic nor vascular. Clinical enlargement alone, with or without abnormalities of liver function tests, is not adequate. Liver biopsy may be used to confirm the presence of liver involvement in a patient with abnormal liver function tests or when imaging assessment is equivocal.

Lung involvement is demonstrated by radiologic evidence of parenchymal involvement in the absence of other likely causes, especially infection. Lung biopsy may be performed to clarify equivocal cases.

Bone involvement is demonstrated using appropriate imaging studies.

CNS involvement is demonstrated by (a) a spinal intradural deposit or spinal cord or meningeal involvement, which may be diagnosed on the basis of the clinical history and findings supported by plain radiology, CSF examination, myelography, CT, and/or MRI (spinal extradural deposits should be carefully assessed, because they may be the result of soft tissue disease that represents extension from bone metastasis or disseminated disease) and (b) intracranial involvement, which will rarely be diagnosed clinically at presentation. It should be considered on the basis of a space-occupying lesion in the face of disease in additional extranodal sites.

Bone marrow involvement is assessed by an aspiration and bone marrow biopsy.

International Prognostic Index (IPI).   The International Non-Hodgkin Lymphoma Prognostic Factors Project used pretreatment prognostic factors in a sample of several thousand patients with aggressive lymphomas treated with doxorubicin-based combination chemotherapy to develop a predictive model of outcome for aggressive non-Hodgkin lymphoma. On the basis of factors identified in multivariate analysis of the above data set, the International Prognostic Index (Table 48.4) was proposed. Five pretreatment characteristics were found to be independent statistically significant factors: age in years (60 vs. >60); tumor stage I or II (localized) versus III or IV (advanced); number of extranodal sites of involvement (1 vs. >1); patient's performance status (0 or 1 vs. >2); and serum LDH level (normal vs. abnormal). With the use of these five pretreatment risk factors, patients could be assigned to one of the four risk groups on the basis of the number of presenting risk factors: low (0 or 1), low intermediate (2), high intermediate (3), and high (4 or 5). When patients were analyzed by risk factors, they were found to have very different outcomes with regard to complete response (CR), relapse-free survival (RFS), and overall survival (OS) (Fig. 48.1–48.7). The outcomes indicated that the low-risk patients had an 87% CR rate and an OS rate of 73% at 5 years in contrast to a 44% CR rate and 26% 5-year survival in patients in the high-risk group. A similar pattern of decreasing survival with a number of adverse factors was observed when younger patients only were considered. The IPI was useful in indolent lymphomas, and the validity of the IPI has been confirmed in a population of patients with T-cell lymphomas.

HODGKIN LYMPHOMA

A TNM classification system for Hodgkin lymphoma is not practical. Because Hodgkin lymphoma arises in lymph nodes and usually spreads in a contiguous fashion to the other lymph nodes and ultimately to visceral sites or bone marrow, the concepts of T and N classifications cannot be applied. On the other hand, the Ann Arbor classification system has served oncology well, with only minor modifications, since its introduction in 1971. Two major innovations of the Ann Arbor system were the concept

TABLE 48.4. Risk Factors in the International Prognostic Index

Age ≥60 years

Ann Arbor Stage III or IV

Elevated LDH

Reduced performance status (such as ECOG ≥2)

≥ Extranodal sites of disease

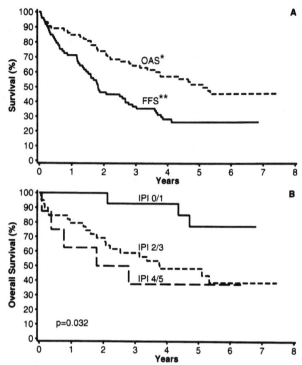

*OAS: Overall Survival
**FFS: Failure Free Survival

Fig 48.1. B-cell chronic lymphocytic leukemia/small lymphocytic lymphoma (B-cell CLL/SLL)

of localized extralymphatic disease (the E designation) and the incorporation of pathologic, as well as clinical, staging into the final stage designation. The E designation remains an important concept, although a precise definition has been elusive. Surgical (laparotomy) staging is now only rarely performed in Hodgkin lymphoma, so the important distinction of clinical versus pathologic staging no longer exists. On the other hand, there is now wide acceptance that the concept of "bulky" disease, especially as it applies to the extent of disease in the mediastinum, is important in staging, because it affects prognosis and treatment selection.

STAGING

Staging is based on the result of multiple clinical evaluations, including history, physical examination, blood analysis, imaging studies, the initial biopsy report, and other biopsies as indicated.

The E Lesion. The Ann Arbor system defined E as extralymphatic. Disease in sites such as Waldeyer's ring, the thymus, and the spleen, although

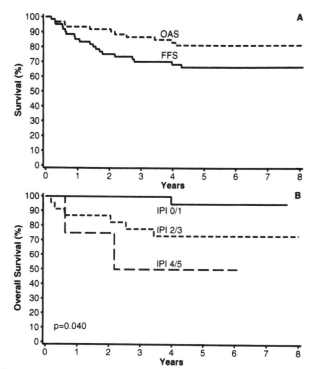

Fig 48.2. Extranodal marginal-zone B-cell lymphoma of mucosa-associated lymphoid tissues (MALT) type (MALT lymphoma)

extranodal, is not extralymphatic and therefore is not considered to be an E lesion. However, the distinction between certain presentations of extralymphatic disease versus Stage IV disease is not explicit in the Ann Arbor system. For the purpose of this revised AJCC staging system, an E lesion is defined as disease that involves extralymphatic site(s) adjacent to site(s) of lymphatic involvement but in which direct extension is not necessarily demonstrable.

Examples of E lesions include extension into pulmonary parenchyma from adjacent pulmonary hilar or mediastinal lymph nodes; extension into the anterior chest wall *and* into the pericardium from a large mediastinal mass (two areas of extralymphatic involvement); involvement of the iliac bone in the presence of adjacent iliac lymph node involvement; involvement of a lumbar vertebral body in conjunction with para-aortic lymph node involvement; involvement of the pleura as an extension from adjacent internal mammary nodes; and involvement of the thyroid with adjacent cervical lymph node involvement. A pleural or pericardial effusion with negative (or unknown) cytology is not an E lesion.

Lymph Node Involvement. For the purpose of staging, lymph node involvement includes disease affecting lymph nodes in any of the major

12

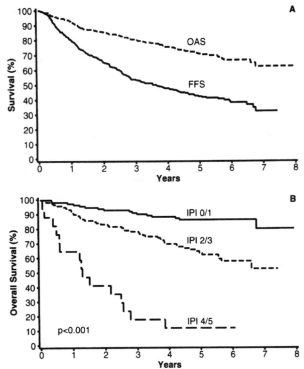

Fig 48.3. Follicular lymphoma

lymph node regions. This may be based on physical examination, imaging studies, or biopsy.

A modification of the Ann Arbor system is to include the "infra-clavicular" region as a part of the axilla, because anatomic landmarks separating these two regions are difficult to define. Other lymphatic structures include the spleen, appendix, Peyer's patches, Waldeyer's ring (the lymphatic tissue of the tonsils, oropharynx, and nasopharynx), and thymus.

Spleen Involvement. Involvement of the spleen is accepted if there is evidence of one or more nodule(s) in the spleen, of any size, on imaging evaluation or if there is histologic involvement documented by biopsy or splenectomy. Splenic enlargement alone (indicated by physical examination or imaging study) is insufficient to support a diagnosis of splenic involvement. Splenic involvement is designated by the letter S.

Hepatic Involvement. Involvement of the liver is accepted if there is evidence of one or more nodule(s) in the liver, of any size, on imaging evaluation or if there is histologic involvement documented by biopsy. Hepatic enlargement alone (indicated by physical examination or imaging

---

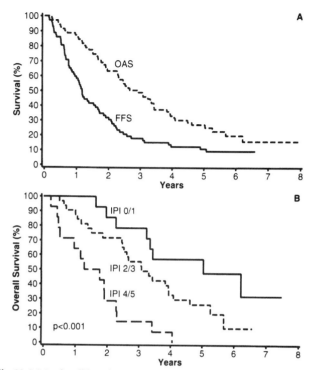

Fig 48.4. Mantle cell lymphoma

study) is insufficient to support a diagnosis of liver involvement. Hepatic involvement is designated by the letter H. Liver involvement is always considered as diffuse extralymphatic disease (Stage IV).

Bone Marrow Involvement.   Suspected bone marrow involvement must be documented by biopsy from a clinically/radiographically uninvolved area of bone. Bone marrow involvement is designated by the letter M. Bone marrow involvement is always considered as diffuse extralymphatic disease (Stage IV).

Lung Involvement.   Lung involvement (one or more lobes) that represents extension from adjacent mediastinal or hilar lymph nodes is considered extralymphatic extension (E lesion). Pulmonary nodular disease (any number of nodules) is considered as diffuse extralymphatic disease (Stage IV). Lung involvement is designated by the letter L.

Detailed Site Information.   Details of specific sites involved are designated by letter subscripts. When the involved sites have been documented by biopsy, a plus (+) sign is added following the letter subscript. If a biopsy has been performed but the tissue/organ is uninvolved, a minus

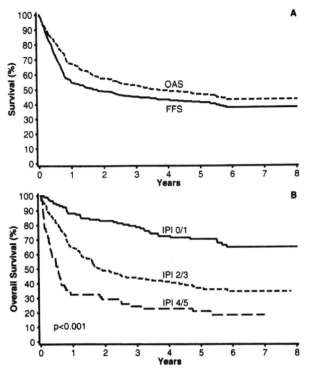

Fig 48.5. Diffuse large B-cell lymphoma

(−) sign is added following the letter subscript. If the tissue/organ is involved clinically but a biopsy has not been performed, neither a plus nor a minus sign is added.

Spleen	S
Pulmonary (lung)	L
Bone marrow	M
Hepatic	H
Pericardium	Pcard
Pleura	P
Waldeyer's (tonsil, naso-oropharynx)	W
Osseous (bone)	O
Gastrointestinal	GI
Skin	D
Soft tissue	Softis
Thyroid	Thy

Stages. Stage I: Involvement of a single lymph node region (I); or localized involvement of a single extralymphatic organ or site in the absence of any lymph node involvement (IE) (rare in Hodgkin lymphoma).

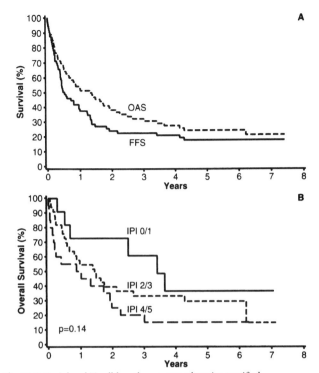

Fig 48.6. Peripheral T-cell lymphoma, not otherwise specified

Stage II: Involvement of two or more lymph node regions on the same side of the diaphragm (II); or localized involvement of a single extralymphatic organ or site in association with regional lymph node involvement with or without involvement of other lymph node regions on the same side of the diaphragm (IIE). The number of regions involved may be indicated by a subscript, as in, for example, II_3.

Stage III: Involvement of lymph node regions on both sides of the diaphragm (III), which also may be accompanied by extralymphatic extension in association with adjacent lymph node involvement (IIIE) or by involvement of the spleen (IIIS) or both (IIIE,S).

Stage IV: Diffuse or disseminated involvement of one or more extralymphatic organs, with or without associated lymph node involvement; or isolated extralymphatic organ involvement in the absence of adjacent regional lymph node involvement, but in conjunction with disease in distant site(s); or any involvement of the liver or bone marrow, or nodular involvement of the lung(s). The location of Stage IV disease is identified further by specifying the site according to the notations listed above.

Bulky Mediastinal Disease. The extent of mediastinal disease is defined by a ratio between the maximum single width of the mediastinal mass on

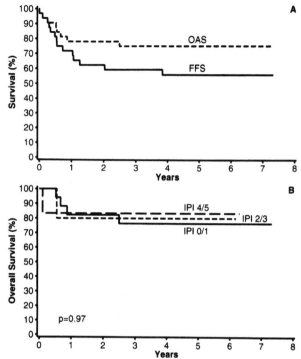

Fig 48.7. Anaplastic large T-cell lymphoma, primary systemic type

a standing PA chest radiograph and the maximum intrathoracic diameter on the same radiograph. A ratio greater than or equal to l/3 defines a large (bulky) mediastinal mass. The presence of a large mediastinal mass is designated by the subscript letter X. The presence of bulky disease in locations other than the mediastinum is not identified.

A and B Classification (Symptoms). Each stage should be classified as either A or B according to the absence or presence of defined constitutional symptoms. These are

1. *Fevers.* Unexplained fever with temperature above 38°C.
2. *Night sweats.* Drenching sweats that require change of bedclothes.
3. *Weight loss.* Unexplained weight loss of more than 10% of the usual body weight in the 6 months prior to diagnosis.

Note: Pruritus alone does not qualify for B classification, nor does alcohol intolerance, fatigue, or a short, febrile illness associated with suspected infections.

Examples. Involvement of the mediastinum and bilateral supraclavicular regions only. The mediastinal mass ratio is 0.25. Weight loss is 15 pounds (usual weight 125 pounds). Bone marrow is involved on biopsy. Stage II_3B_M

Involvement of the mediastinum and bilateral supraclavicular regions. The mediastinal mass ratio is 0.4. There is clinical extension of disease into the anterior chest wall and onto the pericardium. There are no constitutional symptoms. Stage II$_{3XE}$A$_{Pcard, softis}$

Involvement of the right tonsil and right cervical/supraclavicular nodes only. There are no constitutional symptoms. Stage II$_2$A

Involvement of the right cervical/supraclavicular nodes, Para-aortic nodes and spleen. Unexplained fevers to 39°C. A bone marrow biopsy demonstrates involvement. Stage IV$_3$B$_{M+}$

Involvement of the right supraclavicular, mediastinal (ratio = 0.30), and right hilar lymph nodes with extension into the pulmonary parenchyma of the right lung. No constitutional symptoms are present. A bone marrow biopsy indicates no involvement. Stage II$_{3E}$A$_{L,M-}$

Involvement of the right supraclavicular, mediastinal (ratio = 0.30), and right hilar lymph nodes with a pulmonary nodule in the right middle lobe. No constitutional symptoms are present. A bone marrow biopsy indicates no involvement. Stage IV$_3$A$_{L,M-}$

Involvement of bilateral supraclavicular and mediastinal lymph nodes and spleen. No constitutional symptoms are present (ratio = 0.42). A bone marrow biopsy indicates no involvement. Stage III$_{3X}$A$_{S,M-}$

MULTIPLE MYELOMA

Multiple myeloma is a neoplastic disorder characterized by the proliferation of a single clone of plasma cells derived from B-cells. This clone of plasma cells grows in the bone marrow and frequently invades the adjacent bone, producing skeletal destruction that results in bone pain and fractures. Other common clinical findings include anemia, hypercalcemia, and renal insufficiency. Recurrent bacterial infections and bleeding can occur, but the hyperviscosity syndrome is rare. The clone of plasma cells produces monoclonal (M-protein) of IgG or IgM and rarely IgD or IgE or free monoclonal light chains (kappa or lambda) (Bence Jones protein). The diagnosis depends on identification of monoclonal plasma cells in the bone marrow, M-protein in the serum or urine, osteolytic lesions, and a consistent clinical picture with multiple myeloma.

RULES FOR CLASSIFICATION

Diagnosis. Minimal criteria for the diagnosis of multiple myeloma includes a bone marrow containing more than 10% plasma cells or a plasmacytoma plus at least one of the following: (1) an M-protein in the serum (usually > 3 g/dL), (2) an M-protein in the urine, or (3) lytic bone lesions. In addition, the patient must have the usual clinical features of multiple myeloma. Metastatic carcinoma, lymphoma, leukemia, and connective tissue disorders must be excluded in the differential diagnosis. In addition, monoclonal gammopathy of undetermined significance (MGUS) and smoldering multiple myeloma (SMM) must be excluded. MGUS is characterized by the absence of symptoms, M-protein < 3 g/dL, fewer than 10% plasma cells in the bone marrow, and no lytic lesions, anemia,

12

hypercalcemia, or renal insufficiency. Smoldering multiple myeloma is characterized by an M-protein > 3 g/dL and > 10% plasma cells in the bone marrow. These patients have no lytic lesions, anemia, or hypercalcemia. The plasma cell labeling index is helpful in differentiating MGUS and SMM from multiple myeloma. An elevated plasma cell labeling index (PCLI) is a strong indication of active multiple myeloma. However, 40% of patients with symptomatic multiple myeloma have a normal PCLI. Monoclonal plasma cells of the same isotype can be detected in the peripheral blood of 80% of patients with active multiple myeloma. Circulating plasma cells either are absent or are present in only small numbers in MGUS and SMM.

Staging. The Durie-Salmon staging system has been utilized for the past 25 years. Stage I requires hemoglobin > 10.0 g/dL, serum calcium ≤ 12 mg/dL, normal bone X-rays or a solitary bone lesion, IgG < 5 g/dL, IgA < 3 g/dL, and urine M-protein < 4 g/24 h. Stage III includes one or more of the following: hemoglobin < 8.5 g/dL, serum calcium > 12 mg/dL, advanced lytic bone lesions, IgG > 7 g/dL, IgA > 5 g/dL, or urine M-protein > 12 g/24 h. Stage II patients fit neither Stage I nor Stage III. Patients are further subclassed as (A) serum creatinine < 2.0 mg/dL and (B) serum creatinine ≥ 2.0 mg/dL. The median survival is approximately 5 years for those with Stage IA disease and is 15 months for those with Stage IIIB disease. This system primarily measures tumor cell burden and has major limitations. Other staging systems have been proposed, but utilization of independent prognostic factors is more useful.

PROGNOSTIC FACTORS

The plasma cell labeling index (PCLI) and beta-2 microglobulin values are the most important prognostic factors. The PCLI is a measurement of the proliferative activity of the plasma cells in myeloma. The monoclonal antibody (BU-1) that reacts with 5-bromo-2-deoxyuridine identifies the cells that synthesize DNA. This antibody does not require denaturation, so fluorescence-conjugated immunoglobulin antisera (kappa and lambda) identify monoclonal plasma cells and plasmacytoid lymphocytes. The high PCLI predicts poor overall and progression-free survival. In multivariate analysis, the PCLI has consistently demonstrated independent prognostic value. Most investigators use a cutoff PCLI value of 1%.

Beta-2 microglobulin correlates with the myeloma tumor burden. A high value predicts poor survival following both conventional chemotherapy and autologous stem cell transplantation. Cytogenetic abnormalities are of major prognostic significance in multiple myeloma. Abnormalities that involve chromosome 11 or 13 and translocations are the most unfavorable prognostic features. Conventional cytogenetics detects abnormalities in only 40% of patients, whereas fluorescence *in situ* hybridization (FISH) demonstrates abnormalities in approximately 80% of patients. CRP (C-reactive protein) is an acute phase reactant and has been used as a surrogate for measurement for Il-6 levels. Il-6 is a potent growth factor for plasma cells. Soluble interleukin-6 receptor (SII-6R) is an independent predictor of a poor outcome in multiple myeloma. Lactate dehydrogenase

(LDH), when elevated, is an important prognostic factor indicating progressive disease. However, fewer than 10% of patients with multiple myeloma have an elevated LDH level.

Plasmablastic Morphology.   The presence of 2% or more plasmablasts in the bone marrow is an unfavorable prognostic factor. In addition, the presence of $> 3 \times 10^6$ circulating plasma cells in the peripheral blood is associated with a poor prognosis. Bone marrow angiogenesis is increased in multiple myeloma and represents a prognostic factor. The degree of angiogenesis can be determined by using immunohistochemical staining for factor VIII–related antigen to identify microvessels. The overall survival is significantly longer in patients with low-grade angiogenesis compared to those with high-grade angiogenesis. The expression of K-ras gene is associated with a shorter median survival than is observed in patients with N-ras mutations. Other findings that affect survival are age, hemoglobin value, degree of renal insufficiency, plasma cell content of the bone marrow, and level of CD19 + or CD4 + cells in the peripheral blood.

PEDIATRIC LYMPHOID MALIGNANCY

Diagnosis.   Children with NHL usually have Burkitt lymphoma, lymphoblastic lymphoma, or diffuse large B-cell lymphoma. The diagnosis of NHL is most readily established by examination of tissue obtained by open biopsy of the involved area. Histologic, immunophenotypic, cytogenetic, and molecular studies are all helpful in confirming the diagnosis. In cases where the patient is too unstable for general anesthesia, as in the case of a child with a large anterior mediastinal mass, a fine-needle aspiration of the mass may be sufficient to establish the diagnosis. Bone marrow and cerebrospinal fluid examination should be performed early in the workup of a child with suspected NHL, because they may be diagnostic and may preclude the need for more invasive procedures.

Workup.   The workup of a child with newly diagnosed NHL should include a history and physical examination, a complete blood count, and a chemistry panel. Diagnostic imaging studies should include CT scans of chest, abdomen, and pelvis and a bone scan. A gallium scan may be helpful in evaluating residual masses. MRI of the base of the skull should be considered in children with cranial nerve palsies. Examination of the cerebrospinal fluid and bone marrow (bilateral iliac crest bone marrow aspiration and biopsy) should be performed in all patients.

Upon completion of the foregoing workup, the child is usually assigned a disease stage according to the St. Jude system described by Murphy (Table 48.5), which was designed to accommodate the noncontiguous nature of disease spread, predominant extranodal involvement, and involvement of the central nervous system and bone marrow that characterize the pediatric NHLs. Stages I and II are considered to represent limited stage disease, whereas Stages III and IV are considered advanced stages.

12

TABLE 48.5. St. Jude Staging System

Stage I

A single tumor (extranodal) or single anatomic area (nodal), with the exclusion of mediastinum or abdomen

Stage II

A single tumor (extranodal) with regional node involvement

Two or more nodal areas on the same side of the diaphragm

Two single (extranodal) tumors with or without regional node involvement on the same side of the diaphragm

A primary gastrointestinal tract tumor, usually in the ileocecal area, with or without involvement of associated mesenteric nodes only*

Stage III

Two single tumors (extranodal) on opposite sides of the diaphragm

Two or more nodal areas above and below the diaphragm

All primary intrathoracic tumors (mediastinal, pleural, thymic)

All extensive primary intra-abdominal disease*

All paraspinal or epidural tumors, regardless of other tumor site(s)

Stage IV

Any of the above with initial CNS and/or bone marrow involvement**

*A distinction is made between apparently localized GI tract lymphoma and more extensive intra-abdominal disease because of their quite different patterns of survival after appropriate therapy. Stage II disease typically is limited to segment of the gut plus or minus the associated mesenteric nodes only, and the primary tumor can be completely removed grossly by segmental excision. Stage III disease typically exhibits spread to para-aortic and retroperitoneal areas by implants and plaques in mesentery or peritoneum, or by direct infiltration of structures adjacent to the primary tumor. Ascites may be present, and complete resection of all gross tumor is not possible.

**If the marrow involvement is present initially, the number of abnormal cells must be 25% or less in an otherwise normal marrow aspirate with a normal peripheral blood picture.

BIBLIOGRAPHY

Armitage JO, Weisenburger D for the Non-Hodgkin's Lymphoma Classification Project. New approach to classifying non-Hodgkin's lymphomas: clinical features of the major histologic subtypes. J Clin Oncol 16:2780–2795, 1998

Carbone PP, Kaplan HS, Musshoff K, et al: Report of the committee on Hodgkin's disease staging classification. Cancer Res 31:1860–1861, 1971

Durie BGM, Salmon SE. A clinical staging system for multiple myeloma: correlation of measured myeloma cell mass with presenting clinical features, response to treatment, and survival. Cancer 36:842, 1975

Greipp PR, Lust JA, O'Fallon WM, et al: Plasma cell labeling index and beta2-microglobulin predict survival independent of thymidine kinase and C-reactive protein in multiple myeloma. Blood 81:3382, 1993

Harris NL, Jaffe ES, Stein H, et al: A revised European–American classification of lymphoid neoplasms: A proposal from the International Lymphoma Study Group. Blood 84:1361–1392, 1994

Jaffe ES, Harris NL, Stein H, Vardiman JW (Eds.): World Health Organization Classification of Tumours. Pathology and Genetics of Tumours of Haematopoietic and Lymphoid Tissues. IARC Press: Lyon 2001.

The International Non-Hodgkin's Lymphoma Prognostic Factors Project: A predictive model for aggressive non-Hodgkin's lymphoma. N Engl J Med 329:987–994, 1993

Lister T, Crowther D, Sutcliffe S, et al: Report of a committee convened to discuss the evaluation and staging of patients with Hodgkin's disease: Cotswolds meeting. J Clin Oncol 7:1630, 1989

Murphy S, Fairclough D, Hutchison R, et al: NHL of childhood. An analysis of the histology, staging and response to treatment of 338 cases at a single institution. J Clin Oncol 7:186, 1989

The Non-Hodgkin's Lymphoma Classification Project: A clinical evaluation of the International Lymphoma Study Group classification of non-Hodgkin's lymphoma. Blood 89:3909–3918, 1997

HISTOLOGIES—LYMPHOID NEOPLASMS

9590/3	Malignant lymphoma, NOS
9591/3	Malignant lymphoma, non-Hodgkin, NOS
9596/3	Composite Hodgkin and non-Hodgkin lymphoma
9650/3	Hodgkin lymphoma, NOS
9651/3	Hodgkin lymphoma, lymphocyte-rich
9652/3	Hodgkin lymphoma, mixed cellularity, NOS
9653/3	Hodgkin lymphoma, lymphocyte depletion, NOS
9654/3	Hodgkin lymphoma, lymphocyte depletion, diffuse fibrosis
9655/3	Hodgkin lymphoma, lymphocyte depletion, reticular
9659/3	Hodgkin lymphoma, nodular lymphocyte predominance
9661/3	Hodgkin granuloma
9662/3	Hodgkin sarcoma
9663/3	Hodgkin lymphoma, nodular sclerosis, NOS
9664/3	Hodgkin lymphoma, nodular sclerosis, cellular phase
9665/3	Hodgkin lymphoma, nodular sclerosis, grade 1
9667/3	Hodgkin lymphoma, nodular sclerosis, grade 2
9670/3	Malignant lymphoma, small B lymphocytic, NOS
9671/3	Malignant lymphoma, lymphoplasmacytic
9673/3	Mantle cell lymphoma
9675/3	Malignant lymphoma, mixed small and large cell, diffuse
9678/3	Primary effusion lymphoma
9679/3	Mediastinal large B-cell lymphoma
9680/3	Malignant lymphoma, large B-cell, diffuse, NOS
9684/3	Malignant lymphoma, large B-cell, diffuse, immunoblastic, NOS
9687/3	Burkitt lymphoma, NOS
9689/3	Splenic marginal zone B-cell lymphoma
9690/3	Follicular lymphoma, NOS
9691/3	Follicular lymphoma, grade 2
9695/3	Follicular lymphoma, grade 1
9698/3	Follicular lymphoma, grade 3
9699/3	Marginal zone B-cell lymphoma, NOS
9700/3	Mycosis fungoides
9701/3	Sezary syndrome
9702/3	Mature T-cell lymphoma, NOS
9705/3	Angioimmunoblastic T-cell lymphoma
9708/3	Subcutaneous panniculitis-like T-cell lymphoma
9709/3	Cutaneous T-cell lymphoma, NOS
9714/3	Anaplastic large cell lymphoma, T-cell and Null cell type
9716/3	Hepatosplenic γδ (gamma-delta) cell lymphoma
9717/3	Intestinal T-cell lymphoma

12

HISTOLOGIES—LYMPHOID NEOPLASMS (CONT.)

9718/3	Primary cutaneous CD30+ T-cell lymphoproliferative disorder
9719/3	NK/T-cell lymphoma, nasal and nasal-type
9727/3	Precursor cell lymphoblastic lymphoma, NOS
9728/3	Precursor cell lymphoblastic lymphoma, NOS
9728/3	Precursor B-cell lymphoblastic lymphoma
9729/3	Precursor T-cell lymphoblastic lymphoma

PART XIII
Personnel
and Contributors

13

Current Members of the Full Committee of the American Joint Committee on Cancer (2001–2002)

Frederick L. Greene, M.D., *Chair**

David L. Page, M.D., *Vice-Chair**

Charles M. Balch, M.D.*

Michael L. Blute, M.D.

Blake Cady, M.D.

William G. Cance, M.D.

Carolyn C. Compton, M.D.

Myles P. Cunningham, M.D.*

Stephen B. Edge, M.D.

Irvin D. Fleming, M.D.*

April G. Fritz, C.T.R., R.H.I.T.

H. Irene Hall, Ph.D.

Daniel G. Haller, M.D.*

Elizabeth H. Hammond, M.D.

Nancy C. Jackson, C.T.R.

Vencine Kelly, C.T.R.

Nancy C. Lee, M.D.

Raymond E. Lenhard, Jr., M.D.

John R. Lurain III, M.D.

Robert J. Mayer, M.D.

Mack Roach, III, M.D.*

John C. Ruckdeschel, M.D.

David S. Schrump, M.D.

Stephen F. Sener, M.D.

Sudhir Srivastava, Ph.D., M.P.H.*

Joel E. Tepper, M.D.

James Brantley Thrasher, M.D.

Andrea Trotti, III, M.D.

Donald L. Trump, M.D.

Thomas K. Weber, M.D.

Phyllis Wingo, Ph.D.*

W. Douglas Wong, M.D.*

---

*Current members of the AJCC Executive Committee

13

Sixth Edition Site Task Forces

BONE

*Michael A. Simon, M.D., Chair
University of Chicago
Chicago, Illinois

Lee J. Helman, M.D.
National Cancer Institute
Bethesda, Maryland

Mark Krailo, Ph.D.
University of Southern California
Arcadia, California

Brian O'Sullivan, M.D.
Princess Margaret Hospital
Toronto, Canada

Shreyaskumar Patel, M.D.
M. D. Anderson Cancer Center
Houston, Texas

Theola K. Rarick, C.T.R.
University of Iowa Hospital &
    Clinics
Iowa City, Iowa

Andrew Rosenberg, M.D.
Massachusetts General Hospital
Boston, Massachusetts

Murali Sundaram, M.D.
St. Louis University Medical Center
St. Louis, Missouri

BREAST

*Sonja Eva Singletary, M.D., Chair
M. D. Anderson Cancer Center
Houston, Texas

Craig Allred, M.D.
Baylor College of Medicine
Houston, Texas

Pandora Ashley, C.T.R.
Scott and White Memorial Hospital
Temple, Texas

Larry Bassett, M.D.
University of California—Los
    Angeles
Los Angeles, California

Donald Berry, Ph.D.
M. D. Anderson Cancer Center
Houston, Texas

Kirby I. Bland, M.D.
University of Alabama—
    Birmingham
Birmingham, Alabama

Patrick I. Borgen, M.D.
Memorial Sloan-Kettering Cancer
    Center
New York, New York

Gary M. Clark, Ph.D.
Baylor College of Medicine
Houston, Texas

Stephen B. Edge, M.D.
Roswell Park Cancer Institute
Buffalo, New York

Daniel F. Hayes, M.D.
University of Michigan
Ann Arbor, Michigan

Lorie L. Hughes, M.D.
Kennestone Hospital
Atlanta, Georgia

Robert V. P. Hutter, M.D.
Livingston, New Jersey

13

David L. Page, M.D.
Vanderbilt University School of
Medicine
Nashville, Tennessee

Abram Recht, M.D.
Beth Israel Deaconess Medical
Center
Boston, Massachusetts

Richard L. Theriault, D.O.
M. D. Anderson Cancer Center
Houston, Texas

Ann Thor, M.D.
Northwestern University Evanston
Hospital
Evanston, Illinois

Donald L. Weaver, M.D.
Fletcher Allen Health Care
Burlington, Vermont

H. Samuel Wieand, Ph.D.
National Surgical Adjuvant Breast
and Bowel Project
Pittsburgh, Pennsylvania

CENTRAL NERVOUS SYSTEM

*Edward R. Laws, Jr., M.D., Chair
University of Virginia Health
Sciences Center
Charlottesville, Virginia

Howard Fine, M.D.
National Cancer Institute
Bethesda, Maryland

Minesh Mehta, M.D.
University of Wisconsin Hospital
Madison, Wisconsin

Angel Morris, R.N., B.S.N.
University of Virginia Health
Sciences Center
Charlottesville, Virginia

Bernd Scheithauer, M.D.
Mayo Clinic
Rochester, Minnesota

Charles Scott, Ph.D.
American College of Radiology
Philadelphia, Pennsylvania

Linda R. Taylor, C.T.R.
University of New Mexico
Health Sciences Center
Albuquerque, New Mexico

COLORECTAL

J. Milburn Jessup, M.D., Chair
Georgetown University School of
Medicine
Washington, D.C.

Leonard Gunderson, M.D., Vice-
Chair
Mayo Clinic
Rochester, Minnesota

Jaffer Ajani, M.D.
M. D. Anderson Cancer Center
Houston, Texas

Robert W. Beart, Jr., M.D.
University of Southern California
Los Angeles, California

Jacqueline Benedetti, Ph.D.
Southwest Oncology Group
Seattle, Washington

Al B. Benson III, M.D.
Northwestern University Medical
Center
Chicago, Illinois

Alfred M. Cohen, M.D.
Lucille P. Markey Cancer Center
Lexington, Kentucky

Carolyn C. Compton, M.D.
McGill University
Montréal, Canada

Richard Goldberg, M.D.
Mayo Clinic
Rochester, Minnesota

Frederick L. Greene, M.D.
Carolinas Medical Center
Charlotte, North Carolina

Daniel G. Haller, M.D.
University of Pennsylvania Health
System
Philadelphia, Pennsylvania

Stanley R. Hamilton, M.D.
M. D. Anderson Cancer Center
Houston, Texas

Vencine Kelly, C.T.R.
Stony Brook University Hospital
Stony Brook, New York

Bruce D. Minsky, M.D.
Memorial Sloan-Kettering Cancer
　Center
New York, New York

Heidi Nelson, M.D.
Mayo Clinic
Rochester, Minnesota

Stephen Rubesin, M.D.
University of Pennsylvania
Philadelphia, Pennsylvania

Leslie H. Sobin, M.D.
Armed Forces Institute of Pathology
Washington, D.C.

Mark Lane Welton, M.D.
University of California—San
　Francisco
San Francisco, California

DIGESTIVE

*Douglas B. Evans, M.D., Chair
M. D. Anderson Cancer Center
Houston, Texas

Paul Catalano, S.C.D.
Dana Farber Cancer Institute
Boston, Massachusetts

Chuslip Charnsangavej, M.D.
M. D. Anderson Cancer Center
Houston, Texas

Carlos Fernandez-del Castillo, M.D.
Massachusetts General Hospital
Boston, Massachusetts

Yuman Fong, M.D.
Memorial Sloan-Kettering Cancer
　Center
New York, New York

Gregory Y. Lauwers, M.D.
Massachusetts General Hospital
Boston, Massachusetts

John MacDonald, M.D.
St. Vincent's Medical Center
New York, New York

Eileen M. O'Reilly, M.D.
Memorial Sloan-Kettering Cancer
　Center
New York, New York

Susan E. Pater, C.T.R., R.H.I.T.
Children's Hospital Medical Center
Cincinnati, Ohio

Tyvin Rich, M.D.
University of Virginia
Health Sciences Center
Charlottesville, Virginia

J. Nicholas Vauthey, M.D.
M. D. Anderson Cancer Center
Houston, Texas

Mary Kay Washington, M.D.
Vanderbilt University Medical
　Center
Nashville, Tennessee

Christopher G. Willett, M.D.
Massachusetts General Hospital
Boston, Massachusetts

Christian Wittekind, M.D.
Institut für Patholgie der Universitat
Leipzig, Germany

Charles J. Yeo, M.D.
Johns Hopkins Hospital
Baltimore, Maryland

GENITOURINARY

*Ian M. Thompson, Jr., M.D., Chair
University of Texas Health Science
　Center
San Antonio, Texas

Gerald L. Andriole, M.D.
Washington University School of
　Medicine
St. Louis, Missouri

13

Brent Blumenstein, Ph.D.
American College of Surgeons
    Oncology Group
Durham, North Carolina

David G. Bostwick, M.D.
Bostwick Laboratories
Richmond, Virginia

Ruth Etzioni, Ph.D.
Fred Hutchinson Cancer Center
Seattle, Washington

Jeffrey Forman, M.D.
Harper Hospital Karmanos Cancer
    Center
Detroit, Michigan

Mary K. Gospodarowicz, M.D.
Princess Margaret Hospital
Toronto, Canada

Celestia Higano, M.D.
University of Washington Cancer
    Center
Seattle, Washington

Gary Miller, M.D.
University of Colorado Health
    Sciences Center
Denver, Colorado

James E. Montie, M.D.
University of Michigan
Ann Arbor, Michigan

Alan W. Partin, M.D.
Johns Hopkins Hospital
Baltimore, Maryland

Derek Raghavan, M.D.
University of Southern California
    Norris Comprehensive Cancer
    Center
Los Angeles, California

Mack Roach III, M.D.
University of California—San
    Francisco
San Francisco, California

Wael Sakr, M.D.
Wayne State University
Detroit, Michigan

Paul F. Schellhammer, M.D.
Eastern Virginia Graduate School of
    Medicine
Norfolk, Virginia

James Brantley Thrasher, M.D.
University of Kansas Medical Center
Kansas City, Kansas

Dennis Timony, C.T.R.
Mount Sinai Medical Center
New York, New York

Dean Troyer, M.D.
University of Texas Health Science
    Center—San Antonio
San Antonio, Texas

GYNECOLOGIC

*Howard W. Jones III, M.D., Chair
Vanderbilt University Medical
    Center
Nashville, Tennessee

Hervy E. Averette, M.D.
Sylvester Comprehensive Cancer
    Center
Miami, Florida

J. L. Benedet, M.D., F.R.C.S.C.
Vancouver General Hospital
Vancouver, Canada

Larry Copeland, M.D.
Ohio State University
Columbus, Ohio

Patricia J. Eifel, M.D.
M. D. Anderson Cancer Center
Houston, Texas

David M. Gershenson, M.D.
M. D. Anderson Cancer Center
Houston, Texas

Perry W. Grigsby, M.D.
Washington University School of
    Medicine
St. Louis, Missouri

Robert Kurman, M.D.
Johns Hopkins Hospital
Baltimore, Maryland

Helen Lewis, C.T.R.H.
Lee Moffitt Cancer Center
Tampa, Florida

Edward E. Partridge, M.D.
University of Alabama at
Birmingham
Birmingham, Alabama

Lynya Talley, Ph.D.
University of Alabama at
Birmingham
Birmingham, Alabama

Peyton T. Taylor Jr., M.D.
University of Virginia Health
Sciences Center
Charlottesville, Virginia

Charles W. Whitney, M.D.
Christiana Care
Newark, Delaware

HEAD AND NECK

*Jatin P. Shah, M.D., Chair
Memorial Sloan-Kettering Cancer
Center
New York, New York

K. Kian Ang, M.D.
M. D. Anderson Cancer Center
Houston, Texas

Arlene Forastiere, M.D.
Johns Hopkins Oncology Center
Baltimore, Maryland

Adam Garden, M.D.
M. D. Anderson Cancer Center
Houston, Texas

Henry T. Hoffman, M.D.
University of Iowa Hospitals and
Clinics
Iowa City, Iowa

J. Jack Lee, Ph.D.
M. D. Anderson Cancer Center
Houston, Texas

William Lydiatt, M.D.
Nebraska Medical Center
Omaha, Nebraska

Jesus E. Medina, M.D.
University of Oklahoma Health
Sciences Center
Oklahoma City, Oklahoma

Suresh Mukherji, M.D.
University of North Carolina
Chapel Hill, North Carolina

Martha E. Oliva, C.T.R., R.H.I.T.
Jackson Memorial Hospital
Miami, Florida

Brian O'Sullivan, M.D.
Princess Margaret Hospital
Toronto, Canada

Augusto Paulino, M.D.
University of Michigan
Ann Arbor, Michigan

Bhuvanesh Singh, M.D.
Memorial Sloan-Kettering Cancer
Center
New York, New York

Randal Weber, M.D.
University of Pennsylvania Health
System
Philadelphia, Pennsylvania

Ernest Weymuller, M.D.
University of Washington
Seattle, Washington

LUNG AND ESOPHAGUS

*Valerie W. Rusch, M.D., Chair
Memorial Sloan-Kettering Cancer
Center
New York, New York

Henry D. Appelman, M.D.
University of Michigan
Ann Arbor, Michigan

Roger Byhardt, M.D.
Clement J. Zablocki VA Medical
Center
Milwaukee, Wisconsin

Ms. Ellen Edry, C.T.R.
Lowell General Hospital
Lowell, Massachusetts

13

Laurie Gaspar, M.D.
University of Colorado Health
    Sciences Center
Denver, Colorado

Robert J. Ginsberg, M.D.
Toronto General Hospital
Toronto, Canada

James E. Herndon, II, Ph.D.
Duke University Medical Center
Durham, North Carolina

David H. Johnson, M.D.
Vanderbilt Ingram Cancer Center
Nashville, Tennessee

David P. Kelsen, M.D.
Memorial Sloan-Kettering Cancer
    Center
New York, New York

William Mackillop, M.D.
Kingston Regional Cancer Center
Kingston, Ontario, Canada

Steven J. Mentzer, M.D.
Brigham and Women's Hospital
Boston, Massachusetts

Mark B. Orringer, M.D.
Taubman Health Care Center
Ann Arbor, Michigan

Edward Patz, M.D.
Duke University Medical Center
Durham, North Carolina

William D. Travis, M.D.
Armed Forces Institute of Pathology
Washington, DC

Andrew Turrisi, M.D.
Medical University of South
    Carolina
Charleston, South Carolina

LYMPHOMA

*James O. Armitage, M.D., Chair
University of Nebraska Medical
    Center
Omaha, Nebraska

Fernando Cabanillas, M.D.
M. D. Anderson Cancer Center
Houston, Texas

Inez Evans, C.T.R., R.H.I.T.
Wake Forest University
Baptist Medical Center
Winston-Salem, North Carolina

Richard I. Fisher, M.D.
Loyola University Medical Center
Maywood, Illinois

Mary K. Gospodarowicz, M.D.
Princess Margaret Hospital
Toronto, Canada

Nancy Harris, M.D.
Massachusetts General Hospital
Boston, Massachusetts

Richard T. Hoppe, M.D.
Stanford University Hospital
Stanford, California

Robert A. Kyle, M.D.
Mayo Clinic
Rochester, Minnesota

Michael LeBlanc, Ph.D.
Southwest Oncology Group
Seattle, Washington

Andrew Lister, M.D.
St. Bartholomew's Hospital
London, England

John Sandlund, M.D.
St. Jude Children's Research
    Hospital
Memphis, Tennessee

Dennis D. Weisenburger, M.D.
University of Nebraska Medical
    Center
Omaha, Nebraska

John W. Yarbro, M.D.
University of Missouri
Columbia, Missouri

MELANOMA

*Charles M. Balch, M.D., Chair
Johns Hopkins Medical Institutions
Baltimore, Maryland

Michael B. Atkins, M.D.
Beth Israel Deaconess Medical
  Center
Boston, Massachusetts

Antonio C. Buzaid, M.D., Co-Chair,
  ad hoc member
Hospital Sirio Libanes Centro De
  Oncologia
São Paulo, Brazil

Natale Cascinelli, M.D., ad hoc
  member
Istituto Nazionale per lo Studio
Milan, Italy

Alistair Cochran, M.D., ad hoc
  member
University of California—Los
  Angeles
Los Angeles, California

Daniel G. Coit, M.D.
Memorial Sloan-Kettering Cancer
  Center
New York, New York

Jay S. Cooper, M.D., ad hoc member
New York University Medical
  Center
New York, New York

Lyn M. Duncan, M.D., ad hoc
  member
Massachusetts General Hospital
Boston, Massachusetts

Jeffrey E. Gershenwald, M.D.
M. D. Anderson Cancer Center
Houston, Texas

Alan Houghton, Jr., M.D., ad hoc
  member
Memorial Sloan-Kettering Cancer
  Center
New York, New York

Robert V. P. Hutter, M.D.
Livingston, New Jersey

John M. Kirkwood, M.D.
University of Pittsburgh
Pittsburgh, Pennsylvania

Kelly M. McMasters, M.D.
James Graham Brown Cancer
  Center
Louisville, Kentucky

Greg Menaker, M.D., ad hoc member
Evanston Northwestern Health
  Center
Skokie, Illinois

Martin C. Mihm, Jr., M.D.
Massachusetts General Hospital
Boston, Massachusetts

Donald L. Morton, M.D.
John Wayne Medical Institute
Santa Monica, California

Douglas Reintgen, M.D.
H. Lee Moffitt Cancer Center
Tampa, Florida

Merrick I. Ross, M.D.
M. D. Anderson Cancer Center
Houston, Texas

Arthur Sober, M.D.
Massachusetts General Hospital
Boston, Massachusetts

Seng-Jaw Soong, Ph.D.
University of Alabama at
  Birmingham
Birmingham, Alabama

John A. Thompson, M.D.
University of Washington Medical
  Center
Seattle, Washington

John F. Thompson, M.D., F.R.A.C.S.,
  ad hoc member
University of Sydney
Sydney Cancer Centre
Campertown, Australia

13

OPHTHALMIC

*Barrett Haik M.D., Chair
University of Tennessee at Memphis
Memphis, Tennessee

Maj. Darryl J. Ainbinder, M.D.
Madigan Army Medical Center
Tacoma, Washington

Patricia Jo Downing, C.T.R.
Deaconess Hospital
Oklahoma City, Oklahoma

Paul T. Finger, M.D.
The New York Ophthalmic
    Oncology Center
New York, New York

James C. Fleming, M.D.
University of Tennessee Health
    Science Center
Memphis, Tennessee

Hans E. Grossniklaus, M.D.
Emory University
Atlanta, Georgia

J. William Harbour, M.D.
Washington University School of
    Medicine
St. Louis, Missouri

Leonard M. Holbach, M.D.
University Erlangen-Nurenberg
Erlangen, Germany

Zeynel A. Karcioglu, M.D.
Tulane University Medical School
New Orleans, Louisiana

A. Linn Murphree, M.D.
Children's Hospital Los Angeles
Los Angeles, California

SOFT TISSUE SARCOMA

*Raphael E. Pollock, M.D., Chair
M. D. Anderson Cancer Center
Houston, Texas

Laurence H. Baker, D.O.
University of Michigan
    Comprehensive Cancer Center
Ann Arbor, Michigan

Brent Blumenstein, Ph.D.
American College of Surgeons
    Oncology Group
Duke University School of Medicine
Durham, North Carolina

Murray F. Brennan, M.D.
Memorial Sloan-Kettering Cancer
    Center
New York, New York

Tapas K. Das Gupta, M.D.
University of Illinois
Chicago, Illinois

Jeffrey S. Kneisl, M.D.
Carolinas Medical Center
Charlotte, North Carolina

Brian O'Sullivan, M.D.
Princess Margaret Hospital
Toronto, Canada

David Panicek, M.D.
Memorial Sloan-Kettering Cancer
    Center
New York, New York

Peter W. T. Pisters, M.D.
M. D. Anderson Cancer Center
Houston, Texas

Herman D. Suit, M.D., Ph.D.
Massachusetts General Hospital
Boston, Massachusetts

Carol S. Venuti, C.R.T., R.H.I.A.
Massachusetts General Hospital
Boston, Massachusetts

Sharon Weiss, M.D.
Emory University Hospital
Atlanta, Georgia

STATISTICAL

*Seng-Jaw Soong, Ph.D., Chair
University of Alabama at
    Birmingham
Birmingham, Alabama

Jacqueline Benedetti, Ph.D.
Southwest Oncology Group
Seattle, Washington

Donald Berry, M.D.
M. D. Anderson Cancer Center
Houston, Texas

Brent Blumenstein, Ph.D.
American College of Surgeons
    Oncology Group
Durham, North Carolina

Paul Catalano, S.C.D.
Dana Farber Cancer Institute
Boston, Massachusetts

Gary M. Clark, Ph.D.
Baylor College of Medicine
Houston, Texas

William Dupont, Ph.D.
Vanderbilt University Medical
    Center
Nashville, Tennessee

Ruth Etzioni, Ph.D.
Fred Hutchinson Cancer Center
Seattle, Washington

Benjamin F. Hankey, S.C.D.
SEER Program—National Cancer
    Institute
Rockville, Maryland

James E. Herndon II, Ph.D.
Duke University Medical Center
Durham, North Carolina

Mark Krailo, Ph.D.
University of Southern California
Arcadia, California

Michael LeBlanc, Ph.D.
Southwest Oncology Group
Seattle, Washington

J. Jack Lee, Ph.D.
M. D. Anderson Cancer Center
Houston, Texas

Charles Scott, Ph.D.
American College of Radiology
Philadelphia, Pennsylvania

Lynya Talley, Ph.D.
University of Alabama at
    Birmingham
Birmingham, Alabama

H. Samuel Wieand, Ph.D.
National Surgical Adjuvant Breast
    and Bowel Project
Pittsburgh, Pennsylvania

13

Index

A

Abdomen, 221. *See also* specific organs
Abdominal esophagus, 102
Acoustic/vestibular nerve, 417
Actinic keratoses, 232
Adamantinoma, 216
Adjusted survival rates, 20–21
Adnexa, 411
Alpha-fetoprotein, 147, 312, 343, 346
Alveolar ridges, 35
American Joint Committee on Cancer
    (AJCC)
    classification, 3
Ampulla of Vater, 164, 171
Anal canal, 139–144
Anaplastic astrocytoma, 417
Anaplastic carcinoma of the thyroid
    gland, 96
Anaplastic large T-cell lymphoma, 442
Angiosarcoma, 216
Ann Arbor staging system, 430–431,
    435–436
Anorectal lymph nodes, 140
Anterior mediastinum, 221
Anus, 139
Aortic lymph nodes, 192, 338, 356, 362
Aortopulmonary lymph nodes, 104
Appendix, 127
Armed Forces Institute of Pathology, 5
Articular cartilage, 213
Aryepiglottic folds, 47, 62
Arytenoids, 62
Atlas of Tumor Pathology, 5
Autonomic nervous system, 221
Autopsy classification, 8
Axillary lymph nodes, 258–259, 273, 274

B

Barrett's esophagus, 106
Basal cell carcinomas, 232
B-cell lymphocytic leukemia/small
    lymphocytic lymphoma (B-cell
    CLL/SLL), 436
B-cell neoplasms, 430
Beta-2 microglobulin, 444
Bile ducts, extrahepatic, 163–164
Bile ducts, intrahepatic, 145
Biliary tract, 163

Bladder, 367
Bladder, urinary, 367–370
Bone, 213–219
Brain, 417–423
Brain stem, 417
Brain stem glioma, 417
Breast, 257–274
Breast cancer
    outcomes, 270
    SEER data, 17, 18, 19, 20
    survival rates, 272–277, 276
Bronchus, main, 191
BU-1 monoclonal antibody, 444
Buccal mucosa, 35
Buccinator lymph nodes, 28

C

CA-125, 312
Carcinomas
    anal canal, 142
    cervical, 297
    conjunctival, 387–390
    eyelid, 383–386
    hepatocellular, 151
    lacrimal gland, 407–409
    ovarian, 307, 313
    prostatic, 378
    skin, 231–237
    stomach, 109–116
    thyroid gland, 93–96
    uterine, 304
    vaginal, 291
    vulvar, 287
Cardia, 111
Cauda equina, 417
Caval lymph nodes, 146
Cecum, 127, 129
Celiac lymph nodes, 104, 156, 164–165
Censored cases, 16
Central nervous system, 417–423
Central neurocytoma, 417
C-erbB-2, 217
Cerebellum, 417
Cerebral meninges, 417
Cerebrum, 417
Cervical esophagus, 102
Cervical lymph nodes, 338, 387, 391, 397,
    401, 407, 411
Cervix uteri, 293–297

Salivary glands, major, 81–84
    cancer of, 84
Sarcomas
    bone, 216
    orbit, 411–414
    soft tissue, 221–226
Satellite nodules, 195
Scalene lymph nodes, 206, 338
Scalp, 231, 239
Scapula, 213
Schwannoma, 417
Scrotum, 231, 239
Sentinel lymph nodes
    breast, 260, 262, 265–266, 269, 272, 275
    melanoma, 240, 242, 252
Shoulders
    carcinoma of the skin, 231
    melanoma of the skin, 239
    soft-tissue sarcomas, 221
Sigmoid mesenteric lymph nodes, 129
Skeleton. See bone
Skin
    carcinoma of, 231–237
    melanoma of, 239–252
Small cell lung cancer (SCLC), 192–194
    survival rates, 194
Small intestine, 119–125
Smoldering multiple myeloma (SMM), 444
Soft palate, 47
Soft tissue sarcomas, 221–226
Spinal cord, 417–423
Spleen, 428
Splenic lymph nodes, 104
Sputum, 195
Squamous cell carcinomas
    glottis, 68
    head and neck (SCCHN), 30
    hypopharyngeal, 56
    laryngeal, 66
    lip, 42
    nasopharyngeal, 54
    oral cavity, 43
    oropharyngeal, 55
    skin, 232
    subglottis, 69
    supraglottis, 67
St. Jude staging system, 446
Stage groupings, 8–9, 13–14, 151
Staging
    general rules of, 6
    philosophy of, 3–4
    principles of, 3–14
Standard error, 22
Starting points, survival studies, 23
Sternum, 213
Stomach, 111–112
Subcarinal lymph nodes, 104, 192
Subcutaneous tissues, 221
Subglottis, 61, 62, 64, 69
Sublingual glands, 81–84

Submandibular lymph nodes, 28, 81–84, 387, 391, 397, 401, 407, 411
Submental lymph nodes, 28
Sub-occipital lymph nodes, 28
Superficial inguinal lymph nodes, 331
Superior mesenteric lymph nodes, 156, 164–165
Supraclavicular fossa, 51, 53
Supraclavicular lymph nodes, 104, 206, 257, 259, 338
Supraglottis, 61, 63, 67
Suprahyoid epiglottis, 62
Surgical margins, pancreatic, 182–183
Survival, relative, 21
Survival analysis, 15–25
Survival curve, definition, 15
Survival rate analyses
    adjusted, 20–21
    breast cancer, 16–17
    calculation of, 16
    definition of, 15
    regression method, 21–22
    standard error of, 22
    starting points, 23
    statistical significance, 22–23
    subclassification, 18–20
    T classification and, 150
    time intervals, 24
Systematized Nomenclature of Medicine (SNOMED), 5

T

T, definition of, 223
T1 tumor survival rates, 150
T-cell lymphoma, peripheral, 441
T-cell neoplasms, 429, 430
Technitium scintigraphy, 214
Temporal lobe, 417
Terminal events, 23
Testis, 347–352
Thorax, soft-tissue sarcomas, 221
Thyroid cartilage, 48
Thyroid gland, 89–96
    anaplastic carcinoma of, 96
    follicular adenocarcinoma of, 94
    medullary carcinoma of, 95
    papillary adenocarcinoma of, 93
TNM system, 10
    general rule of, 6–9
    philosophy of, 3–4
    subdivisions of, 10–12
Tongue, 35
    base of, 47
    oral, 36
Tonsillar fossa, 47
Tonsillar pillar, 47
Tonsils, 47
Tracheobronchial lymph nodes, 104
Trigone of bladder, 367
Trophoblastic tumors, gestational, 323–326